MW00511643

Pediatric Imaging

The Fundamentals

Pediatric Imaging
The Fundamentals

Lane F. Donnelly, MD

Radiologist-in-Chief, Department of Radiology
Cincinnati Children's Hospital Medical Center
Professor of Radiology and Pediatrics
University of Cincinnati College of Medicine
Cincinnati, Ohio

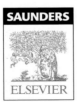

SAUNDERS

ELSEVIER

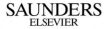

1600 John F. Kennedy Blvd.
Suite 1800
Philadelphia, Pennsylvania 19103-2899

PEDIATRIC IMAGING ISBN: 978-1-4160-5907-3
Copyright © 2009, by Saunders, an imprint of Elsevier Inc.

All rights reserved. No part of this publication may be reproduced or transmitted in any form or by any means, electronic or mechanical, including photocopying, recording, or any information storage and retrieval system, without permission in writing from the publisher. Permissions may be sought directly from Elsevier's Rights Department: phone: (+1) 215 239 3804 (US) or (+44) 1865 843830 (UK); fax: (+44) 1865 853333; e-mail: healthpermissions@elsevier.com. You may also complete your request on-line via the Elsevier website at http://www.elsevier.com/permissions.

Notice

Knowledge and best practice in this field are constantly changing. As new research and experience broaden our knowledge, changes in practice, treatment, and drug therapy may become necessary or appropriate. Readers are advised to check the most current information provided (i) on procedures featured or (ii) by the manufacturer of each product to be administered to verify the recommended dose or formula, the method and duration of administration, and contraindications. It is the responsibility of the practitioner, relying on his or her own experience and knowledge of the patient, to make diagnoses, to determine dosages and the best treatment for each individual patient, and to take all appropriate safety precautions. To the fullest extent of the law, neither the publisher nor the author assumes any liability for any injury and/or damage to persons or property arising out of or related to any use of the material contained in this book.

The Publisher

Library of Congress Cataloging-in-Publication Data (in PHL)
Donnelly, Lane F.
    Pediatric imaging: the fundamentals/Lane F. Donnelly. – 1st ed.
        p. ;   cm.
    Includes bibliographical references.
    ISBN 978-1-4160-5907-3
1. Pediatric diagnostic imaging. I. Title.
    [DNLM: 1. Diagnostic Imaging–methods. 2. Child. 3. Infant. WN 240 D685p 2009]
    RJ51. D5D66 2009
    618.92'00754–dc22   2008038937

Senior Acquisitions Editor: Rebecca S. Gaertner
Developmental Editor: Elizabeth Hart
Publishing Services Manager: Tina K. Rebane
Designer: Steve Stave
Marketing Manager: Catalina Nolte

Printed in China.

Working together to grow
libraries in developing countries

www.elsevier.com | www.bookaid.org | www.sabre.org

ELSEVIER   BOOK AID
            International   Sabre Foundation

Last digit is the print number: 9 8 7 6 5 4 3 2 1

For my wife, Carolina V. Guimaraes, MD. You are everything to me.

Preface

I know that as a resident, I retained more useful information when I read short and basic books over and over than when I read longer, more detailed texts once. The intention of this book is to serve as a basic introductory text on pediatric imaging. The book is written in prose, rather than as an outline, and is intended to be readable. The emphasis is on commonly encountered imaging scenarios and pediatric diseases. The topics included reflect questions that I am commonly asked by residents on the pediatric radiology service, important issues that the rotating residents often seem not to know about, and commonly made mistakes. The book is intended to serve as an excellent introduction or review for a resident or medical student who is about to begin a rotation in pediatric radiology or prepare for radiology oral boards. This book may also serve as a review for a general radiologist who wishes to brush up on pediatric radiology. Pediatric residents or pediatricians who want to learn more about pediatric radiology may also benefit from reading this book.

Lane F. Donnelly, MD

Acknowledgments

I would like to thank Marlena Tyre for help with proofreading; Judy Racadio, MD, for her help with medical editing and proofreading; James Leach, MD, for his help with the advanced neuroimaging section; and Glenn Minnano for his help with the diagrams. The information in this book is a summation of the material that was taught to me by numerous radiologists, and I would like to thank them for their time and efforts. The case material in this book is the result of the hard work of the faculty, technologists, and trainees in the Department of Radiology at Cincinnati Children's Hospital Medical Center and the referring physicians who care for these patients. I would like to acknowledge their efforts, without which this book would not be possible.

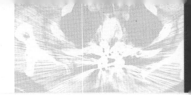

Contents

CHAPTER ONE

Special Considerations in Pediatric Imaging

PEDIATRIC RADIOLOGY AS A POTENTIAL CAREER

Most pediatric radiologists are very happy with both their jobs and their career choice. I know that I am. There are a number of attractive aspects about pediatric radiology. First, one of the most important elements of job satisfaction is the quality of the interactions you have with the people with whom you work. In general, the physicians who choose to go into pediatric subspecialties, as well as health care workers who choose to work at pediatric institutions in general, tend to be nice, gentle people. Aggressive, power-hungry people tend not to want to work with children. This makes a huge difference in the quality of daily life. Also, pediatric subspecialists seem to rely on the opinions of pediatric radiologists more than many of their adult subspecialist counterparts. Similarly, pediatric radiology does not seem to have the same number of turf battles that many adult-oriented departments have.

Another unique feature of pediatric radiology is that you get to be a "general specialist." Pediatric radiology is a small part of medical imaging overall and in this sense, the pediatric radiologist is very much a subspecialist. Compared to general radiologists who must have a working knowledge of a daunting amount of information, I believe that most pediatric radiologists feel comfortable that they have an adequate command of the knowledge they need in order to provide outstanding care. At the same time, pediatric radiologists are generalists in the sense that many pediatric radiologists deal with all modalities and organ systems. They get the best of both worlds. It is also possible in pediatric radiology to become a sub-subspecialist, such as a pediatric neuroradiologist, pediatric interventional radiologist, pediatric cardiac imager, or pediatric fetal imager.

The most powerful and fulfilling aspect of becoming a pediatric health care provider is probably the satisfaction that comes from working with and for children. Few activities are more rewarding than helping children and their families. There are many other attractive aspects of pediatric care. First, most kids recover from their illnesses, as compared to elderly adults. Most pediatric illnesses are not self-induced. Pediatric diseases are highly varied and interesting. In addition, pediatric conditions are being increasingly recognized as important precursors to adult illnesses that cause significant mortality rates—obesity, osteoporosis, and glucose intolerance. Finally, children and their families are highly appreciative of pediatricians' help.

Finally, and importantly, there are plenty of jobs available in pediatric radiology. It is the radiology subspecialty with the greatest workforce shortage. Currently, there are pediatric radiology opportunities in almost any city in North America and there is no sign that this will change in the near future.

INTRODUCTION: SPECIAL CONSIDERATIONS IN PEDIATRIC IMAGING

Many issues are unique to the imaging of children as compared to that of adults. Imaging examinations that are easily carried out in adults require special adjustments to be successfully achieved in children. The rotating resident on a pediatric imaging rotation and the general radiologist who occasionally images children must be prepared to deal with these issues and to adjust imaging techniques so as to safely and successfully obtain the imaging examination. In this introductory chapter, several of the general issues that can arise when imaging children are addressed briefly.

Relationship Between Imager and Parents

In both pediatric and adult patient care situations, there are family members with whom the imager must interact. However, in the pediatric setting, there are several unique features in the relationship among imager, patient, and family. When caring for children, communication more often takes place between the radiologist and the parent than between the radiologist and the patient. Obviously, communication directly with the child is also paramount to success. In addition, the degree of interaction between the imager and the child-parent unit may be greater in the pediatric than in the adult setting because of associated issues, such as the potential need for sedation, the need for consent from the parent rather than the child (if the child is a minor), and the need for intense explanation of the procedure on the levels of both the child and the parent. People are also much more inquisitive and protective when their children are involved. Because of these reasons, descriptions of what to expect during the visit to the imaging area may have to be more detailed when dealing with pediatric patients and their parents.

The stress level of parents when their child is or may be ill is immense, and such stress often brings out both the best and the worst in people. Because of the intense bonds between most parents and their children, the relationship between imager and parents is most successful when the radiologist exercises marked empathy, patience, professionalism, and effective communication.

Professionalism and Effective Communication

It is interesting to note that in pediatric health care, most of the complaints by parents and families are not related to technical errors; they are more commonly related to issues of professionalism and communication. Of reported parent complaints 30% are related to poor communication and unprofessional behavior. In addition, practicing effective communication has been shown to have multiple positive outcomes, including better patient outcome, decreased cost, increased patient and family satisfaction, and decreased chance of litigation in the presence of adverse events.

Although we are referred to as health care "professionals," historically, physicians have not received formal training in professionalism and communication, have had poor role models, and have been seen as individual practitioners rather than as members of health care teams. Radiology departments and individual radiologists must be proactive in making improvements in this area. As part of our program to improve and standardize our interactions with families, our department has a professionalism booklet that is given to all radiology faculty and rotation trainees. The booklet outlines the types of behaviors that are expected, such as introducing ourselves to patients and families and stating our positions and roles in the upcoming procedure, as well as behaviors to avoid, such as stating that the patient's ordering physician does not know how to order or that you do not have time to talk to a referring physician because you are too busy.

Inability to Cooperate

Infants and young children are commonly unable to cooperate with requirements that typically are easily met by adults. For example, they may be unable to keep still, remain in a certain position, concentrate for more than a brief moment, or breath-hold. Children of various ages have unique limitations. Infants and toddlers are unable to stay still, whereas 3-year-olds are more apt to refuse to cooperate. These limitations affect almost all pediatric imaging examinations: radiography, fluoroscopy, ultrasound, computed tomography (CT), magnetic resonance imaging (MRI), nuclear imaging, and interventional radiology. There are a number of potential solutions and tricks that can be helpful in these situations. Commonly employed techniques include distracting the child, providing child-friendly surroundings (Figs. 1-1, 1-2, 1-3), immobilization, and sedation.

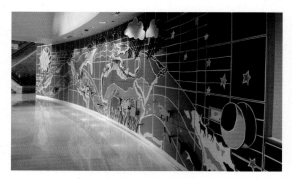

FIGURE 1-1. Colorful, child-friendly décor in corridor leading to radiology area.

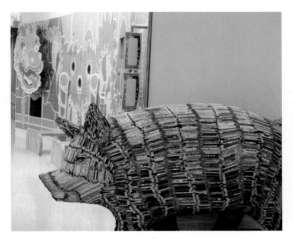

FIGURE 1-2. Child-friendly waiting area with pencil pig and colorful mural.

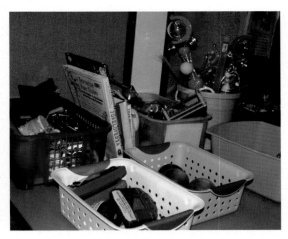

FIGURE 1-4. Supply of toys and other tools to distract and comfort children in fluoroscopy area.

Distracting the child with something other than the procedure is often a simple and easy tactic to employ. The Department of Radiology at Cincinnati Children's Hospital Medical Center (CCHMC) keeps a stock of rattles and noise-making toys (Fig. 1-4) to distract infants. Talking to older children about school and other activities can be helpful. Our department has certified child-life specialists to help coach and distract the children. We have video players in all of our ultrasound, fluoroscopy, and CT rooms (Fig. 1-5) and video goggles (Fig. 1-6) in our MRI scanners. Children are encouraged to bring their own movies or choose from the department's stock. It is amazing how cooperative many children will be when they are able to watch television. Using a combined program that includes the introduction of a child-life specialist and the installation of magnetic resonance video goggles, a video player on a multijoint arm for watching videos in various potential patient positions in CT, a color-light-show device that projects on the CT gantry (Fig. 1-7) to calm infants and young children, and the promotion of a culture change, avoiding sedation whenever possible can be effective. By these means, the Department of Radiology at CCHMC has been able to achieve a reduction from baseline in the frequency of sedation in children less than 7 years of age of 34.6% for MRI and 44.9% for CT.

Providing child-friendly surroundings may help to ease a young child's anxiety and cause him or her to be more cooperative. Paintings on the walls and equipment and cartoonish figures in the examination rooms can be helpful. Eliminating or minimizing painful portions of the examination can also be very helpful in keeping a young child cooperative. The placement of

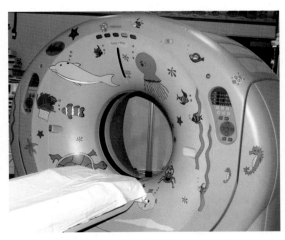

FIGURE 1-3. CT scanner decorated with child-friendly stickers.

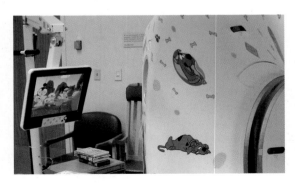

FIGURE 1-5. Flat-screen video monitor on multijointed mechanical arm adjacent to CT scanner with child-friendly decorations. The video screen is designed so that a child can watch a video regardless of his or her position in the CT scanner.

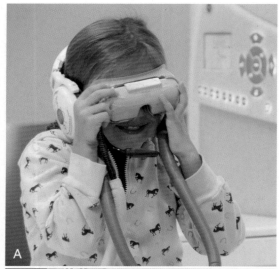

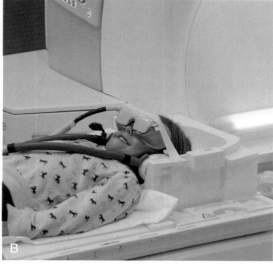

FIGURE 1-6. Video goggles can help young children cooperate for MR examination, thus avoiding sedation. **A,** Video goggles on a child preparing for an MR examination. **B,** Video goggles with audio headphones in place as child is slid into scanner. Note happy demeanor.

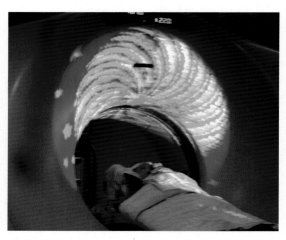

FIGURE 1-7. Color light show projected on gantry of CT scanner distracting young child so that a CT scan can be obtained without sedation.

an intravenous line often causes a great deal of patient anxiety and renders the child uncooperative for a subsequent imaging study such as a CT scan. Using topical analgesia to decrease the pain of the IV placement commonly makes this portion of the examination less traumatic. Also, it is helpful to schedule appropriate sequencing of imaging examinations so that the most difficult exam is performed last. For example, it can be much easier to perform a renal ultrasound prior to

rather than after the child has experienced a voiding cystourethrogram.

Immobilization is also a helpful technique. Infants who are bundled or papoosed in a blanket are more apt to stay still than infants who are not. This may make the difference between needing or not needing sedation to obtain a CT examination. There are also a number of commercially available immobilization devices that are helpful when performing certain examinations, such as the use of an octagon board when obtaining fluoroscopic studies of young children. There are also other devices that enhance proper positioning for specific modalities such as chest radiographs. Imaging departments that image children should consider making such equipment available.

In certain situations, distraction and immobilization may not be successful, and sedation or general anesthesia may be necessary to obtain imaging studies. Many children younger than 6 years of age require sedation for MRI studies because of the prolonged nature of the examination and the need for the patient to be completely still. Sedation is needed less often now than in the past for children undergoing CT examination because of the increased speed of acquisition by the newer CT scanners and the previously mentioned sedation reduction program. Other procedures that might require sedation include some nuclear medicine studies and most interventional procedures.

Standards of care for conscious sedation are required by the Joint Commission of Accreditation of Health Care Organizations and are based on standards published by several organizations, including the Committee on Drugs, American Academy of Pediatrics. Any imaging department planning to sedate children must have a defined sedation program that is in concordance with these guidelines. The sedation program must have protocols for presedation preparation, sedative agents utilized, monitoring during sedation and during postsedation recovery, and discharge criteria. There has been a national shift concerning who provides sedation for pediatric imaging studies in pediatric radiology departments. In the 1990s, most pediatric radiology sedation programs were run by radiologists. Now, multiple factors have led such programs' being run by anesthesiologists, emergency physicians, or intensive care physicians. At many institutions, such physicians have access to sedatives that are better for imaging sedation, such as propofol. In the Department of Radiology at CCHMC, the Department of Anesthesia now provides sedation services for imaging procedures.

Variable Size and Physiology

Because of the size variability from infant to adult-sized children, many adaptations must be considered for pediatric imaging studies in relation to size. The doses of contrast and drugs utilized in imaging examinations need to be adjusted according to a child's size, often on a per-weight (mg/kg) basis. For example, in CT, the standard dose of intravenous contrast may be 2 ml/kg. Oral contrast dosing is also based on patient weight or age. To continue using CT as an illustrative example, other variables may be affected by patient size as well. In small children, the largest possible IV may be very small, often 22- or 24-gauge. The IV may be placed in the foot or hand. The length of the region of interest to be imaged is variable, and the lengths of the patient's veins are variable. Physiologic parameters such as the patient's cardiac output are also more variable in children than in adults. These factors affect parameters such as the time between contrast injection and the onset of scanning as well as choices in contrast administration technique (hand bolus versus power injector). Slice thickness should be smaller in

younger children because of the smaller anatomic parts. Similar adjustments must be considered in all other imaging modalities when applied to children. Radiation dose reduction is discussed in Patient Safety.

Age-Related Changes in Imaging Appearance

Another factor that makes imaging in children different from that in adults is the continuous changes in the imaging appearance of multiple organ systems during normal childhood development. The normal imaging appearance of certain aspects of organ systems can be different both at varying ages during childhood and between children and adults. For example, the kidneys look different on ultrasound in neonates from the way they look in a 1-year-old child. The developing brain demonstrates differences in signal at varying ages on MRI, which is related to changes in myelination. A large mediastinal shadow related to the thymus may be normal or severely abnormal depending upon the child's age. The skeleton demonstrates marked changes at all ages of childhood; this is related to the maturation of apophyses and epiphyses and the progressive ossification of structures. Knowledge of the normal age-related appearances of these organ systems is vital to appropriate interpretation of imaging studies. Lack of this knowledge is one of the more common causes of mistakes in pediatric radiology.

Age-Related Differential Diagnoses

The types of diseases that affect children are vastly different from those that commonly affect adults. Therefore, the differential diagnosis of and the significance of a particular imaging finding in a child is dramatically different from the identical imaging finding when it is seen in an adult. In addition, the diseases that affect specific age groups of children are different. Therefore, the differential diagnosis and significance of a particular imaging finding in a 2-month-old infant may differ dramatically from those determined by the identical imaging finding in a 10-year-old child.

Patient Safety

A lot of national attention has been paid to patient safety initiatives since the 1999 Institute of Medicine's report stating that somewhere between 44,000 and 98,000 deaths per year are caused by medical errors in the United States alone. This poor safety record would be the equivalent of the airline industry's having a large passenger plane crash in the United States every single day! If this were the case, we would probably think twice about flying. However, this is what our patients potentially face when they enter the current health care system. If looked at from the patients' perspective, even more important to them than "Heal me" (quality of care) and "Be nice to me" (customer service) is the plea "Don't harm me" (patient safety). No higher priority exists than patient safety.

Many institutions have developed programs to improve patient safety, but they have shown mixed results. At CCHMC, our patient safety improvement strategy stresses error-prevention training for all clinical employees. Such training has previously been successful in markedly reducing errors in high-performance industries such as aviation and nuclear power. This training emphasizes three behavioral expectations: (1) make a personal commitment to safety; (2) communicate clearly; (3) pay attention to detail. For each expectation, the employees are taught behavioral techniques to aid them in error reduction.

Several cultural changes are involved in improving safety. The first is dispelling the notion that physicians are "independent practitioners" rather than key components of an integrated care-providing team. No other industry in which there must be outstanding safety performance allows this type of behavior. Second, we need to create a culture in which people are expected to and encouraged to speak up in the face of uncertainty. The old culture of a medical hierarchy in which the physician is in charge and is not to be questioned does not promote safety. Medical staff, trainees, and even family members need to feel comfortable "stopping the line" and asking for clarification if things don't seem right. In most of the serious safety events we have had historically at CCHMC, there was almost always someone who stated that he or she had thought things were not right but had not felt empowered to speak up. This situation must be transformed culturally.

RADIATION SAFETY

Safety issues specific to radiology include radiation safety, MRI safety, and correct and effective communication of the information in and the interpretation of imaging examinations for the referring physician. We will touch here on radiation safety because it is germane to pediatric radiology. Children are much more sensitive to the potential harmful effects of radiation than are adults, and they also have a longer expected life span during which to develop potential complications of radiation such as cancer. Therefore, attention to radiation safety in all areas of pediatric radiology is paramount. CT delivers higher doses of radiation than other diagnostic imaging modalities. The exact radiation risk in CT examinations and even whether a risk absolutely exists are controversial topics. However, some researchers estimate the increased risk that a young child might develop cancer related to an abdominal CT scan is in the magnitude of 1:1000. In other words, for every 1000 CT scans of the abdomen you perform in children, you will be causing cancer in one child. Given the number of CT scans performed in children, that number, if true, is astounding! Therefore, it is essential for all radiologists to practice dose-reduction techniques in pediatric CT. Such tactics include avoiding CT when unnecessary; using alternative diagnostic methods that do not utilize radiation, such as ultrasound, when possible; and adjusting CT parameters to minimize dose when CT is performed. Because children are smaller than adults and need less radiation to create the same signal-to-noise ratios, the tube current (mA) can be greatly reduced when imaging a small child. Other techniques include reducing kVp; using in-plane shielding for areas such as the eye, thyroid, and breasts; increasing beam pitch; and picking a CT manufacturer that has put effort into dose-reducing technology.

Suggested Readings

Chung T, Kirks DR: Techniques. In Kirks DR, editor: *Practical pediatric imaging of infants and children,* ed 3, Philadelphia, Lippincott-Raven, 1998.

Donnelly LF, editor: *Diagnostic imaging: pediatric,* Salt Lake City, AMIRSYS, 2005.

Donnelly LF, Strife JL: How I do it: establishing a program to promote professionalism and effective communication in radiology, *Radiology* 283:773-779, 2006.

Donnelly LF, Strife JL: Performance-based assessment of radiology faculty: a practical plan to promote improvement and meet JCAHO standards, *AJR* 184:1398-1401, 2005.

Frush DP, Bisset GS III: Pediatric sedation in radiology: the practice of safe sleep, *AJR* 167:1381-1387, 1996.

Institute of Medicine: *Crossing the quality chasm: a new health system for the 21st century,* Washington, DC, National Academy Press, 2001.

Khan JJ, Donnelly LF, Koch BL, et al: A program to decrease the need for pediatric sedation, *Appl Radiol* 4:30-33, 2007.

Pichert JW, Miller CS, Hollo AH, et al: What health professionals can do to identify and resolve patient dissatisfaction. *Jt Comm J Qual Improv* 124:303-312, 1998.

Thrall JH: Quality and safety revolution in health care, *Radiology* 233:3-6, 2004.

CHAPTER TWO

Airway

It has been said that one of the differentiating features between a pediatric and a general radiologist is that a pediatric radiologist remembers to look at the airway. Problems with the airway are much more common in children than in adults. For practical purposes, abnormalities of the airway can be divided into acute upper airway obstruction, lower airway obstruction (extrinsic compression, intrinsic obstruction), obstructive sleep apnea (OSA), and congenital high airway obstruction syndrome (CHAOS).

Clinically, children with acute upper airway obstruction (above the thoracic inlet) tend to present with inspiratory stridor, whereas children with lower airway obstruction (below the thoracic inlet) are more likely to present with expiratory wheezing. However, the categorization of a child with noisy breathing into one of these two groups is commonly more difficult than we are led to believe. The primary imaging evaluation of the pediatric airway for acute conditions should include frontal and lateral high-kilovolt radiography of the airway and frontal and lateral views of the chest.

ACUTE UPPER AIRWAY OBSTRUCTION

Acute stridor in a young child is the most common indication for imaging the pediatric airway. The most common causes of acute upper airway obstruction in children include inflammatory disorders and foreign bodies. Common inflammatory disorders include croup, epiglottitis, exudative tracheitis, and retropharyngeal cellulitis/abscess. Anatomic structures that are especially important to evaluate on radiographs of children with acute upper airway obstruction include the epiglottis, aryepiglottic folds, subglottic trachea, and retropharyngeal soft tissues.

Croup

Croup (acute laryngotracheobronchitis) is the most common cause of acute upper airway

obstruction in young children. Croup is a disease of infants and young children; the peak incidence occurs between 6 months and 3 years of age. The mean age at presentation of croup is 1 year of age. In children older than 3 years, other causes of airway obstruction should be suspected. Croup is viral in cause and is usually a benign, self-limited disease. Redundant mucosa in the subglottic region becomes inflamed, swells, and encroaches upon the airway. The children present with a barky ("croupy") cough and intermittent inspiratory stridor. It usually occurs following or during other symptoms of lower respiratory tract infection. Most children with croup are managed supportively as outpatients, and the parents are managed by reassurance. Inhaled corticosteroids are becoming a popular therapy in children with croup. They have been shown to reduce the length and severity of illness.

The purpose of obtaining radiographs in a patient with suspected croup is not to document the diagnosis but rather to exclude other, more serious, causes of upper airway obstruction that require intervention. However, characteristic radiographic findings that indicate croup are best seen on frontal radiographs. With croup, there is loss of the normal shoulders (lateral convexities) of the subglottic trachea secondary to symmetric subglottic edema (Fig. 2-1A, B). Normally, the subglottic trachea appears rounded, with "shoulders" that are convex outward (Fig 2-2). In croup, the subglottic trachea becomes long and thin, with the narrow portion extending more inferiorly than the level of the pyriform sinuses. The appearance has been likened to an inverted V or a church steeple (see Fig. 2-1). I have found the term *church steeple* confusing because some steeples look like croup and some are shaped like the normal subglottic airway (Fig. 2-3). Lateral radiographs may demonstrate a narrowing or loss of definition of the lumen of the subglottic trachea (see Fig. 2-1) or hypopharyngeal overdistention. The epiglottis and aryepiglottic folds appear normal.

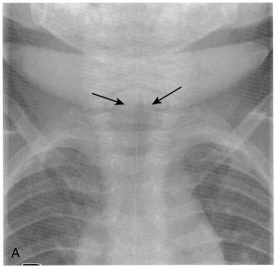

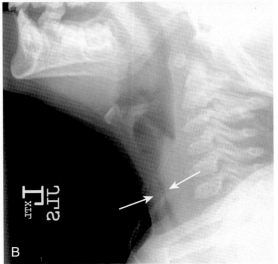

FIGURE 2-1. Croup. **A,** Frontal radiograph showing symmetric subglottic narrowing *(arrows)* with loss of normal shouldering. The narrowing extends more inferiorly than the piriform sinuses. **B,** Lateral radiograph showing subglottic narrowing *(arrows)*. Note normal-appearing epiglottis.

Epiglottitis

In contrast to croup, epiglottitis is a life-threatening disease that could potentially require emergent intubation. The possibility that a child with epiglottitis might arrive in a deserted radiology department was once a constant source of anxiety for on-call radiology residents. However, most cases of epiglottitis are caused by *Hemophilus influenzae* and are now preventable by immunization (HiB vaccine), so the incidence of epiglottitis has dramatically decreased. I think caregivers should be more nervous

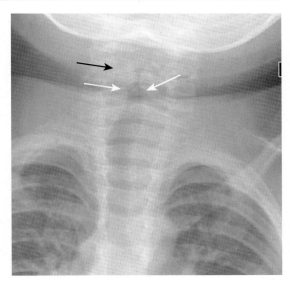

FIGURE 2-2. Normal frontal radiograph of the airway. The subglottic airway demonstrates rounded shoulders *(white arrows)* that are convex outward. Note the appearance and location of the pyriform recess *(black arrow on right pyriform recess)*.

about epiglottitis now because health care workers are less used to dealing with patients with this disorder. Children with epiglottitis are usually toxic appearing and present with an abrupt onset of stridor, dysphagia, fever, restlessness, and an increase in respiratory distress when recumbent. The patients are typically older than those with croup; the classically described peak incidence occurs at age 3.5 years. However, since the introduction of the HiB vaccine, some reports have shown a marked increase in the mean age of presentation to 14.6 years. Because of the risk for complete

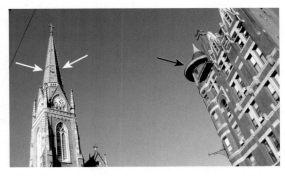

FIGURE 2-3. Steeple sign. I find the term *steeple sign* confusing. It is meant to denote the pointed configuration of the subglottic trachea on a frontal radiograph of the airway when subglottic edema has effaced the normally convex lateral shoulders in this region. However, some steeples look like croup *(white arrows)* and some look like a normal subglottic airway *(black arrow)*.

airway obstruction and respiratory failure, no maneuvers should be performed that make the patient uncomfortable. If the diagnosis is not made on physical examination, a single lateral radiograph of the neck should be obtained, usually with the patient erect or in whatever position that allows the patient to breathe comfortably. Children with epiglottitis should never be made to lie supine against their will in order to obtain a radiograph because it can result in acute airway obstruction and, potentially, death.

On the lateral radiograph, there is marked enlargement of epiglottis. The swollen epiglottis has been likened to the appearance of a thumb. There is also thickening of the aryepiglottic folds (Fig. 2-4A-C). The aryepiglottic folds are the soft tissues that extend from the epiglottis

anterosuperiorly to the arytenoid cartilage posteroinferiorly and normally are convex downward. When the aryepiglottic folds become abnormally thickened, they appear convex superiorly. An obliquely imaged, or so-called omega-shaped, epiglottis may artifactually appear wide because both the left and right sides of the epiglottis are being imaged adjacent to each other. This should not be confused with a truly enlarged epiglottis. The presence or absence of thickening of the aryepiglottic folds can be helpful in making this differentiation. On lateral view, a normal epiglottis has a very thick appearance. Often both the left and right walls of the epiglottis are visible (Fig. 2-5). Symmetric subglottic narrowing, similar to croup, may be seen on frontal radiography (if obtained); do not let that confuse you.

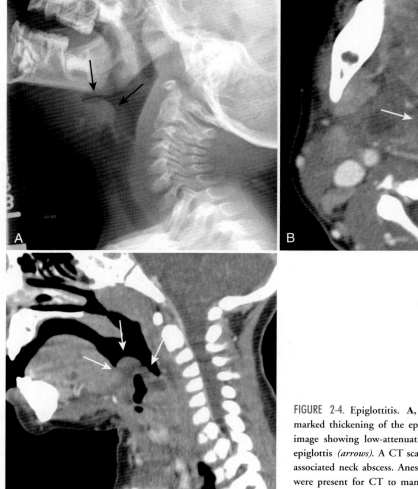

FIGURE 2-4. Epiglottitis. **A,** Lateral radiograph showing marked thickening of the epiglottis *(arrows).* **B,** Axial CT image showing low-attenuation swelling of the C-shaped epiglottis *(arrows).* A CT scan was obtained because of an associated neck abscess. Anesthesiology and otolaryngology were present for CT to manage airway. **C,** Sagittal reconstructed CT image shows markedly swollen epiglottis *(arrows)* and aryepiglottic folds.

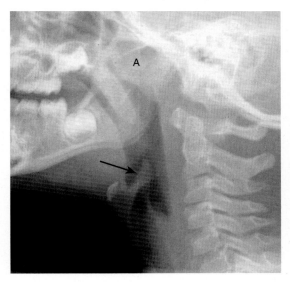

FIGURE 2-5. Normal epiglottis. Lateral radiograph showing thick-appearing epiglottis *(arrow)*. Incidentally, note appearance of enlarged adenoid tonsils *(A)*.

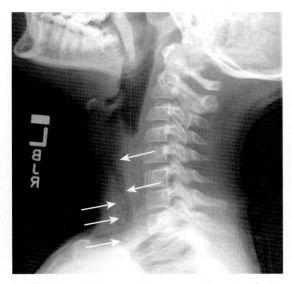

FIGURE 2-6. Exudative tracheitis. Lateral radiograph showing irregular plaquelike filling defects and airway wall irregularities *(arrows)* within trachea. Again, note the normal appearance of the nonthickened epiglottis in this patient.

Exudative Tracheitis

Exudative tracheitis (also know as bacterial tracheitis, membranous croup, or membranous laryngotracheobronchitis) is another uncommon but potentially life-threatening cause of acute upper airway obstruction. The disorder is characterized by a purulent infection of the trachea in which exudative plaques form along the tracheal walls (much like those seen in diphtheria). Affected children are usually older and more ill than those with standard croup; typically their ages range from 6 to 10 years. Although initial reports described most cases to be secondary to infection by *Staphylococcus aureus*, other reports have noted multimicrobial infections. It is unclear whether the disease is a primary bacterial infection or a secondary bacterial infection that occurs following damage to the respiratory mucosa by a viral infection. A linear soft tissue filling defect (a membrane) seen within the airway on radiography is the most characteristic finding. A plaquelike irregularity of the tracheal wall is also highly suspicious (Fig. 2-6). Nonadherent mucus may mimic a membrane radiographically. In cooperative patients, having them cough and then repeating the film may help to differentiate mucus from a membrane. Other findings include symmetric or asymmetric subglottic narrowing in a child too old typically to have croup and irregularity or loss of definition of the tracheal wall.

Membranes and tracheal wall irregularities may be seen on frontal or lateral radiographs, and often seen on one but not the other, so it is therefore important to get both views.

If one of these exudative "membranes" is sloughed into the lumen, it can lead to airway occlusion and respiratory arrest. Therefore, children who are suspected to have exudative tracheitis should be evaluated endoscopically, the exudative membranes stripped, and elective endotracheal intubation performed.

A number of controversies regarding exudative tracheitis exist. First, it is seen with great frequency at some institutions and not at all at others. Second, although it is considered a life-threatening condition, to my knowledge, no patient has ever died at home of this disease. Both of these points raise the question of the validity of this diagnosis. My take is that there are definitive cases of this disease, but it is probably overdiagnosed and overtreated at some institutions.

Retropharyngeal Cellulitis and Abscess

Retropharyngeal cellulitis is a pyogenic infection of the retropharyngeal space that usually follows a recent pharyngitis or upper respiratory tract infection. Children present with sudden onset of fever, stiff neck, dysphagia, and occasionally stridor. Most affected children are young, with more than half of the cases occurring between 6 and 12 months of age. On lateral radiography, there is thickening of the retropharyngeal soft tissues (Figs. 2-7A, B, 2-8A-C). In an infant or young child, the soft tissues between the posterior aspect of the aerated pharynx and the anterior aspect of the vertebral column should not exceed the anterior to posterior diameter of the cervical vertebral bodies. However, in infants, who have short necks, it is common to see

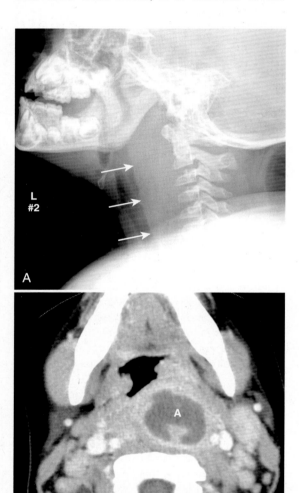

FIGURE 2-7. Retropharyngeal abscess. A, Lateral radiograph showing marked thickening of the retropharyngeal soft tissues *(arrows),* which are wider than the adjacent vertebral bodies. Note the anterior convexity of soft tissues. **B,** Contrast-enhanced CT shows a low attenuation region with enhancing rim *(A),* suggestive of a drainable abscess.

pseudothickening of the retropharyngeal soft tissues when the lateral radiograph is obtained without the neck's being well-extended (Fig. 2-9A, B). Apex anterior convexity of the retropharyngeal soft tissues provides supportive evidence that there is true widening of the retropharyngeal soft tissues (see Fig. 2-7). If it is unclear on the initial lateral radiograph whether the soft tissues are truly versus artifactually widened, it is best to repeat the lateral radiograph with the neck placed in full extension (see Fig. 2-9). The only radiographic feature that can differentiate abscess from cellulitis is the identification of gas within the retropharyngeal soft tissues. Computed tomography (CT) is commonly performed to define the extent of disease and to help predict cases in which a drainable fluid collection is present (see Figs. 2-7, 2-8). On CT, a low-attenuation, well-defined area with an enhancing rim is suspicious for a drainable fluid collection (see Fig. 2-7). Cellulitis without abscess (see Fig. 2-8) is actually more common than a drainable abscess.

LOWER AIRWAY OBSTRUCTION

The most common cause of wheezing in children is small airway inflammation such as is caused by asthma and viral illness (bronchiolitis). When the wheezing persists, presents at an atypical age for asthma, or is refractory to treatment, other reasons for lower airway obstruction are entertained. Other causes of lower airway obstruction can be divided into those that are intrinsic to the airway (such as bronchial foreign body, tracheomalacia, or intrinsic masses) and those that cause extrinsic compression of the trachea (such as vascular rings). The initial radiologic screening procedure for wheezing is frontal and lateral radiography of the airway and chest. Radiographs are used to exclude acute causes of upper airway obstruction, to evaluate for other processes that can cause wheezing such as cardiac disease, and to help categorize the abnormality as being more likely to be an intrinsic or an extrinsic airway process. Important findings to look for on the radiographs include evidence of tracheal narrowing, position of the aortic arch, asymmetric lung aeration, radiopaque foreign body, and lung consolidation. When tracheal compression is present on radiography, it is important to note both the superior to inferior level of the

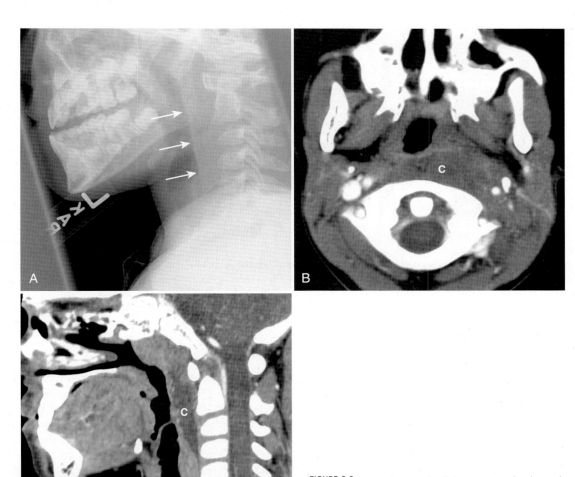

FIGURE 2-8. Retropharyngeal cellulitis. **A,** Lateral radiograph showing increased thickness of the retropharyngeal soft tissues *(arrows).* **B** and **C,** Contrast-enhanced CT in axial (**B**) and sagittal (**C**) planes showing low attenuation edema *(C)* in retropharyngeal soft tissues. There is no focal collection with enhancing rim to suggest drainable fluid.

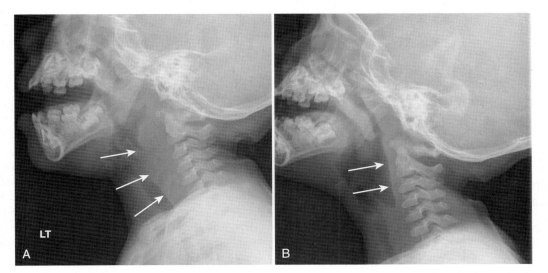

FIGURE 2-9. Pseudoretropharyngeal soft tissue thickening secondary to lack of extended neck positioning. **A,** Initial lateral radiograph showing apparent thickening of retropharyngeal soft tissues mimicking potential retropharyngeal abscess *(arrows).* **B,** Repeat lateral radiograph with neck extended, showing normal thickness of retropharyngeal soft tissues, much narrower in thickness than adjacent vertebral bodies *(arrows).*

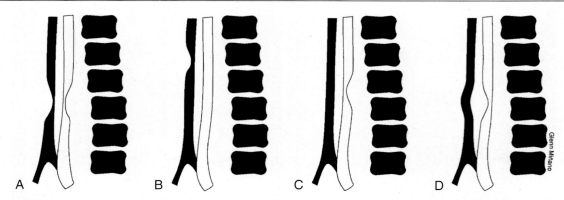

FIGURE 2-10. Patterns of compression of the trachea and esophagus in common vascular rings. The diagrams are comparable to a lateral radiograph of the chest. The trachea is black; the esophagus is white. **A,** Double aortic arch. The trachea is compressed on its anterior aspect, and the esophagus is compressed on its posterior aspect. **B,** Innominate artery compression. The trachea is compressed on its anterior aspect. The level of compression is just below the thoracic inlet, higher than other vascular causes of compression. **C,** Left arch with aberrant right subclavian artery or right arch with aberrant left subclavian artery. There is compression of the posterior aspect of the esophagus. The trachea is not compressed. **D,** Aberrant left pulmonary artery (pulmonary sling). The trachea is compressed on its posterior aspect and the esophagus is compressed on its anterior aspect.

compression and whether the compression comes from the anterior or posterior aspect of the trachea because various vascular rings present with different patterns of tracheal compression (Fig. 2-10).

If the radiographs suggest an intrinsic abnormality, bronchoscopy is the next procedure of choice. If the radiographs suggest an extrinsic compression, cross-sectional imaging is performed. There has been a shift from using primarily magnetic resonance imaging (MRI) for the evaluation of extrinsic airway compression in the 1990s to using predominantly CT now. This shift is related to the rapid acquisition times of the newer multidetector CT scanners. The advantages of CT over MRI are that most infants can be scanned without sedation on CT (which is a significant factor in an infant with airway difficulties) and that better evaluation of the lungs is possible. The disadvantages of CT are the radiation exposure and the dependence upon IV contrast.

Extrinsic Lower Airway Compression

Almost any process that causes either a space-occupying mass within the mediastinum or the enlargement or malposition of a vascular structure can lead to compression of the airway. The classically described vascular causes of lower airway compression include double aortic arch, anomalous left pulmonary artery, and innominate artery compression syndrome. However, other causes of airway compression include middle mediastinal masses, such as a bronchogenic cyst (Fig. 2-11A-C) or large anterior mediastinal masses (Fig. 2-12); enlargement of the ascending aorta such as is seen in Marfan syndrome; enlargement of the pulmonary arteries, as in congenital absence of the pulmonary valve; malposition of the descending aorta, as in midline-descending aorta-carina-compression syndrome; enlargement of the left atrium; or abnormal chest wall configuration such as a narrow thoracic inlet. On axial imaging, the trachea is normally rounded in configuration (Fig. 2-13), sometimes with a flattened posterior wall related to the noncartilaginous portion. A normal trachea is never oblong, with a greater left-to-right than anterior-to-posterior diameter (never "pancake-shaped").

DOUBLE AORTIC ARCH

Double aortic arch is a congenital anomaly related to the persistence of both the left and right fourth aortic arches. It is the most common symptomatic vascular ring. Usually an isolated lesion, it typically presents with symptoms early in life (soon after birth). Anatomically, the two arches surround and compress the trachea anteriorly and the esophagus posteriorly. Typically, the right arch is dominant, both larger and positioned more superiorly (Fig. 2-14). In such cases, the left arch is ligated by performing a left thoracotomy. When the left arch is dominant, a right thoracotomy is

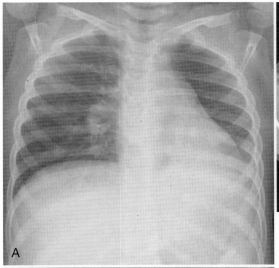

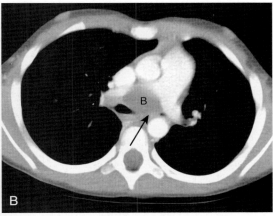

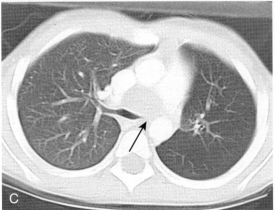

FIGURE 2-11. Bronchogenic cyst causing compression of left main bronchus. **A,** Chest radiograph showing left lower lobe, retrocardiac density, and asymmetric hyperlucency of left upper lobe. Similar findings were present on radiography on multiple occasions. **B** and **C,** CT showing mediastinal (**B**) and lung (**C**) windows, which show a well-defined, low-attenuation mass *(B),* which is consistent with a bronchogenic cyst. The lesion is adjacent to the carina and is compressing the left main bronchus *(arrow).*

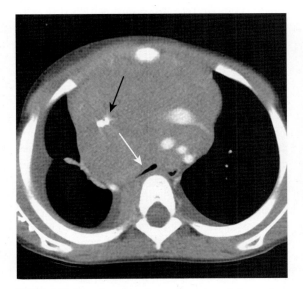

FIGURE 2-12. Lymphoma causing compression of the trachea. CT shows a large anterior mediastinal mass with posterior displacement and severe compression of the trachea *(white arrow).* The superior vena cava is also compressed *(black arrow).* There is a small amount of right pleural thickening.

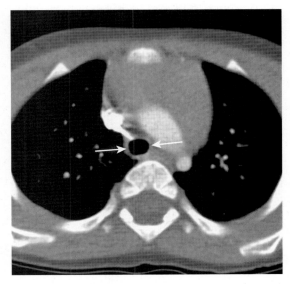

FIGURE 2-13. Normal configuration of trachea on cross-sectional imaging is rounded *(arrows).* An oval or pancake-shaped intrathoracic trachea is not normal. Note the prominence of the normal thymus in this infant.

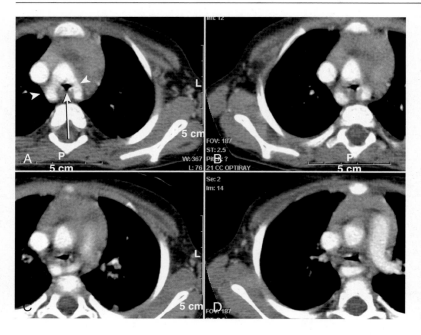

FIGURE 2-14. Double aortic arch. Sequential axial CT images showing right and left arches *(arrowheads)* surrounding a small compressed trachea *(arrow)*. The arches rejoin to form the descending aorta posteriorly. The right arch is only slightly larger than the left.

performed and the right arch ligated. Determining the dominant arch is one of the goals of performing cross-sectional imaging. The level of compression is the mid to lower intrathoracic trachea. On CT, there is symmetric take-off of four great arteries from the superior aspect of the arches.

Pulmonary Sling

In cases of anomalous origin of the left pulmonary artery (pulmonary sling), the left pulmonary artery arises from the right pulmonary artery rather than from the main pulmonary artery and passes between the trachea and esophagus as it courses toward the left lung. The resultant sling compresses the trachea. Pulmonary sling is the only vascular anomaly to course between the trachea and esophagus (Fig. 2-15A, B). Therefore, compression of the posterior aspect of the trachea and the anterior aspect of the esophagus on lateral imaging is characteristic. It is the only vascular cause of airway compression that is associated with asymmetric lung inflation on chest radiographs (see Fig 2-15). Pulmonary sling can be associated with congenital heart disease, complete tracheal rings (Fig. 2-16) (an additional cause of airway problems), and anomalous origin of the right bronchus. On CT, the trachea is compressed at the level of the sling and appears flattened in the anterior to posterior direction—like a pancake. If complete tracheal rings are present, the rings are typically superior to the pulmonary sling,

and the trachea appears very small in caliber and round at the level of the rings (Fig. 2-16).

Right Aortic Arch with Aberrant Left Subclavian Artery

Right aortic arch with an aberrant left subclavian artery (RAA-ALSCA) is another arch anomaly that can be associated with airway compression (Fig. 2-17A-D). Airway compression typically occurs when there is a persistent ductus ligament completing the ring. However, you cannot see or know whether this is the case by imaging. There are several mechanisms by which RAA-ALSCA contributes to airway compression in addition to compression by the completed ring. Often, there is dilatation of the subclavian artery at the origin from the right aorta (called a Kommerell diverticulum), which can contribute to airway compression. In addition, the descending aorta may lie in the midline, immediately anterior to the vertebral bodies, if the descending aorta passes from right to left as it descends (see Fig. 2-17). This midline descending aorta can contribute to airway compression as the result of the abnormal stacking of anatomic structures in the limited space between the sternum and vertebral bodies.

Innominate Artery Compression Syndrome

The innominate artery passes immediately anterior to the trachea just inferior to the level of the thoracic inlet. In infants, in whom the innominate artery arises more to the left than in adults

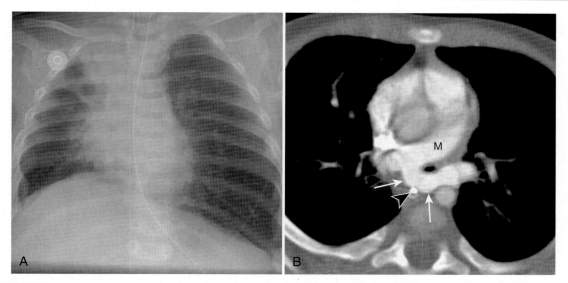

FIGURE 2-15. Pulmonary sling. **A,** Frontal radiograph showing asymmetric aeration of the lungs, often seen in pulmonary sling but rarely in other causes of extrinsic tracheal compression. **B,** CT showing anomalous origin of left pulmonary artery *(arrows)* from the right pulmonary artery rather than from the main pulmonary artery *(M)*. The pulmonary sling wraps around and compresses the trachea (small low-attenuation area) as it passes into the left hemithorax. Note the enteric tube in the esophagus *(arrowhead)*, posterior to the sling.

and in whom the mediastinum is crowded by the relatively large thymus, there can be narrowing of the trachea at this level. There is a spectrum from normal to severe narrowing; the term *syndrome* is reserved for cases that are symptomatic. The compression and resultant symptoms decrease with time as the child grows, and surgical therapy is reserved for cases in which symptoms are severe. On lateral radiography, there is indentation of the anterior aspect of the trachea at or just below the thoracic inlet (Fig. 2-18). CT demonstrates the abnormality as anterior compression of the trachea at the level of the crossing of the innominate artery and also excludes other causes of the airway compression.

Intrinsic Lower Airway Obstruction

Intrinsic abnormalities of the lower airway include dynamic processes, such as tracheomalacia, tracheal stenosis, foreign bodies, and focal masses. Tracheomalacia is tracheal wall softening related to abnormality of the cartilaginous rings of the trachea. It can be a primary or secondary condition and results in intermittent collapse of the trachea. The diagnosis cannot be made on a single static radiograph. However, lateral fluoroscopy or endoscopy can demonstrate dynamic changes in the caliber of the trachea, and they are diagnostic.

The most common soft tissue masses in the trachea are hemangiomas, which most commonly occur in the subglottic region, are often associated with facial hemangiomas in a beard distribution, and appear on frontal radiographs with asymmetric subglottic narrowing.

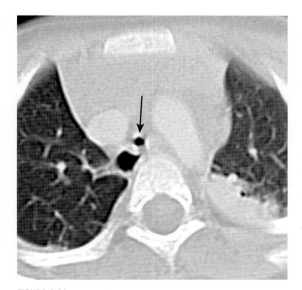

FIGURE 2-16. Complete tracheal rings. CT shows the very small caliber and rounded appearance *(arrow)* of the midtrachea.

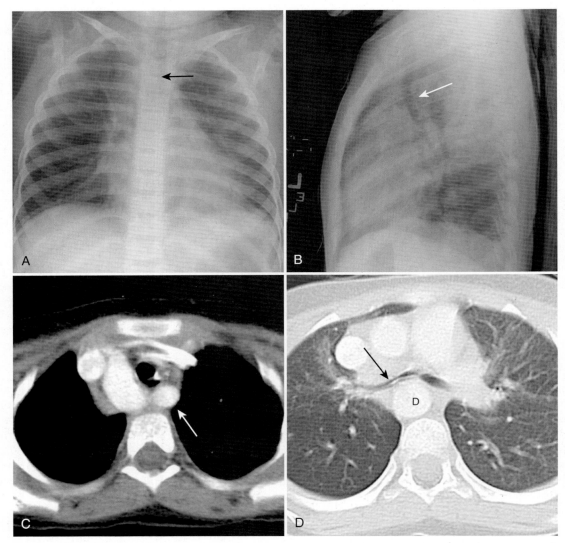

FIGURE 2-17. Right-sided aortic arch with aberrant left subclavian artery and associated airway compression. **A,** Frontal radiograph showing trachea deviated leftward, with soft tissue impression in the rightward aspect of the trachea, consistent with right aortic arch. **B,** Lateral radiograph showing trachea *(arrow)* to be bowed anteriorly and to be compressed. **C,** CT showing right-sided aortic arch with aberrant left subclavian artery *(arrow).* The trachea is not compressed at this level. **D,** CT at more inferior level showing compression of right main bronchus *(arrow)* secondary to midline position of descending aorta *(D),* associated with descending aorta starting on right superiorly and crossing over to left more inferiorly. Abnormal stacking leads to airway compression.

Other tracheal masses include tracheal papilloma and tracheal granuloma.

AIRWAY FOREIGN BODY

Infants and toddlers explore their environments with their mouths and will put almost anything into them. When such foreign bodies are aspirated, the bronchus is the most common site of lodgment. The aspiration commonly is not witnessed, and symptoms may be indolent, leading to an occult presentation. Radiographic findings of bronchial foreign bodies include asymmetric lung aeration, hyperinflation, oligemia, atelectasis, lung consolidation, pneumothorax, and pneumomediastinum. The vast majority of bronchial foreign bodies (as much as 97%) are nonradiopaque. Inspiratory films alone can be normal in as much as one third of patients in whom bronchial foreign bodies are present. Because the volume of the affected lung segments can be normal, increased, or decreased, the key radiographic feature is the

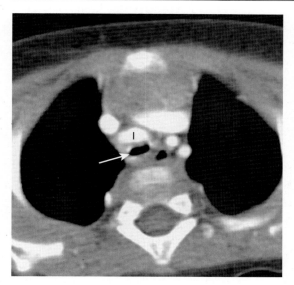

FIGURE 2-18. Innominate artery compression syndrome. CT shows innominate artery *(I)* compressing the trachea *(arrow)*. The trachea is oblong. Normally, the trachea is round at this level.

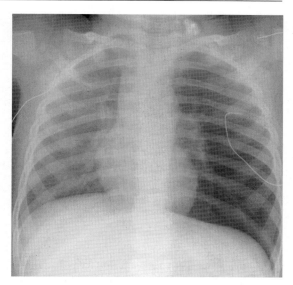

FIGURE 2-19. Bronchial foreign body. Radiograph showing slight asymmetry in lung volumes, with the left being larger and more lucent. Decubitus films documented left air-trapping.

lack of change in lung volume demonstrated at different phases of the respiratory cycle (Fig. 2-19). Evaluation at varying phases of the respiratory cycle is easily accomplished in cooperative children by taking expiratory and inspiratory films. In infants and uncooperative children, the population most at risk for foreign body aspiration, air trapping can be detected in bilateral decubitus views of the chest or by fluoroscopy. Some articles propose non-contrast-enhanced CT for the diagnosis of bronchial foreign bodies, but it is not a widespread practice at this time. The differential diagnoses for an asymmetric lucent lung include bronchial foreign body, Swyer-James syndrome, and pulmonary hypoplasia.

Laryngeal or tracheal foreign bodies are far less common than bronchial foreign bodies and usually present with abrupt stridor or respiratory distress. Radiographic findings include a radiopaque foreign body, soft tissue density within the airway, and loss of visualization (silhouetting) of the airway wall contours. Foreign bodies lodged within the proximal esophagus may also present with airway compression.

Obstructive Sleep Apnea (OSA)

One of the most common clinical problems involving the pediatric airway is the presence of OSA. This disorder affects 3% of children (millions in the United States alone) and is increasingly being associated with significant morbidities, such as poor performance in school, attention deficit disorder, excessive daytime sleepiness, and failure to thrive. Most children with OSA are otherwise healthy children in whom there is enlargement of the adenoid and palatine tonsils, causing OSA. When the

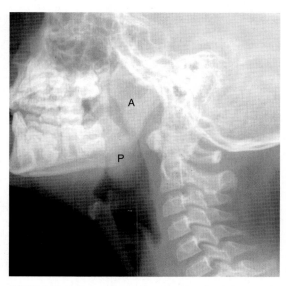

FIGURE 2-20. Enlargement of the adenoid and palatine tonsils. Lateral radiograph showing enlargement of the palatine *(P)* and adenoid *(A)* tonsils, with near obstruction of the nasopharynx.

adenoid and palatine tonsils are removed, the OSA-related symptoms typically resolve. In these children, imaging is limited to a lateral radiograph of the airway preoperatively. The palatine tonsils can be evaluated on physical examination. The lateral radiograph is obtained to evaluate the adenoid tonsils. On radiography, enlarged adenoids appear as a convex soft tissue mass in the posterior nasopharynx and are greater than 12 mm in diameter (Fig. 2-20). Markedly enlarged adenoid tissues may completely obstruct the posterior nasopharynx. Enlarged palatine tonsils can also be seen radiographically; they appear as a large soft tissue mass projecting over the posterior aspect of the soft palate on lateral radiography (see Fig 2-20).

Certain children have more complicated airway issues. In these children, an MR sleep study may be helpful in planning future management. Such studies have been shown to influence management decisions and help to plan surgical interventions in the majority of cases. Sequences performed include T1-weighted (for anatomy) and T2-weighted images with fat-saturation (depicts tonsillar tissue as bright on a dark background), as well as fast-gradient echo images that can be displayed in a cine, or movie, fashion to depict patterns of airway motion and collapse. Indications for MR sleep studies include persistent OSA despite previous airway surgery (most commonly tonsillectomy and adenoidectomy); predisposition to multilevel obstruction such as in Down and other syndromes; OSA and

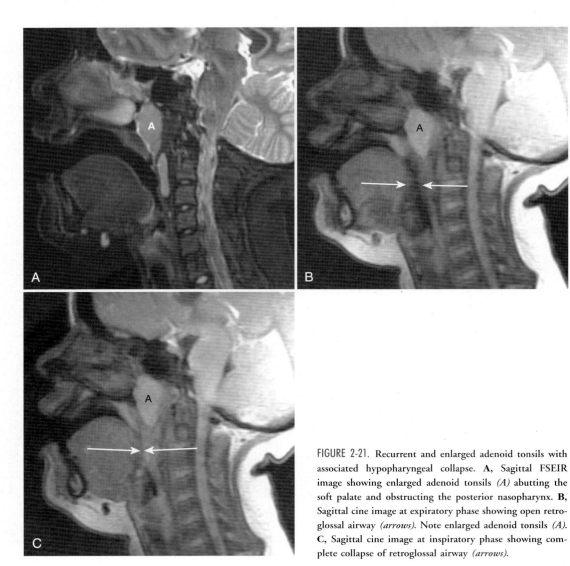

FIGURE 2-21. Recurrent and enlarged adenoid tonsils with associated hypopharyngeal collapse. **A,** Sagittal FSEIR image showing enlarged adenoid tonsils *(A)* abutting the soft palate and obstructing the posterior nasopharynx. **B,** Sagittal cine image at expiratory phase showing open retroglossal airway *(arrows)*. Note enlarged adenoid tonsils *(A)*. **C,** Sagittal cine image at inspiratory phase showing complete collapse of retroglossal airway *(arrows)*.

severe obesity; and preoperative evaluation prior to complex airway surgery. Commonly encountered diagnoses include recurrent enlarged adenoid tonsils, enlarged palatine tonsils, enlarged lingual tonsils, glossoptosis, hypopharyngeal collapse, and abnormal soft palate.

Recurrent and Enlarged Adenoid Tonsils

The adenoid tonsils are absent at birth, rapidly proliferate during infancy, and reach their maximal size when children are between 2 and 10 years of age. During the second decade of life, they begin to decrease in size. One of the things I have been surprised by is how commonly the adenoids can grow back. It is one of the most common causes of recurrent OSA after tonsillectomy and adenoidectomy. Adenoid tonsils are considered to be recurrent and enlarged (Fig. 2-21A-C) if they are greater than 12 mm in anterior to posterior diameter and are associated with intermittent collapse of the posterior nasopharynx on cine images. There may also be associated collapse of the hypopharynx because the relatively superior obstruction generates negative pressure in the hypopharynx during inspiration. On axial images, the postsurgical appearance of a V-shaped defect in the midportion of the adenoid tonsil is typically seen (Fig. 2-22).

Enlarged Palatine Tonsils

Unlike the adenoid tonsils, which commonly grow back after surgical removal, the palatine tonsils do not. Therefore, because most MR sleep studies are performed after tonsillectomy, absence of the palatine tonsils is depicted in most cases. When present and enlarged (Fig. 2-23), the palatine tonsils appear as round, high T2-signal structures in the palatine fossa, and they bob inferiorly and centrally, intermittently obstructing the airway. There is no published range of normal size for palatine tonsils on imaging.

Enlarged Lingual Tonsils

Enlargement of the lingual tonsils is being recognized as a common cause of persistent OSA following previous tonsillectomy and adenoidectomy. In such patients, the lingual tonsils can become quite large and obstruct the retroglossal airway. Enlarged lingual tonsils appear as high-signal masses (Fig. 2-24A, B) that are

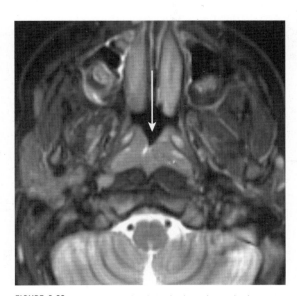

FIGURE 2-22. Recurrent and enlarged adenoid tonsils shown on axial FSEIR MR image. Note wedge-shaped central defect (*arrow*) in adenoid tonsil, typical of postoperative appearance.

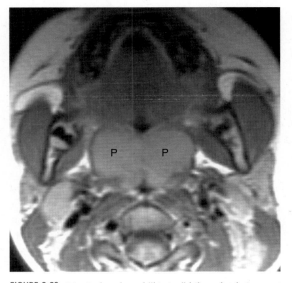

FIGURE 2-23. Massively enlarged "kissing" bilateral palatine tonsils. Axial proton-density image showing bilateral markedly enlarged palatine tonsils (*P*) touching in the midline and obstructing airway.

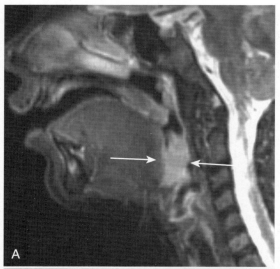

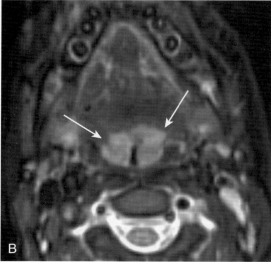

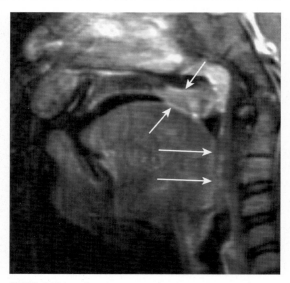

FIGURE 2-25. Glossoptosis and edematous soft palate. Sagittal FSEIR showing large tongue with posterior aspect of tongue *(large arrows)* abutting the posterior pharyngeal wall and obstructing the retroglossal airway. Note the high signal and thickening of soft palate *(small arrows)*, consistent with edematous soft palate, a sign of significant OSA. Normally, the soft palate produces the same signal intensity as the musculature of the tongue.

Glossoptosis

Glossoptosis is defined as posterior motion of the tongue during sleep. The posterior aspect of the tongue intermittently falls posteriorly and abuts the posterior pharyngeal wall, obstructing the retroglossal airway (Fig. 2-25). It is associated with large tongues (macroglossia), small jaws (micrognathia), and decreased muscular tone. It is most commonly seen in children with Down syndrome, Pierre-Robin sequence, and neuromuscular disorders such as cerebral palsy. On imaging, intermittent posterior motion of the tongue in the anterior to posterior direction is depicted on cine images.

FIGURE 2-24. Enlarged lingual tonsils. **A,** Sagittal FSEIR image showing enlarged lingual tonsils *(arrows)* completely obstructing the retroglossal pharynx. **B,** Axial FSEIR showing enlarged bilateral lingual tonsils *(arrows)* as a dumbbell-shaped area of high signal intensity posterior to tongue.

round or that have grown together and appear as a single dumbbell-shaped mass immediately posterior to the tongue. It is an important diagnosis to make on imaging because it is not readily seen on physical examination and is one of the more easily surgically curable causes of persistent OSA. Enlargement of the lingual tonsils appears to be particularly common after tonsillectomy and adenoidectomy in obese children and in children with Down syndrome.

Hypopharyngeal (Retroglossal) Collapse

Hypopharyngeal collapse can be a primary phenomenon caused by decreased muscle tone, or it may occur secondary to negative pressure generated by a more superior obstruction (typically enlarged adenoid tonsils). With hypopharyngeal collapse, there is cylindrical collapse of the retroglossal airway, with the anterior,

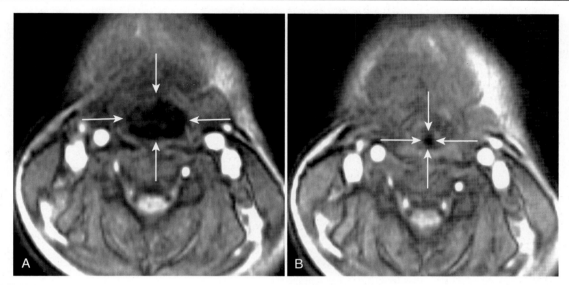

FIGURE 2-26. **Hypopharyngeal (retroglossal) collapse. A,** Axial cine image during expiration showing open retroglossal airway *(arrows)*. **B,** Axial cine image during inspiration showing complete collapse of the retroglossal airway *(arrows)*. Note that lateral left and right, anterior, and posterior walls all collapse cylindrically to the center of airway, in contrast to tongue moving posteriorly, as seen in glossoptosis.

posterior, left, and right walls of the airway all collapsing centrally (Fig. 2-26A, B). In contrast, with glossoptosis, the tongue moves anteriorly and posteriorly, and the lateral diameter of the airway remains unchanged. This differentiation is easiest to observe on axial cine images at the level of the midportion of the tongue, from superior to inferior. It is important to characterize the pattern of collapse of the retroglossal airway as hypopharyngeal collapse or glossoptosis because the surgical options for the two groups of patients are quite different.

Abnormal Soft Palate

A prominent soft palate is one of the contributing factors in some cases of OSA, and there are surgical procedures that decrease the size of the soft palate. As you can imagine, there are no published criteria for abnormal soft palate enlargement. If the soft palate is prominent in size, is draped over the tongue and hangs more inferiorly than the midportion of the tongue, and is associated with intermittent collapse of the posterior nasopharynx or retroglossal airway, we consider it enlarged.

The soft palate can be edematous as seen on physical examination in patients with significant OSA. This is thought to be related to the repeated trauma of snoring. On T2-weighted MR sequences, the edema is depicted as an increased signal throughout the soft palate (see Fig. 2-25); in patients without OSA, the soft palate is similar in signal to that of the musculature of the tongue.

CONGENITAL AIRWAY OBSTRUCTION

With the increase in fetal surgery centers and associated fetal ultrasound and MRI, pediatric radiologists are beginning to see an increasing number of cases of congenital obstruction of the airway, although it remains a rare entity. Congenital high airway obstruction syndrome (CHAOS) is the term given to a constellation of findings resulting from this form of airway obstruction. Causes of the airway obstruction include in utero laryngeal atresia, subglottic stenosis, and head and neck masses obstructing the upper airway, most commonly lymphatic malformations or teratomas. Fetal imaging findings in CHAOS (Fig. 2-27A-C) include massive increases in lung volumes, flattened or everted hemidiaphragms, hydrops, and polyhydramnios. Infants with airway obstruction secondary to masses (Fig. 2-28A, B) or other causes, with or without associated CHAOS findings, may be delivered via an ex utero intrapartum treatment (EXIT). In an EXIT, the head of the infant is delivered via a cesarean section, and the airway is established by tracheotomy or intubation prior to the child's

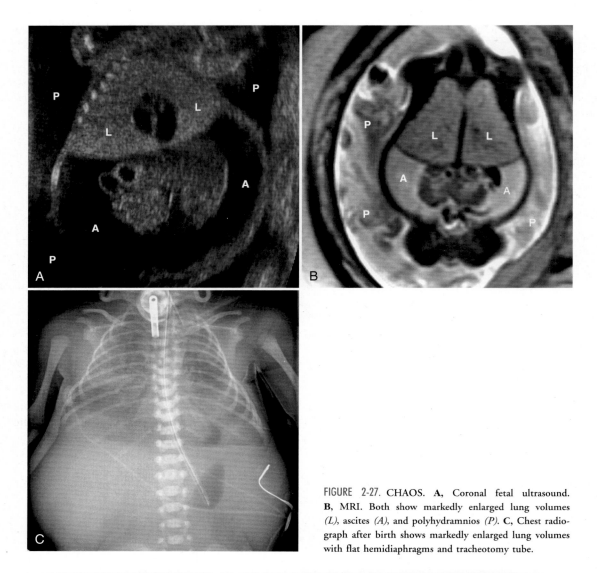

FIGURE 2-27. CHAOS. **A,** Coronal fetal ultrasound. **B,** MRI. Both show markedly enlarged lung volumes *(L)*, ascites *(A)*, and polyhydramnios *(P)*. **C,** Chest radiograph after birth shows markedly enlarged lung volumes with flat hemidiaphragms and tracheotomy tube.

FIGURE 2-28. Teratoma of the neck. **A,** Fetal MRI sagittal to fetal head and neck showing large mass *(arrows)* in the region of the neck. Note the well-defined area of increased signal centrally in lesion *(H)*, consistent with proteinacious fluid. **B,** Photograph during EXIT procedure: head of baby is delivered via cesarean section and airway is established while baby is still on placental blood supply. Note the large mass adjacent to the baby's head.

being taken off placental circulation. Once the airway has been established, the child can be completely delivered.

Suggested Readings

Berdon WE, Baker DH: Vascular anomalies and the infant lung: rings, slings, and other things, *Semin Roentgenol* 7:39-63, 1972.

Capitanio MA, Kirkpatrick JA: Obstruction of the upper airway in infants and children, *Radiol Clin North Am* 6:265-277, 1968.

Donnelly LF, Strife JL, Bisset GS III: The spectrum of extrinsic lower airway compression in children: MR imaging, *AJR* 168:59-62, 1997.

Donnelly LF, Frush DP, Bisset III GS: The multiple presentations of foreign bodies in children, *AJR* 170:471-477, 1998.

Donnelly LF: OSA in pediatric patients: evaluation with cine MR sleep studies, *Radiology* 236:768-778, 2005.

Dunbar JS: Upper respiratory tract obstruction in infants and children, *AJR* 109:227-246, 1970.

Hedrick MH, Ferro MM, Filly RA, et al: Congenital high airway obstruction syndrome (CHAOS): a potential for perinatal intervention, *J Pediatr Surg* 29:271-274, 1994.

Heyer CM, Nuesslein TY, Jung D, et al: Tracheobronchial anomalies and stenoses: detection with low-dose multi-detector CT with virtual tracheobronchoscopy: comparison with flexible tracheobronchoscopy, *Radiology* 242:542-549, 2007.

John SD, Swischuk KE: Stridor and upper airway obstruction in infants and children, *Radiographics* 12:625-643, 1992.

Pacharn P, Poe SA, Donnelly LF: Low-tube-current CT for children with suspected extrinsic airway compression, *AJR* 179:1523-1527, 2002.

CHAPTER THREE

Chest

The chest radiograph is one of the most commonly obtained examinations in pediatric imaging. It is also the examination most likely to be encountered by radiology residents, pediatric residents, general radiologists, and pediatricians. Therefore, topics such as chest imaging in neonates and the evaluation of suspected pneumonia are discussed in detail.

NEONATAL CHEST

Causes of respiratory distress in newborn infants can be divided into those that are secondary to diffuse pulmonary disease (medical causes) and those that are secondary to a space-occupying mass compressing the pulmonary parenchyma (surgical causes).

Diffuse Pulmonary Disease in the Newborn

Diffuse pulmonary disease causes respiratory distress much more commonly than surgical diseases, particularly in premature infants, who make up the majority of cases of respiratory distress in the newborn. A simple way to evaluate these patients and try to offer a limited differential diagnosis is to evaluate the lung volumes and to characterize the pulmonary opacities.

Lung volumes can be categorized as high, normal, or low. Normally, the apex of the dome of the diaphragm is expected to be at the level of approximately the tenth posterior rib. Lung opacity, if present, can be characterized as streaky, perihilar (central) densities that have a linear quality or as diffuse, granular opacities that have an almost sandlike character. Classically, cases fall into one of the following two categories: (1) cases with high lung volumes and streaky perihilar densities and (2) cases with low lung volumes and granular opacities (Table 3-1). This is more of a guideline, rather than a rule, because many neonates with diffuse pulmonary disease have normal lung volumes. The differential diagnosis for cases with high lung volumes and streaky perihilar densities includes meconium aspiration, transient tachypnea of the newborn, and neonatal pneumonia. Most of the neonates in this group are term. The differential for cases with low lung volumes and granular opacities includes surfactant deficiency and β-hemolytic streptococcal pneumonia. Most of these neonates are premature.

Meconium Aspiration Syndrome

Meconium aspiration syndrome results from intrapartum or intrauterine aspiration of meconium. It usually occurs secondary to stress, such as hypoxia, and more often occurs in term or postmature neonates. The aspirated meconium causes both obstruction of small airways secondary to its tenacious nature and also chemical pneumonitis. The degree of respiratory failure can be severe. Radiographic findings include hyperinflation (high lung volumes), which may be asymmetric and patchy, and asymmetric lung densities that tend to have a ropy appearance and a perihilar distribution (Fig. 3-1). Commonly there are areas of hyperinflation alternating with areas of atelectasis. Pleural effusions can be present. Because of the small-airway obstruction by the meconium, air-block complications are common, with pneumothorax occurring in 20% to 40% of cases. Meconium aspiration syndrome is relatively common; 25,000 to 30,000 cases occur in the United States annually.

Transient Tachypnea of the Newborn

Transient tachypnea of the newborn (TTN) is also referred to by a variety of other names, including wet lung disease and transient respiratory distress. It occurs secondary to delayed clearance of fetal lung fluid. Physiologically, the clearing of fetal lung fluid is facilitated by the "thoracic squeeze" during vaginal deliveries; therefore, most cases of TTN are related to

TABLE 3-1. **Differential Diagnosis of Diffuse Pulmonary Disease in the Newborn**

High lung volumes, streaky perihilar densities	Low lung volumes, granular opacities
Meconium aspiration syndrome Transient tachypnea of the newborn Neonatal pneumonia	Surfactant deficiency β-hemolytic streptococcal pneumonia

cesarean section in which the thoracic squeeze is bypassed. Other causes include maternal diabetes and maternal sedation. The hallmark of TTN is a benign course. Respiratory distress develops by 6 hours of age, peaks at 1 day of age, and is resolved by 2 to 3 days. There is a spectrum of radiographic findings similar to those seen with mild to severe pulmonary edema. There is a combination of airspace opacification, coarse interstitial markings, prominent and indistinct pulmonary vasculature, fluid in the fissures, pleural effusion, and cardiomegaly (Fig. 3-2). Lung volumes are normal to increased.

Neonatal Pneumonia

Neonatal pneumonia can be caused by a large number of infectious agents that can be acquired intrauterine, during birth, or soon after birth. With the exception of β-hemolytic streptococcal pneumonia, which will be discussed separately, the radiographic appearance of neonatal

pneumonia is that of patchy, asymmetric perihilar densities and hyperinflation (Fig. 3-3). Pleural effusions may be present (Fig. 3-4). Such cases of neonatal pneumonia may have a similar radiographic appearance to and be indistinguishable from meconium aspiration syndrome when using imaging alone.

Surfactant-Deficient Disease

Surfactant-deficient disease (SDD; also referred to as respiratory distress syndrome or hyaline membrane disease) is a common disorder, with approximately 40,000 new cases annually in the United States. It is primarily a disease of premature infants, affecting up to 50% of them, and it is the most common cause of death in live newborns. SDD is related to the inability of premature type II pneumocytes to produce surfactant. Normally, surfactant coats the alveolar surfaces and decreases surface tension, allowing for the alveoli to remain open. As a result of the lack of surfactant, there is alveolar collapse, resulting in noncompliant lungs. The radiographic findings reflect these pathologic changes (Fig. 3-5A, B).

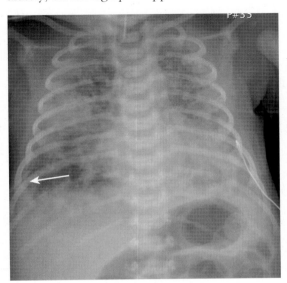

FIGURE 3-1. **Meconium aspiration syndrome.** Newborn chest radiograph shows normal to large lung volumes, increased perihilar markings, and bilateral, coarse, ropy markings. Note right pleural effusion *(arrow)*.

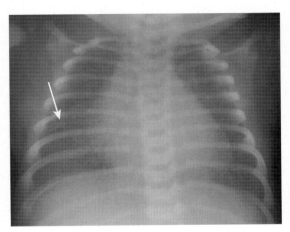

FIGURE 3-2. **Transient tachypnea of the newborn.** Newborn chest radiograph shows normal lung volumes, cardiomegaly, indistinct pulmonary vascularity, and fluid in the minor fissure *(arrow)*. Within 24 hours the patient was asymptomatic.

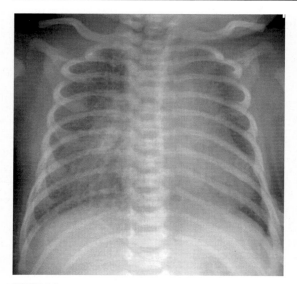

FIGURE 3-3. Neonatal pneumonia. Newborn chest radiograph shows large lung volumes and coarse, bilateral perihilar markings.

Lung volumes are low. There are bilateral granular opacities that represent collapsed alveoli interspersed with open alveoli. Because the larger bronchi do not collapse, there are prominent air bronchograms. When the process is severe enough and the majority of alveoli are collapsed, there may be coalescence of the granular opacities, resulting in diffuse lung opacity.

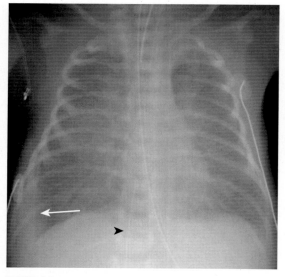

FIGURE 3-4. Neonatal pneumonia. Newborn chest radiograph shows large lung volumes and coarse, bilateral perihilar markings. Note right pleural effusion *(arrow)*. Also note umbilical venous catheter with tip into right atrium. Tip should be at the junction of the right atrium and inferior vena cava.

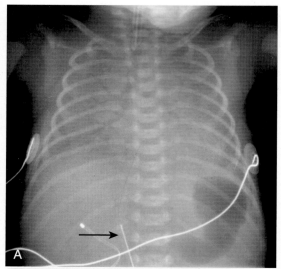

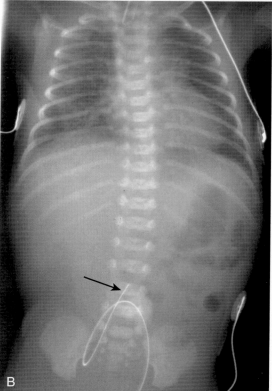

FIGURE 3-5. Surfactant-deficient disease responding to surfactant therapy. **A,** Radiograph shortly after birth shows low lung volumes, confluent densities, and prominent air bronchograms. Note the umbilical venous catheter *(arrow)* with tip in intrahepatic intravenous catheter. **B,** Radiograph obtained immediately following surfactant administration shows increased lung volumes and decreased lung opacities. The umbilical venous catheter was removed in the interim. Note the umbilical venous catheter *(arrow)* in "low"-type position, with tip at L4.

A normal film at 6 hours of age excludes the presence of SDD.

Surfactant Replacement Therapy

One of the therapies for SDD is surfactant administration. Surfactant can be administered via nebulized or aerosol forms. It is administered into the trachea via a catheter or an adapted endotracheal tube. The administration of surfactant in neonates with SDD has been shown to be associated with decreased oxygen and ventilator setting requirements, decreased air-block complications, decreased incidence of intracranial hemorrhage and bronchopulmonary dysplasia, and decreased death rate. However, there is an associated increased risk for development of patent ductus arteriosus and pulmonary hemorrhage, and there can be an acute desaturation episode in response to surfactant administration. Surfactant administration can be given on a rescue basis when premature neonates develop respiratory distress or can be given prophylactically in premature infants who are at risk. Prophylactic administration is commonly given immediately after birth and is becoming a more common practice. In response to surfactant administration, radiography may demonstrate complete, central, or asymmetric clearing of the findings of SDD (see Fig. 3-5). There is usually an increase in lung volumes. Neonates without radiographic findings of a response to surfactant have poorer prognoses than those who have radiographic evidence of a response. A pattern of alternating distended and collapsed acini may create a radiographic pattern of bubblelike lucencies that can mimic pulmonary interstitial emphysema. Knowledge of when surfactant has been administered is helpful in rendering accurate interpretation of chest radiographs taken in the neonatal intensive care unit (NICU).

β-Hemolytic Streptococcal Pneumonia

β-hemolytic (group B) streptococcal pneumonia is the most common type of pneumonia in neonates. The infection is acquired during birth, and at least 25% of women in labor are colonized by the organism. Premature infants are more commonly infected than are term infants. In contrast

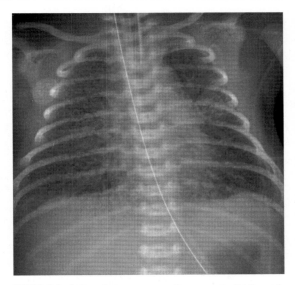

FIGURE. 3-6. β-Hemolytic streptococcal pneumonia. Radiograph shows low lung volumes and diffuse granular opacities, similar in appearance to cases of surfactant deficiency.

to the other types of neonatal pneumonias, the radiographic findings include bilateral granular opacities and low lung volumes (Fig. 3-6), the identical findings in surfactant-deficient disease. The presence of pleural fluid is a helpful differentiating factor because it is very uncommon in surfactant deficiency but has been reported in between 25% and 67% of cases of β-hemolytic streptococcal pneumonia.

Persistent Pulmonary Hypertension in the Neonate

Persistent pulmonary hypertension in the neonate, also referred to as persistent fetal circulation, is a term often used in the NICU and is addressed here because it can be a source of confusion. The high pulmonary vascular resistance that is normally present in the fetus typically decreases during the newborn period. When this fails to happen, the pulmonary pressures remain abnormally high, and the condition is referred to as persistent pulmonary hypertension. It is a physiologic finding rather than a specific disease. It can be a primary phenomenon or it can occur secondary to causes of hypoxia, such as meconium aspiration syndrome, neonatal pneumonia, or pulmonary hypoplasia associated with congenital diaphragmatic hernia. These patients are quite ill. The radiographic patterns are variable and are more often reflective of the underlying cause of hypoxia than the presence of persistent pulmonary hypertension.

Neonatal Intensive Care Unit Support Apparatus

One of the primary roles of chest radiography in the NICU is to monitor support apparatus. They include endotracheal tubes, enteric tubes, central venous lines, umbilical arterial and venous catheters, and extracorporeal membrane oxygenation (ECMO) catheters. The radiographic evaluation of many of these tubes is the same as that seen in adults and is not discussed here. When evaluating the positions of endotracheal tubes in premature neonates, it is important to consider that the length of the entire trachea may be only about 1 cm. Keeping the endotracheal tube in the exact center of such a small trachea is an impossible task for caregivers, and phone calls and reports suggesting that the tube needs to be moved 2 mm proximally may be more annoying than helpful. Direct phone communication may be more appropriately reserved for times when the tube is in a main bronchus or above the thoracic inlet. There is an increased propensity to use esophageal intubation in neonates compared to its use in adults. Although it would seem that esophageal intubation would be incredibly obvious clinically, this is not always the case. I have seen cases in which a child has in retrospect been discovered to have been esophageally intubated for more than 24 hours. Therefore, the radiologist may be the first to recognize esophageal intubation. Obviously, when the course of the endotracheal tube does not overlie the path of the trachea, the use of esophageal intubation is fairly obvious. Other findings of esophageal intubation include a combination of low lung volumes, gas within the esophagus, and gaseous distention of the bowel (Fig. 3-7).

Umbilical Arterial and Venous Catheters

Umbilical arterial and venous catheters are commonly used in the NICU. Umbilical arterial catheters pass from the umbilicus inferiorly into the pelvis via the umbilical artery to the iliac artery. The catheters then turn cephalad within the aorta (see Fig. 3-5). These catheters

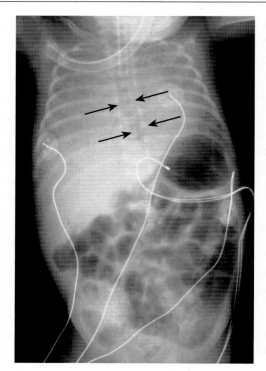

FIGURE 3-7. Esophageal intubation in a 6-day-old girl. Chest radiograph obtained after reintubation shows the endotracheal tube overlying the expected location of the midtrachea. However, there are low lung volumes, gas within the esophagus (*arrows*), and multiple air-filled and distended bowel loops.

can be associated with thrombosis of the aorta and its branches. Therefore, it is important to avoid positioning the catheter with the tip at the level of the branches of the aorta (celiac, superior mesenteric, and renal arteries). There are two acceptable umbilical arterial catheter positions: *high lines* have their tips at the level of the descending thoracic aorta (T8-T10; see Fig. 3-9); *low lines* have their tips below the level of L3 (see Fig. 3-5). The catheter tip should not be positioned between T10 and L3 because of the risk for major arterial thrombosis. There is no clear consensus as to whether a high or a low umbilical artery catheter line is better, and both positions are still currently used.

The pathway of the umbilical venous catheter is umbilical vein to left portal vein to ductus venosus to hepatic vein to inferior vena cava (Fig. 3-8). In contrast to umbilical arterial catheters, the course is in the superior direction from the level of the umbilicus. The ideal position of an umbilical venous catheter is with its tip at the junction of the right atrium and the inferior vena cava at the level of the hemidiaphragm

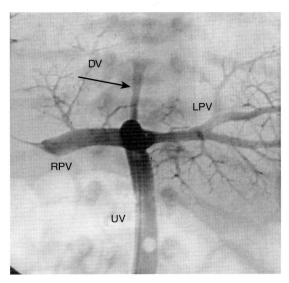

FIGURE 3-8. Anatomy of the course of the umbilical vein *(UV)* catheter as demonstrated by contrast injection of umbilical catheter performed because of inability to advance UV catheter. Note course of umbilical vein to portal vein to ductus venosus *(DV; arrow)*. LPV, left portal vein; RPV, right portal vein.

(see Figs. 3-4, 3-5). The umbilical venous catheter may occasionally deflect into the portal venous system rather than passing into the ductus venosus. Complications of such positioning can include hepatic hematoma or abscess.

Peripherally Inserted Central Catheters in Children

One of the more common lines now seen in children, as in adults, is peripherally inserted central catheters (PICCs). In contrast to adults, in whom some of the PICCs can be as large as 6F, the PICC lines used in children, particularly infants, are often small in caliber (2F or 3F) so that they can be placed into their very small peripheral veins. These small caliber PICCs can be very difficult to see on chest radiography, so some of them must be filled with contrast to be accurately visualized. The tip of the PICC line that enters the child from the upper extremity or scalp should be positioned with the tip in the midlevel of the superior vena cava (see Fig. 3-27). It is essential that PICC lines not be left in place with the tip well into the right atrium. Particularly with the small-caliber lines, the atrium can be lacerated, leading to pericardial tamponade, free hemorrhage, or death.

Many such cases have been reported nationally. Also, the PICC should not be too proximal in the superior vena cava because the distal portion of the line can flip from the superior vena cava into the contralateral brachiocephalic or jugular vein. At Cincinnati Children's Hospital Medical Center, the PICC lines are inserted in a dedicated interventional radiology suite by a team of nurses, with supervision by pediatric interventional radiologists. Ultrasound is often used to guide vein cannulation and certified Child Life Specialists coach most kids through the procedure without having to sedate them. Fluoroscopy is utilized at the end of the procedure to adjust and document tip position in the mid-superior vena cava.

EXTRACORPOREAL MEMBRANE OXYGENATION

ECMO is a last-resort therapy usually reserved for respiratory failure that has not responded to other treatments. ECMO is essentially a prolonged form of circulatory bypass of the lungs and is used only in patients who have reversible disease and a chance for survival. The majority of neonates who are treated with ECMO have respiratory failure as a result of meconium aspiration, persistent pulmonary hypertension (resulting from a variety of causes), severe congenital heart disease, or congenital diaphragmatic hernia. ECMO seems to be used less commonly now than it was in the 1990s.

There are two types of ECMO: arteriovenous and venovenous. In ateriovenous ECMO, the right common carotid artery and internal jugular veins are sacrificed. The arterial catheter is placed via the carotid and positioned with its tip overlying the aortic arch. The venous catheter is positioned with its tip over the right atrium (Fig. 3-9). One of the main roles of a chest radiograph of children on ECMO is to detect any potential migration of the catheters. Careful comparison with previous studies to make sure that the catheters are not coming out or moving too far in is critical. These patients have many bandages and other items covering the external portions of the catheters, so migration may be hard to detect on physical examination. Note that there are various radiographic appearances of the ECMO catheters. Some catheters end where the radiopaque portion of the tube ends, and others have a radiolucent portion with a small metallic marker at the tip (see Fig. 3-9). It is common to see white-out of the lungs soon after a patient is placed on ECMO as a result of decreased ventilator settings and

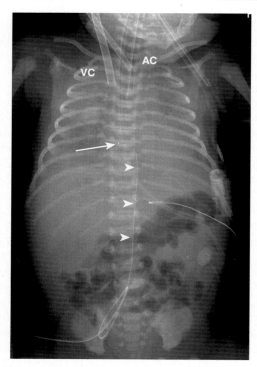

FIGURE 3-9. ECMO catheter placement for meconium aspiration syndrome (same child as in Fig. 3-1). Note venous ECMO catheter *(VC)* has a radiopaque proximal portion and a lucent distal portion. The tip of the venous catheter is marked by a small radiopaque metallic marker *(arrow)* and is actually in the right atrium. Note the arterial ECMO catheter *(AC)* with tip in region of aortic arch. Also, note "high"-type umbilical arterial catheter with tip overlying descending aorta at the level of T8.

third-space shifting of fluid (see Fig. 3-9). Patients on ECMO are anticoagulated and are therefore at risk for hemorrhage.

Types of Ventilation: High-Frequency Oscillator vs. Conventional Ventilation

High-frequency oscillators are commonly used to treat neonates in the NICU. In contrast to conventional ventilation, high-frequency oscillators use supraphysiologic rates of ventilation with very low tidal volumes. Conventional ventilation has been likened to delivering a cupful of air approximately 20 times a minute. In contrast, high-frequency oscillation is like delivering a thimbleful of air approximately 1000 times per minute. The air is vibrated in and out of the lung. The mechanism of oscillators is poorly understood. In conventional ventilation, the diaphragm moves up and down, whereas during high-frequency ventilation the diaphragm stays parked at a certain anatomic level. This level can be adjusted by changing the mean airway pressure of the oscillator. Caregivers usually like to maintain the diaphragm at approximately the level of the 10th posterior ribs. In general, the radiographic appearance of neonatal pulmonary diseases is not affected by whether the patient is being ventilated by conventional or high-frequency ventilation.

Complications in the Neonatal Intensive Care Unit

As in adult intensive care units, major complications detected by chest radiographs include those related to air-block complications, lobar collapse, or acute diffuse pulmonary consolidation. Another type of complication seen in neonates is the development of bronchopulmonary dysplasia. Imaging findings of lobar collapse and air-block complications such as pneumothorax, pneumomediastinum, and pneumopericardium are similar in neonates and in adults. One type of air-block complication that is unique to neonates is pulmonary interstitial emphysema.

Pulmonary Interstitial Emphysema

In patients with severe surfactant deficiency, ventilatory support can result in marked increases in alveolar pressure, leading to perforation of alveoli. The air that escapes into the adjacent interstitium and lymphatics is referred to as pulmonary interstitial emphysema (PIE). PIE appears on radiographs as bubblelike or linear lucencies and can be focal or diffuse (Fig. 3-10). The involved lung is usually noncompliant and is seen to have a static volume on multiple consecutive films. The finding is typically transient. The importance of detecting PIE is that it serves as a warning sign for other impending air-block complications such as pneumothorax, and its presence can influence caregivers in decisions such as switching from conventional to high-frequency ventilation.

It can be difficult to differentiate diffuse PIE from the bubblelike lucencies that are associated with developing bronchopulmonary dysplasia. When encountering this scenario, the patient's age can help to determine which is more likely. Most cases of PIE occur in the first week

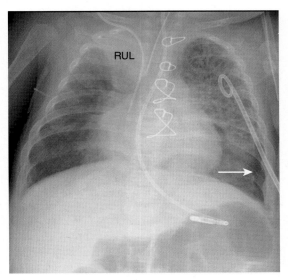

FIGURE 3-10. Pulmonary interstitial emphysema in a premature infant with congenital heart disease. Chest radiograph shows asymmetric bubblelike lucencies within the left upper lobe consistent with PIE. Note left pneumothorax *(arrow)* and right upper lobe collapse *(RUL)*.

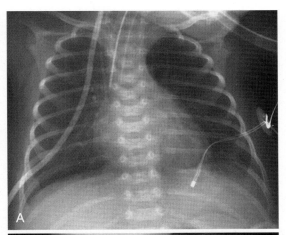

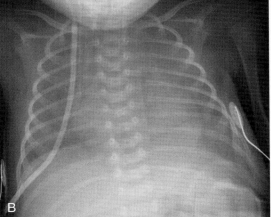

FIGURE 3-11. Patent ductus arteriosus *(PDA)* leading to congestive heart failure in a 1-week-old premature neonate. A, Prior to development of PDA, radiograph shows normal-sized heart and clear lungs; B, After development of PDA, radiograph shows cardiac enlargement and bilateral lung consolidation.

of life, a time at which bronchopulmonary dysplasia is very unlikely. In patients older than 2 weeks, bronchopulmonary dysplasia is more likely. Also, in patients who have undergone a series of daily films, PIE may be noted to occur abruptly, whereas bronchopulmonary dysplasia tends to occur gradually. As previously mentioned, SDD partially treated by surfactant replacement can cause a pattern of lucencies that may mimic PIE as well.

Rarely, PIE can persist and develop into an expansive, multicystic mass. The air cysts can become large enough to cause mediastinal shift and compromise pulmonary function. Often, the diagnosis is indicated by sequential radiography showing evolution of the cystic mass from original findings typical of PIE. In unclear cases, CT demonstrates that the air cysts are in the interstitial space by showing the bronchovascular bundles being positioned within the center of the air cysts. The bronchovascular bundles appear as linear or nodular densities in the center of the cysts.

Causes of Acute Diffuse Pulmonary Consolidation

Acute diffuse pulmonary consolidation is nonspecific in neonates, as it is in adults, and can represent blood, pus, or water. In the neonate, the specific considerations include edema, which may be secondary to the development of patent ductus arteriosus (Fig. 3-11); pulmonary hemorrhage, to which surfactant therapy predisposes; worsening surfactant deficiency (during the first several days of life but not later); or developing neonatal pneumonia (Table 3-2). Diffuse microatelectasis is another possibility because neonates have the propensity to artifactually demonstrate diffuse lung opacity on low lung volume films (expiratory technique; Fig. 3-12A. B); this should not be mistaken for another cause of consolidation. Such radiographs showing low lung volumes offer little information concerning the pulmonary status of the patient and should be repeated when clinically indicated.

TABLE 3-2. Causes of Acute Diffuse Pulmonary Consolidation in Neonates

Edema: patent ductus arteriosus
Hemorrhage
Diffuse microatelectasis: artifact
Worsening surfactant deficiency (only during first days of life)
Pneumonia

Bronchopulmonary Dysplasia

Bronchopulmonary dysplasia (BPD) is also referred to as chronic lung disease of prematurity. It is a common complication seen in premature infants and is associated with significant

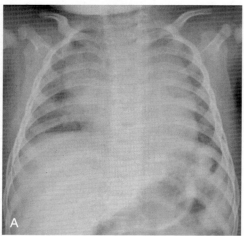
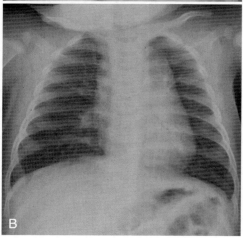

FIGURE 3-12. Expiratory chest radiograph mimicking heart failure in infant. **A,** Initial radiograph shows prominent size of cardiothymic silhouette, indistinctness of pulmonary vascularity, and low lung volumes. **B,** Repeat radiograph obtained immediately after A shows clear lungs and normal heart size.

morbidity rates. It is uncommon in children born at greater than 32 weeks of gestational age, but it occurs in more than 50% of premature infants born at less than 1000 g. BPD is the most common chronic lung disease of infancy.

BPD is related to injury to the lungs that is thought to result from some combination of mechanical ventilation and oxygen toxicity. Although four discrete and orderly stages of the development of BPD were originally described, they are not seen commonly and are probably not important to know. BPD typically occurs in a premature infant who requires prolonged ventilator support. At approximately the end of the second week of life, persistent hazy density appears throughout the lungs. Over the next weeks to months, a combination of coarse lung markings, bubblelike lucencies, and asymmetric aeration can develop (Fig. 3-13). Eventually, focal lucencies, coarse reticular densities, and bandlike opacities develop. In childhood survivors of BPD, many of these radiographic findings decrease in prominence over the years and only hyperaeration may persist. The radiographic findings may completely resolve. Clinically, many children with severe BPD during infancy may eventually improve to normal pulmonary function or may only have minor persistent problems such as exercise intolerance, predisposition to infection, or asthma.

Wilson-Mikity syndrome is a confusing and controversial term. It refers to the development of BPD in the absence of mechanical ventilation. Some people debate whether this disease exists, whereas others think it is a variant of BPD. Certainly, there are cases in which BPD findings develop with minimal ventilator support or develop earlier than is typically expected.

Focal Pulmonary Lesions in the Newborn

In contrast to diffuse pulmonary disease in newborns, focal masses can present with respiratory distress due to compression of otherwise normal lung. Most of these focal masses are related to congenital lung lesions. Congenital lung lesions may appear solid, as air-filled cysts, or mixed in appearance. The differential for a focal lung lesion can be separated on the basis of whether the lesion is lucent or solid appearing on chest radiography (Table 3-3). The most likely

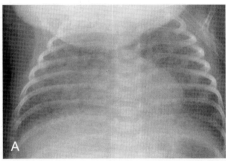

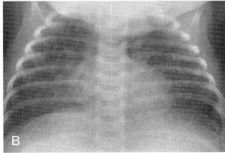

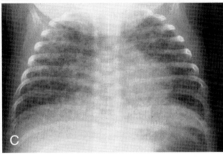

FIGURE 3-13. Bronchopulmonary dysplasia in a premature neonatal girl. **A,** Chest radiograph at 14 days of life shows persistent bilateral lung opacities. **B,** Chest radiograph at 20 days of life shows coarsening of the lung markings. **C,** Chest radiograph at 28 days of life shows increased coarse lung markings and development of diffuse bubblelike lucencies.

considerations for a lucent chest lesion in a newborn are congenital lobar emphysema, congenital cystic adenomatoid malformation, persistent pulmonary interstitial emphysema, and congenital diaphragmatic hernia. CT may be helpful in differentiating among these lesions by demonstrating whether the abnormal lucency

is related to air in distended alveoli, in the interstitium, or in abnormal cystic structures. Lesions that typically appear solid during the neonatal period include sequestration and bronchogenic cyst. Many of these lesions can present in children beyond the neonatal period, and those aspects of these entities are also discussed here.

The following sections are divided into specific congenital lesions. However, it has been increasingly recognized that there can be "mixed" lesions, which show characteristics of more than one type of lesions (see Fig. 3-16). The most common mixed lesions are those that show characteristics of both congenital cystic adenomatoid malformation and sequestration.

It is also worth mentioning that there has been a change in the way these lesions present that is related to the increased use of prenatal ultrasound and magnetic resonance (MR) imaging. Historically, congenital lung lesions were identified only when the infant became symptomatic. Many, if not most, of the congenital lung lesions we currently see are picked up and followed through fetal life, with additional postnatal imaging obtained shortly after birth. A significant number of these children are asymptomatic. This has raised issues related to when and whether to perform surgical treatment in infants with asymptomatic lesions.

Congenital Lobar Emphysema

Congenital lobar emphysema is related to overexpansion of alveoli, but the mechanism is debated. Some reports suggest a ball-valve type of anomaly in the bronchus leading to the affected lung, which causes progressive air trapping. Most cases present with respiratory distress during the neonatal period; 50% present within the first month, and 75% present within the first 6 months of life. There can be associated

TABLE 3-3. **Focal Lung Lesions in Neonates on Radiography**

Lucent Lesions	Solid Lesions
Congenital lobar emphysema	Sequestration
Congenital cystic adenomatoid malformation	Bronchogenic cyst
Persistent pulmonary interstitial emphysema	Congenital cystic adenomatoid
Congenital diaphragmatic hernia	malformation

anomalies, usually cardiac, but they occur in the minority of patients with congenital lobar emphysema. There is a lobar predilection; the most common site is the left upper lobe (43%), followed by the right middle lobe (35%) and right lower lobe (21%), with less than 1% in each of the other lobes. On chest radiography, a hyperlucent, hyperexpanded lobe is seen (Fig. 3-14A, B). On initial radiographs, the lesion may appear to be a soft tissue density because of retained fetal lung fluid. This density resolves and is replaced by progressive hyperlucency. On CT, the air is in the alveoli, so the

interstitial septa and bronchovascular bundles are at the periphery (not the center) of the lucency (see Fig. 3-14). The air spaces are larger than those in the adjacent normal lung, and the pulmonary vessels appear attenuated. The treatment is lobectomy.

Congenital Cystic Adenomatoid Malformation

Congenital cystic adenomatoid malformation (CCAM) is a congenital adenomatoid proliferation that replaces normal alveoli. The majority are detected prenatally or are present with respiratory distress at birth. Most involve only one lobe and, in contrast to congenital lobar emphysema, there is no lobar predilection. CCAMs are divided into three types on the basis of how large the cysts appear at imaging or pathology. Type 1 lesions (50%) have one or more large (2 to 10 cm) cysts. Type 2 lesions (40%) have numerous small cysts of uniform size. Type 3 lesions (10%) appear solid on gross inspection and imaging but have microscopic cysts. There are some who are now advocating the nomenclature congenital *pulmonary airway* malformation and a new classification with five subtypes. Who are these people and don't they have anything better to do?

The classification system has no clinical relevance except that it helps us remember that CCAM can have multiple appearances when imaged. The imaging appearance reflects the type. CCAMs communicate with the bronchial tree at birth and therefore fill with air within the first hours to days of life. On radiography and CT, a completely cystic, mixed cystic and solid, or completely solid mass is seen depending on the number and size of cysts and whether those cysts contain air or fluid (Figs. 3-15A-C, 3-16A-C). The management of symptomatic CCAM is surgical resection. The management of asymptomatic CCAM is currently somewhat controversial. However, most caregivers advocate elective resection because these lesions are at increased risk for infection and, rarely, may develop malignancy.

A scenario encountered with increasing frequency is a prenatally diagnosed lung mass that becomes less prominent on serial prenatal ultrasounds or MR examinations and demonstrates only subtle findings or is not detected on a chest radiograph obtained soon after birth.

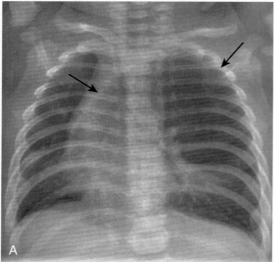

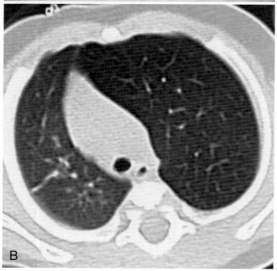

FIGURE 3-14. Congenital lobar emphysema. A, Radiograph obtained at 1 day of age shows diffuse lucency and enlargement of left upper lobe *(arrows)*. B, CT scan shows hyperlucent and enlarged left upper lobe with asymmetric attenuation of vascular structures and increased space between interstitial septa.

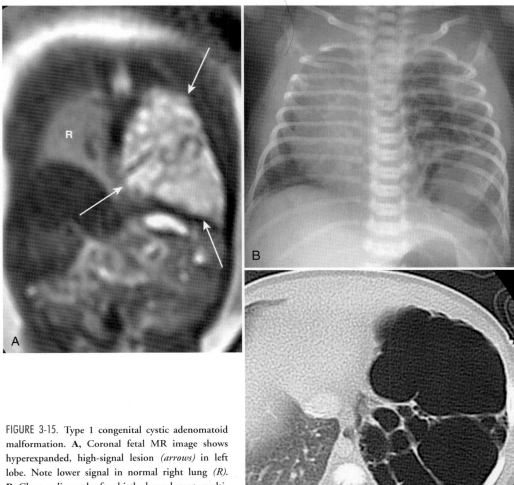

FIGURE 3-15. Type 1 congenital cystic adenomatoid malformation. **A,** Coronal fetal MR image shows hyperexpanded, high-signal lesion *(arrows)* in left lobe. Note lower signal in normal right lung *(R)*. **B,** Chest radiograph after birth shows lucent, multicystic lesion in left lung with rightward mediastinal shift. **C,** CT soon after birth shows large, lucent, multicystic lesion in left lung.

Almost all such lesions are type 2 CCAMs and demonstrate abnormalities on CT, even in light of a normal chest radiograph.

Many CCAMs identified prenatally are followed with MR imaging (see Fig. 3-15), and much has been learned about the nature of these lesions. CCAMs tend to increase in size until approximately 25 weeks of gestation. The mass of the CCAMs then tends to regress over time, sometimes dramatically. Compression of the contralateral lung by a large mass and development of fetal hydrops are associated with high mortality rates. Fetal intervention is typically reserved for cases with hydrops; management options include dominant cyst aspiration and fetal surgery with resection of the lesion. Recently, trials using maternal steroids have shown promise in shrinking the CCAM volumes and avoiding other interventions.

Congenital Diaphragmatic Hernia

Congenital diaphragmatic hernias (CDHs) are usually secondary to posterior defects in the diaphragm (Bochdalek hernia) and are more common on the left side by a ratio of 5 to 1. Most infants with CDHs present at birth with severe respiratory distress. The hernia may contain stomach, small bowel, colon, or liver. The radiographic appearance depends on the hernia contents and on whether there is air within the herniated viscera. On initial radiographs, prior to the introduction of air into the viscera, the appearance may be radiopaque.

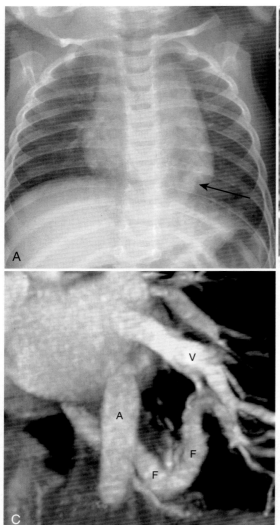

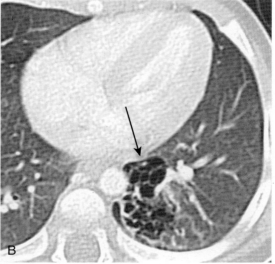

FIGURE 3-16. Mixed lesion with components of both CCAM and sequestration seen at pathology. **A,** Chest radiograph obtained for multiple infections in young child shows bandlike opacity *(arrow)* in left lower lobe. It had been present on multiple radiographs. **B,** CT scan shows multicystic, air-filled lesion *(arrow)* in left lower lobe, suggestive of CCAM. **C,** CT reformat shows systemic arterial feeder *(F)* arising from aorta *(A)* and extending into lesion. Findings are characteristic of sequestration. Note draining pulmonary vein *(V).*

Later, and more commonly, the herniated viscera contain air and the hernia appears as an air-containing cystic mass. Less air-filled viscera in the abdomen than expected and an abnormal position of support apparatus, such as a nasogastric tube within a herniated stomach, are obvious clues that support the diagnosis (Fig. 3-17). Often a nasogastric tube becomes lodged at the esophagogastric junction because of the acute turn in the herniated stomach. This can be a supportive finding of the diagnosis.

The diagnosis of CDH is commonly made prenatally by ultrasound and further evaluated by fetal MR imaging (Fig. 3-18A, B). The mortality rate for CDH is related to the degree of pulmonary hypoplasia. Systems of calculating lung volumes and predicting mortality have

been devised for use with fetal ultrasound, fetal MR imaging, and postnatal radiography. Radiographic predictors of poor prognoses include lack of aerated ipsilateral lung, low percentage of aerated contralateral lung, and severe mediastinal shift. Treatment includes support of respiratory failure, often by high-frequency ventilation or ECMO and surgical repair. The reported mortality rates associated with CDH range from 12% to 50%. One factor contributing to mortality is the presence of associated abnormalities, which are reported in a high percentage of infants born with CDH. One report suggests that as many as 50% of patients with CDH have associated congenital heart disease. By the nature of the herniated bowel into the chest, most patients with CDH have associated malrotation.

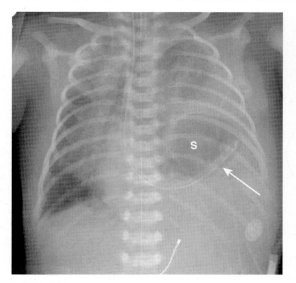

FIGURE 3-17. Congenital diaphragmatic hernia. Radiograph shows stomach *(S)* containing tip of nasogastric tube *(arrow)* in left hemithorax. There is no visualized aerated bowel in the upper abdomen. There is mediastinal shift to the right. Contralateral lung is well-aerated.

Sequestration

The term *pulmonary sequestration* refers to an area of congenital abnormal pulmonary tissue that does not have a normal connection to the bronchial tree. The characteristic imaging feature of sequestration is the demonstration of an anomalous arterial supply to the abnormal lung via a systemic artery arising from the aorta (Fig. 3-19A-C). All modalities that can demonstrate this abnormal systemic arterial supply, including MR imaging, helical CT, ultrasound, and arteriography, have been advocated in making the diagnosis of sequestration. However, contrast-enhanced helical CT is preferred because it both visualizes the systemic arterial supply when a sequestration is present (see Fig. 3-19) and further characterizes the lung abnormality if a sequestration is not present.

Sequestration most commonly presents with recurrent pneumonia, usually in late childhood. Other presentations include a prenatally diagnosed lung mass or respiratory distress in the newborn period. Because sequestrations do not communicate with the bronchial tree unless they become infected, they usually appear as radiopaque masses during the neonatal period. After infection has occurred, air may be introduced and sequestration may appear as

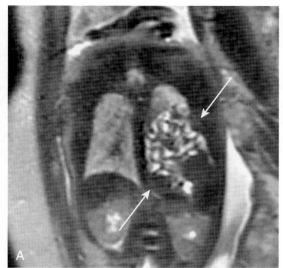

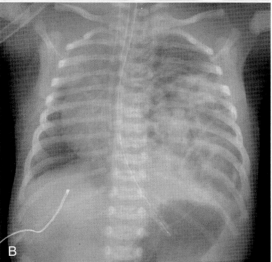

FIGURE 3-18. Congenital diaphragmatic hernia. **A,** Fetal MR image in coronal plane shows high signal content in multiple bowel loops *(arrows)* in left hemithorax. **B,** Chest radiograph after birth shows multiple bubblelike lucencies in left hemithorax. Note that in this case the stomach and nasogastric tube tip are not in the hernia. There is mediastinal shift to the right. The left upper lobe and right lung are well-aerated.

a multiloculated cystic mass. The most common location is within the left lower lobe.

There has been much discussion concerning differentiation between intralobar and extralobar sequestrations. Extralobar sequestrations have a separate pleural covering, whereas intralobar sequestrations, which are more common, do not; however, the presence or absence of an extrapleural covering cannot be determined at imaging. Extralobar sequestrations are associated with other abnormalities in 65% of

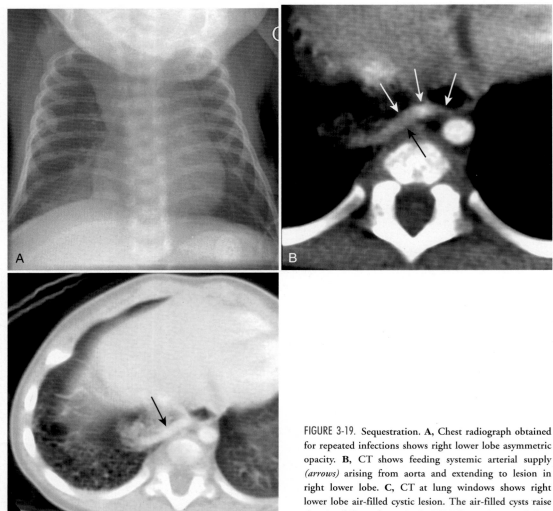

FIGURE 3-19. Sequestration. **A,** Chest radiograph obtained for repeated infections shows right lower lobe asymmetric opacity. **B,** CT shows feeding systemic arterial supply *(arrows)* arising from aorta and extending to lesion in right lower lobe. **C,** CT at lung windows shows right lower lobe air-filled cystic lesion. The air-filled cysts raise the possibility of a mixed CCAM/sequestration lesion. Again noted is the systemic arterial supply *(arrow).*

cases, whereas intralobar sequestrations are not. Differences in venous drainage patterns between intra- and extralobar sequestrations have been emphasized as a differentiating factor but are actually variable with both types. The differentiation between intra- and extralobar sequestration cannot be made at imaging and does not affect surgical management. Visualization of the supplying systemic artery is the characteristic finding and is the documentation the surgeons are looking for prior to surgically removing the lesion.

Bronchogenic Cyst

Bronchogenic cysts occur secondary to abnormal budding of the tracheobronchial tree during development and occur in the lung parenchyma or the middle mediastinum. Mediastinal lesions are reportedly more common, making up between 65% and 90% of cases of bronchogenic cysts. When bronchogenic cysts occur in the lungs, they are most commonly central in location, often in a perihilar distribution. Bronchogenic cysts are almost always solitary lesions; multiple bronchogenic cysts are very uncommon. Because of the propensity for middle mediastinal and perihilar locations, compression of the distal trachea or bronchi is not an uncommon presentation. Air trapping in the lung distal to the lesion can occur. Like sequestrations, they do not contain air until they become infected and therefore may appear as well-defined soft tissue attenuation or cystic air-fluid-containing masses (see Fig. 2-11).

They can be quite large. They appear as well-defined cystic structures on imaging (see Fig. 2-11).

ROLES OF IMAGING IN PEDIATRIC PNEUMONIA

Respiratory tract infection is the most common cause of illness in children and continues to be a significant cause of morbidity and mortality. Evaluation of suspected community-acquired pneumonia is one of the most common indications for imaging in children. Because of the frequency with which this scenario arises, knowledge of the issues concerning the imaging of children with community-acquired pneumonia is important. The roles of imaging in these children are multiple: confirmation or exclusion of pneumonia, characterization and prediction of infectious agents, exclusion of other cause of symptoms, evaluation when there is failure to resolve, and evaluation of related complications.

Confirmation or Exclusion of Pneumonia

Making the diagnosis of pneumonia and consequently deciding on treatment and disposition is a common but complex and difficult issue. The symptoms and physical findings in children with pneumonia are sometimes nonspecific, especially in infants and young children. Many children present with nonrespiratory symptoms, such as fever, malaise, irritability, headaches, chest pain, abdominal pain, vomiting, or decreased appetite. Findings on physical examination are also less reliable in children than in adults because young children are less cooperative with exams and have smaller anatomy and smaller respiratory cycles. Because of the inaccuracy of physical examination, radiography is often requested to evaluate children with suspected pneumonia. Several studies have shown that in a large percentage of cases, findings on chest radiography change caregivers' diagnoses and treatment plans (antibiotics, bronchodilators, and patient disposition) for children being evaluated for potential pneumonia. At our institution, we obtain both a frontal and a lateral film in the evaluation of a child with suspected pneumonia. It has been shown that obtaining both views increases the negative predictive value

of chest radiography for pneumonia. In addition, some findings such as hyperinflation in an infant are much more easily evaluated on the lateral than on the frontal views (Fig. 3-20A, B).

Characterization and Prediction of Infectious Agent

The historic emphasis in textbooks and articles concerning pneumonia has been on radiographic patterns that suggest a specific infectious

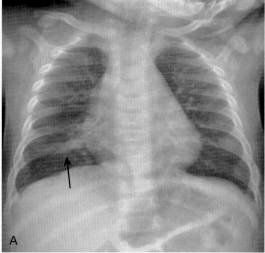

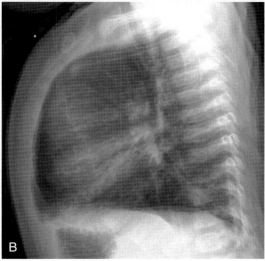

FIGURE 3-20. Viral lower respiratory infection in a young child. **A,** Frontal view shows increased perihilar markings and bandlike density *(arrow)* in right middle lobe, representing subsegmental atelectasis. **B,** Lateral view better shows marked hyperinflation with flattened hemidiaphragms, increased anterior-to-posterior diameter of the chest (chest is wider than it is tall), and barrel shape of chest. Increased perihilar markings make hila appear prominent.

agent, such as staphylococcal or streptococcal pneumonia. However, because of the limited ways in which the lung can respond to inflammation, findings suggestive of a specific diagnosis are usually not encountered in the radiograph of a child with suspected community-acquired pneumonia. The more general issue in the evaluation of suspected pneumonia is whether the infectious agent is likely to be bacteria or viral, which determines whether the patient should be placed on antibiotics. To answer this question it is helpful to review the epidemiology of lower respiratory infections in children, the classic radiographic patterns of viral and bacterial pneumonia in children, and what is known about the accuracy of chest radiography in differentiating viral from bacterial infection.

The common causal agents of lower respiratory tract infections in children vary greatly with age. In all age groups, viral infections are much more common than bacterial infections. In infants and preschool-age children (4 months to 5 years of age), viruses cause 95% of all lower respiratory tract infections. The epidemiology is much different in school-age children (6 to 16 years of age). In school-age children, although viral agents remain the most common cause of lower respiratory tract infections, the incidence of bacterial infection by *Streptococcus pneumoniae* increases. What is most striking is that *Mycoplasma pneumoniae*, which is an uncommon cause of pneumonia in preschool infants and children, is the cause of approximately 30% of lower respiratory tract infections in school-age children. Therefore, the odds that a child should be administered antibiotics for a respiratory tract infection are greatly influenced by the child's age. In addition, there has been a recent increase in the incidence of pneumonia secondary to multidrug-resistant *Staphylococcus aureus* infections. These can occur at any age.

Viral infections affect the airways, causing inflammation of the small airways and peribronchial edema. This peribronchial edema appears on radiography as increased peribronchial opacities—symmetric course markings that radiate from the hila into the lung (Fig. 3-21A, B; and see Fig. 3-20A, B). The central portions of the lungs appear to be "dirty" or "busy." It is one of the most subjective findings in radiology. In addition, the combination of the bronchial wall edema, narrowed airway lumen, and

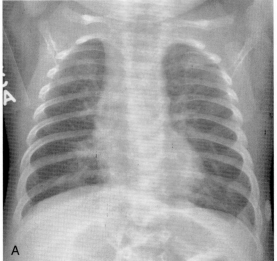

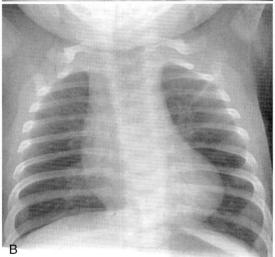

FIGURE. 3-21. Viral lower respiratory illness in a young child. A, Chest radiograph at peak of illness shows ropy increased perihilar markings and areas of subsegmental atelectasis. B, Radiograph 5 days earlier in same child shows clear lungs with absence of increased perihilar markings. Note the difference between the two radiographs.

necrotic debris and mucus in the airway leads to small airway occlusion. This results in both hyperinflation and areas of subsegmental atelectasis. Hyperinflation is evident on chest radiographs in children in the presence of hyperlucency, the depression of the hemidiaphragm to more than 10 posterior ribs, and the increased anterior-to-posterior chest diameter. Hyperinflation is often much better appreciated on lateral than on frontal radiographs in infants and small children (see Fig. 3-20). Subsegmental atelectasis appears as wedge-shaped areas of density, most commonly in the lower and mid lung (see Fig. 3-20A, B). There are several anatomic differences that render small children more predisposed to air trapping and collapse secondary to viral infection than adults: small airway luminal diameter, poorly developed collateral pathways of ventilation, and more abundant mucus production. The misinterpretation of areas of atelectasis as focal opacities suspicious for bacterial pneumonia is thought to be one of the more common misinterpretations in pediatric radiology.

In contrast to the airway involvement in viral pneumonia, bacterial pneumonia occurs secondary to inhalation of the infectious agent into the air spaces. There is a resultant progressive development of inflammatory exudate and edema within the acini, resulting in consolidation of the air spaces. On chest radiography, localized air space consolidation (Fig. 3-22) occurs with air bronchograms. The typical distribution is either lobar or segmental, depending on when in the course of development of the pneumonia the radiograph is obtained. Associated pleural effusions are not uncommon. Also, there is a propensity for pneumonia to appear "round" in younger children (Fig. 3-23). Round pneumonia is more common in children younger than 8 years of age and is most often caused by *S. pneumoniae*. The occurrence of this pattern is thought to be related to poor development of pathways of collateral ventilation. Round pneumonia tends to be solitary and occurs more commonly posteriorly and in the lower lobes. When such a lung mass is seen in a child with cough and fever, round pneumonia should be suspected. The child should be treated with antibiotics and the chest radiograph repeated. It is best to avoid unnecessary CT examination in this clinical scenario. When a round opacity is seen in a child older than 8 years of age, other pathology should be suspected.

Do these classic patterns of viral and bacterial infections accurately differentiate between children who have bacterial infection and need antibiotics and those who do not? Studies have shown that these radiographic patterns do have a high negative predictive value (92%) for excluding bacterial pneumonia. But the positive predictive value is low (30%). In other words, 70% of children who have radiographic findings of bacterial infection actually have viral infection. In regard to decisions about administering antibiotics to children with suspected pneumonia, the goals are to treat all children who have bacterial pneumonia with antibiotics while minimizing the treatment of children with viral illnesses. Therefore, the high negative predictive value of chest radiography for bacterial pneumonia is useful in identifying those children who do not need antibiotics.

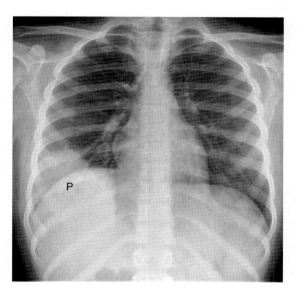

FIGURE 3-22. Bacterial pneumonia. Radiograph shows focal lung consolidation (P) in lateral aspect of right lower lobe, consistent with bacterial pneumonia.

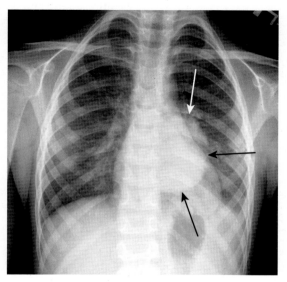

FIGURE 3-23. Round pneumonia. Radiograph shows rounded opacity overlying the left hilum. This is the location of the superior segment of the left lower lobe.

Exclusion of Other Pathologic Processes

Many of the presenting symptoms of pneumonia in children are nonspecific, and the spectrum of presentations overlaps with a number of other pathologic processes involving the chest or other anatomic regions. Therefore, one of the other roles of chest radiography in the evaluation of a child who potentially has pneumonia is the exclusion of other processes. Two areas that are often blind spots for radiologists and may be involved by conditions that mimic pneumonia are the airway and the chest wall. Processes that cause extrinsic compression of the trachea and bronchi can mimic pneumonia by causing noisy breathing, lobar collapse, and recurrent infection. Evaluation of the diameter of the airway should be stressed as a routine part of evaluating radiographs. Rib abnormalities may be evidence that a lung opacity seen on chest radiography does not represent pneumonia. The presence of rib erosion or asymmetric intercostal spaces helps to differentiate neuroblastoma from chest opacity secondary to pneumonia.

Failure to Resolve

Unlike in adults, in whom postobstructive pneumonia secondary to bronchogenic carcinoma is a concern, follow-up radiography to ensure resolution of radiographic findings is not routinely necessary in an otherwise healthy child. There is a tendency to obtain follow-up radiographs both too early and too often. Follow-up radiographs should be reserved for children who have persistent or recurrent symptoms and those who have an underlying condition such as immunodeficiency. The radiographic findings of pneumonia can persist for 2 to 4 weeks, even when the patient is recovering appropriately clinically. When follow-up radiographs are indicated, it is ideal to avoid obtaining them until at least 2 to 3 weeks have passed, if clinical symptoms allow.

Causes of failure of suspected pneumonia to resolve include infected developmental lesions, bronchial obstruction, gastroesophageal reflux and aspiration, and underlying systemic disorders. The most common developmental lung masses that may become infected and present as recurrent or persistent pulmonary infection include sequestration and cystic adenomatoid

malformation. These entities have been discussed previously.

Complications of Pneumonia

The evaluation of complications related to pneumonia can be divided into several clinical scenarios: primary evaluation of parapneumonic effusions, evaluation of a child who has persistent or progressive symptoms despite medical or surgical therapy, and the chronic sequelae of pneumonia.

PRIMARY EVALUATION OF PARAPNEUMONIC EFFUSIONS

Parapneumonic effusions occur commonly in patients who have bacterial pneumonia. Multiple therapeutic options are available in the management of parapneumonic effusions, including antibiotic therapy alone, repeated thoracentesis, chest tube placement, thrombolytic therapy, and thoracoscopy with surgical débridement. Great differences in opinion exist among caregivers regarding the timing and aggressiveness of management of parapneumonic effusions. Traditionally, the aggressiveness of therapy has been based on categorizing parapneumonic effusions as empyema or transudative effusion as determined by needle aspiration and analysis of the pleural fluid.

Several imaging modalities have been advocated to differentiate empyema from transudative effusion without the use of an invasive diagnostic thoracentesis, including decubitus radiographs, ultrasound, and CT. If there is a significant change in the position and appearance of the pleural fluid on the decubitus images as compared to the upright radiograph, the fluid is considered to be free flowing and nonloculated. If there is no change in position of the pleural fluid, the fluid is considered to be loculated (Fig. 3-24A-C). In my experience, these decubitus radiographs have been more confusing than helpful, and we do not advocate the use of decubitus radiographs to evaluate pleural effusions at our institution. On CT, findings such as thickening or enhancement of the parietal pleura and thickening or increased attenuation of the extrapleural fat were previously thought to favor empyema over transudative effusion, but this has been shown to be inaccurate (Fig. 3-25A, B; and see Fig. 3-29). Ultrasound has also been advocated as an aid

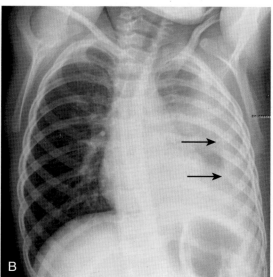

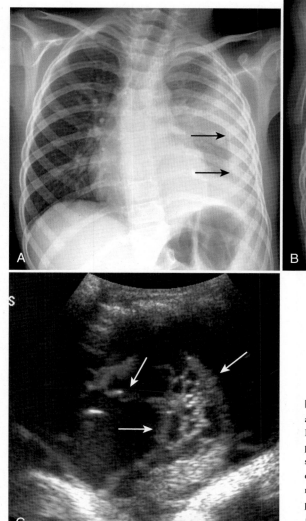

FIGURE 3-24. Parapneumonic effusion (empyema) evaluated by decubitus radiographs and ultrasound. **A,** Radiograph shows pleural effusion *(arrows)* in child with pneumonia. **B,** Decubitus radiograph with left side down shows no change in pleural effusion *(arrows),* I think. Lack of change is supposed to suggest loculation, but is probably not that helpful a diagnostic tool. **C,** Ultrasound of left pleural fluid demonstrating multiple areas of septations *(arrows)* and debris—a high-grade effusion, predictive of benefit from aggressive drainage.

in making therapeutic decisions for parapneumonic effusions. In one study, parapneumonic effusions were categorized as low grade (anechoic fluid without internal heterogeneous echogenic structures) or high grade (fibrinopurulent organization demonstrated by the presence of fronds, septations, or loculations) (see Figs. 3-24, 3-25). In children in whom effusions were high grade, hospital stay was reduced by nearly 50% when operative intervention was performed. The length of hospital stay in children with low-grade effusions was not affected by operative intervention. Therefore, ultrasound may play a more useful role than CT in the early evaluation of parapneumonic effusions. It is not uncommon for ultrasound to show multiple septations and in the same

case to show no evidence of septations on CT (see Fig. 3-25). We currently advocate ultrasound, rather than CT or decubitus radiographs, in the primary evaluation of parapneumonic effusions.

EVALUATION OF PERSISTENT OR PROGRESSIVE SYMPTOMS

When children exhibit persistent or progressive symptoms (fever, respiratory distress, sepsis) despite appropriate medical management of pneumonia, there is commonly an underlying suppurative complication. Potential suppurative complications include parapneumonic effusions such as empyema, inadequately drained effusions, and persistent effusion due to malpositioned chest tube; parenchymal complications,

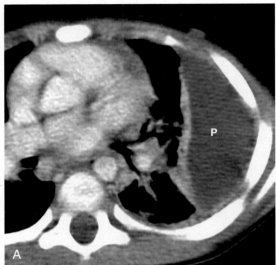

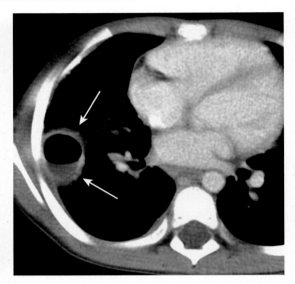

FIGURE 3-26. Lung abscess. Contrast-enhanced CT shows well-defined cavity *(arrows)* with enhancing wall and containing air-fluid level.

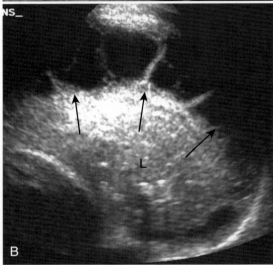

FIGURE 3-25. Parapneumonic effusion (empyema) evaluated by CT and ultrasound. **A,** CT shows left parapneumonic effusion. There are no findings to suggest empyema on CT. There are no septations seen by CT, which is typical. **B,** Ultrasound shows consolidated lung *(L)* with surrounding band of pleural fluid *(arrows).* Note multiple echogenic septations consistent with complex effusion.

such as cavitary necrosis or lung abscess; and purulent pericarditis. Although chest radiography is the primary imaging modality for detecting such complications, a significant percentage of them are not demonstrated by radiography. In a child who has had a noncontributory radiograph and who has not responded appropriately to therapy, contrast-enhanced CT has been shown to be useful in detecting clinically significant suppurative complications. CT can help to differentiate whether there is a pleural or a

parenchymal reason for persistent illness. Administration of intravenous contrast is vital to maximize the likelihood of detection and the characterization of both parenchymal and pleural complications.

LUNG PARENCHYMAL COMPLICATIONS

On contrast-enhanced CT, both noncompromised consolidated lung parenchyma and atelectasis enhance diffusely. Large areas of decreased or absent enhancement are indicative of underlying parenchymal ischemia or impending infarction. Suppurative lung parenchymal complications include a spectrum of abnormalities, such as cavitary necrosis, lung abscess, pneumatocele, bronchopleural fistula, and pulmonary gangrene. The name given to the suppurative process is determined by several factors, including the severity, distribution, condition of the adjacent lung parenchyma, and temporal relationship with disease resolution. Lung abscess represents a dominant focus of suppuration surrounded by a well-formed fibrous wall. Lung abscess is actually uncommon in otherwise healthy children and typically occurs in children who are immunocompromised. On contrast-enhanced CT, lung abscesses appear as fluid- or air-filled cavities with definable enhancing walls (Fig. 3-26). Typically, there is no evidence of necrosis in the surrounding lung. *Pneumatocele* is a term given to thin-walled cysts seen at imaging and may represent

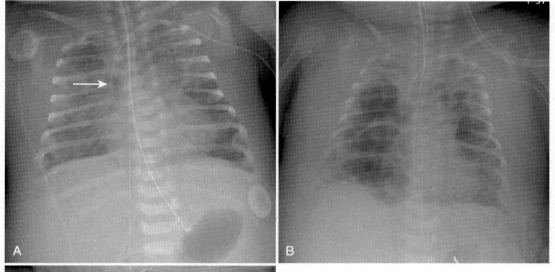

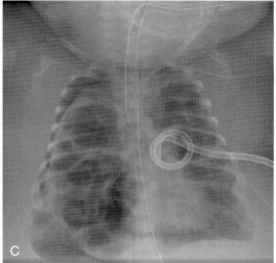

FIGURE 3-27. Rapid development of necrosis and pneumatocele formation in an infant with multi-drug-resistant *S. aureus* pneumonia. **A**, Radiograph obtained in the intensive care unit after intubation for respiratory failure shows patchy bilateral lung consolidation. Note position of PICC with tip in inferior aspect of superior vena cava *(arrow)*. Note widening of soft tissues, consistent with anasarca. **B**, Radiograph 3 days later shows interval development of multiple bilateral areas of necrosis and cyst formation. There is progressive anasarca. **C**. Radiograph taken 2 days after that shown in B shows progressive development of necrosis and cyst formation. Not that it matters, but because many of the cysts are thin-walled and without surrounding opacification, *pneumatocele* is acceptable terminology. Note the development of bilateral pneumothorax with left chest tube placement and progressive anasarca.

a later or less severe stage of resolving or healing necrosis (Fig. 3-27A-C).

Cavitary necrosis is the most commonly encountered suppurative complication. It is characterized by a dominant area of necrosis of a consolidated lobe that is associated with a variable number of thin-walled cysts (Fig. 3-28). CT findings of cavitary necrosis include loss of normal lung architecture, decreased parenchymal enhancement, loss of the lung-pleural margin, and multiple thin-walled cavities containing air or fluid and lacking an enhancing border (Fig. 3-29). Although historically described as a complication of staphylococcal pneumonia, cavitary necrosis was much more commonly seen as a complication of streptococcal pneumonia during the last decade. Cavitary necrosis in association with multi-drug-resistant

S. aureus infection has been occurring with increased frequency recently (see Fig. 3-27). The presence of cavitary necrosis is indicative of an intense and prolonged illness. However, unlike in adults in whom the mortality rate in cavitary necrosis is high, and early surgical removal of the affected lung has been advocated, the long-term outcome for children with cavitary necrosis is favorable in most cases with medical management alone. It is amazing that in children with cavitary necrosis, follow-up radiographs obtained more than 40 days after the acute illness are most often normal or show only minimal scarring.

It may sometimes be difficult on a single imaging study to differentiate a suppurative lung parenchymal complication of pneumonia from an underlying cystic congenital lung

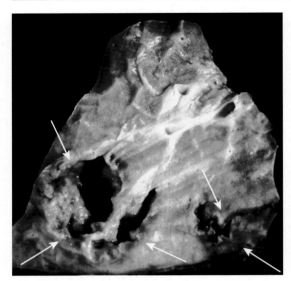

FIGURE 3-28. Cavitary necrosis. Photograph of surgical specimen shows consolidated lung (tan area) with areas of necrosis and cavity formation *(arrows)*.

lesion that has become secondarily infected. Infected congenital cystic adenomatoid malformations may appear very similar to cavitary necrosis. Obviously, historical imaging studies showing a lack of a cystic lesion exclude

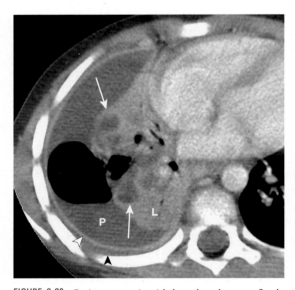

FIGURE 3-29. Cavitary necrosis with bronchopulmonary fistula formation. CT shows consolidation of the right lung. Portions of the lung demonstrate cavitary necrosis *(arrows)*. There are also areas of consolidated lung that enhance *(L)* and are not compromised. There is a pleural effusion *(P)* that contains both air and fluid. There is thickening and enhancement of the parietal pleura *(white arrowhead)* and thickening of the extrapleural space *(black arrowhead)*, both findings that claimed to be suggestive of empyema rather than transudative effusion but were shown to be inaccurate.

underlying CCAM, but such historical examinations often do not exist or are not available. Observable resolution of the cystic lesion on follow-up studies ensures that the lesion is no longer clinically relevant and makes cavitary necrosis much more likely. However, some CCAMs have been reported to scar down and resolve after becoming infected.

CHRONIC LUNG COMPLICATIONS OF PNEUMONIA

Acute pneumonia can lead to parenchymal damage and long-term sequelae. The most common sequelae of acute pneumonia are bronchiectasis and Swyer-James syndrome. Bronchiectasis is enlargement of the diameter of the bronchi that is related to damage to the bronchial walls. It is best demonstrated by high-resolution CT, where the diagnostic finding is that the bronchus in question is larger in diameter than the adjacent pulmonary artery (Fig. 3-30). Swyer-James syndrome is characterized by unilateral lung hyperlucency that is thought to be secondary to a virus-induced necrotizing bronchiolitis that leads to an obliterative bronchiolitis (see Fig. 3-30). Radiography shows a hyperlucent and enlarged lung with a static lung volume. The pulmonary vessels are less prominent than on the normal side.

Tuberculosis

The incidence of tuberculosis in children has been increasing. Children with primary tuberculosis can present with pulmonary consolidation within any lobe. It is often associated with

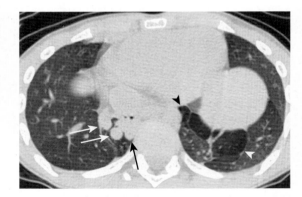

FIGURE 3-30. Chronic complications related to recurrent pneumonias. CT shows multiple round, soft tissue density lesions in medial right lower lobe *(arrows)* consistent with bronchiectasis with mucus plugging. In the left lower lobe, there is an area of air trapping *(arrowheads)* consistent with obliterative bronchiolitis. This area remained hyperlucent on expiratory images.

hilar lymphadenopathy or pleural effusion. Therefore, when lung consolidation is seen with associated lymphadenopathy or effusion in a child who is not acutely ill, there should be a high suspicion for tuberculosis. Most of the cases of pulmonary tuberculosis that I have seen have demonstrated unilateral hilar lymphadenopathy (Fig. 3-31A, B). Such cases should be considered tuberculosis until proven otherwise.

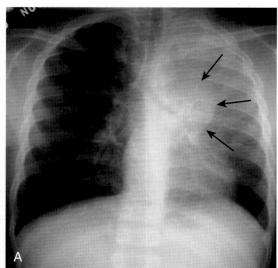

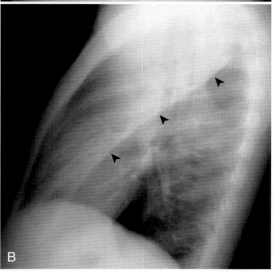

FIGURE 3-31. Tuberculosis in a 7-year-old boy. **A** and **B,** Frontal and lateral radiographs of the chest demonstrate a left hilar mass *(arrows)* consistent with unilateral lymphadenopathy. There is also left upper lobe collapse. Note displaced major fissure on lateral view *(arrowheads).*

COMMON CHRONIC OR RECURRENT PULMONARY PROBLEMS IN SPECIAL POPULATIONS

In children with certain underlying conditions, the clinical scenarios and differential diagnoses differ greatly from those seen in the general population. Commonly encountered scenarios include the evaluation of pneumonia in immunocompromised children, acute chest syndrome in children with sickle cell anemia, and pulmonary complications in children with cystic fibrosis.

Pneumonia in Immunodeficient Children

Children can be immunocompromised for a variety of reasons, including cancer therapy, bone marrow transplantation, solid organ transplantation, primary immunodeficiency, and AIDS. This is a population that continues to increase. Acute pulmonary processes are a common cause of morbidity and mortality in these patients. As with immunocompetent children, radiography is the primary modality used to confirm or exclude pneumonia. However, because many of the chest radiographs obtained in these children are portable and because of the consequences of missing an infection, CT plays a greater role in evaluating for an acute pulmonary process when chest radiographs are noncontributory. I would guess that in many tertiary institutions the number of chest CTs obtained in immunocompromised children is greater than the number of those obtained in immunocompetent children.

In immunocompetent children, the main question is whether a pulmonary process is viral or bacterial; in immunocompromised children, there are many more possible causes of acute pulmonary processes They include alveolar hemorrhage, pulmonary edema, drug reaction, idiopathic pneumonia, lymphoid interstitial pneumonitis, bronchiolitis obliterans, bronchiolitis obliterans with organizing pneumonia, and chronic graft-versus-host disease. The CT findings for many of these entities are overlapping and nonspecific. A clinical question often posed is this: Is there evidence of fungal infection? The hallmark CT finding indicating fungal infection is the presence of nodules

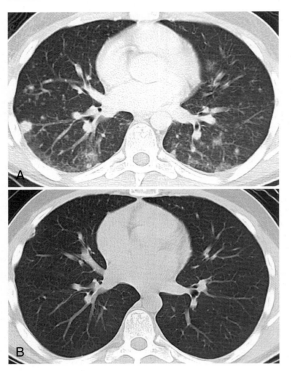

FIGURE 3-32. Fungal pneumonia in child after bone marrow transplantation for aplastic anemia. **A,** CT shows poorly defined nodules and associated ground-glass opacity. **B,** A CT taken earlier shows clear lungs. Note the striking change since this baseline study.

(Figs. 3-32A, B, 3-33). They are commonly clustered and may exhibit poorly defined margins, cavitation, or a surrounding halo that has the opacity of ground glass. However, many of these findings are also nonspecific. In these cases CT does aid in directing potential interventions, such as bronchoscopy or percutaneous lung biopsy, to high yield areas.

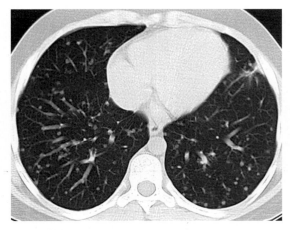

FIGURE 3-33. Histoplasmosis infection. CT shows multiple nodules bilaterally. There is a biopsy site on the left, anteriorly.

Acute Chest Syndrome in Sickle Cell Anemia

Children with sickle cell anemia can develop acute chest syndrome, which is manifested by fever, chest pain, hypoxia, and pulmonary opacities on chest radiographs (Fig. 3-34). Acute chest syndrome is much more common in children than adults with sickle cell anemia. It occurs most commonly between 2 and 4 years of age and is the leading cause of death (25% of deaths) and the second most common cause of hospitalization in those affected with sickle cell anemia. Although it is debated whether the cause of such episodes is more often related to infection or infarction, many believe the lung opacities are related to rib infarction, splinting, and subsequent areas

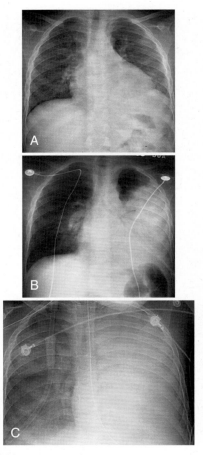

FIGURE 3-34. Acute chest syndrome in a 6-year-old boy with sickle cell anemia. **A,** Chest radiograph obtained at admission shows low lung volumes and minimal focal opacity within the left lower lobe. **B,** Chest radiograph obtained 1 day later shows consolidation of a large portion of the left lung. **C,** Chest radiograph obtained 2 days after **A** shows complete left lung opacification.

of atelectasis. Radiography often shows segmental to lobar pulmonary opacities but can also be normal. There can be an associated increase in cardiomegaly. Bone scans may show rib infarcts. The children are treated with oxygen, antibiotics, and pain control, and the pulmonary opacities are commonly monitored by radiography.

Cystic Fibrosis

Cystic fibrosis is a genetic disease that most commonly affects the respiratory and gastrointestinal tracts. In the respiratory system, abnormally viscous mucus leads to airway obstruction and infection that causes bronchitis and bronchiectasis. Children may initially present with recurrent respiratory tract infections. Radiography may be normal at young ages but eventually demonstrates hyperinflation, increased peribronchial markings, mucus plugging, and bronchiectasis. The hilar areas can become prominent because of a combination of lymphadenopathy secondary to the chronic inflammation and enlarged central pulmonary arteries related to the development of pulmonary arterial hypertension. Chest radiography is used to monitor the disease and evaluate for complications during acute exacerbations. Such complications include focal pneumonia, pneumothorax, and pulmonary hemorrhage. To monitor the progression of disease, some institutions use high-resolution CT, which demonstrates findings such as bronchiectasis and bronchial wall thickening in greater detail and earlier than does radiography (Fig. 3-35).

HIGH-RESOLUTION CT IN CHILDREN WITH QUESTIONED CHRONIC ASPIRATION

One of the more common indications for high-resolution CT in the pediatric population is questioned chronic aspiration. Often this issue arises in children with neurologic abnormalities such as cerebral palsy or chronic tracheotomy tubes when decisions about methods of feeding are being entertained. High-resolution CT findings of chronic aspiration include bronchiectasis, tree-in-bud opacities (Fig. 3-36A, B), and increased interstitial linear opacities. Findings more often occur in lower lobes.

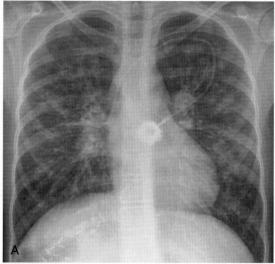
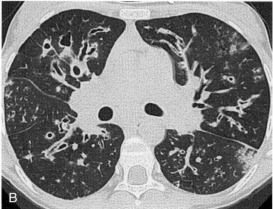

FIGURE 3-35. Cystic fibrosis. **A,** Radiograph shows areas of bronchial wall thickening and bronchiectasis, most prominent in the right upper lobe. **B,** High-resolution CT shows diffuse bronchiectasis and bronchial wall thickening within the upper lobes. There are also multiple areas of poorly defined opacities, particularly in the peripheral portions of the left upper lobe. These have a tree-in-bud appearance.

Trauma

RIB FRACTURES AND LUNG CONTUSION

There is a greater component of cartilage than bone within the chest walls of children, so there is more compliance than there is in the chest walls of adults. Because of this increased compliance, the sequelae of trauma to the pediatric chest are unique in several ways. First, the incidence of rib fractures after high-speed motor vehicle accidents is lower in children than in adults. Second, the deceleration forces of high speed collisions are more likely to be dispersed into the lung in children, resulting in lung contusion. Children with lung contusions have been

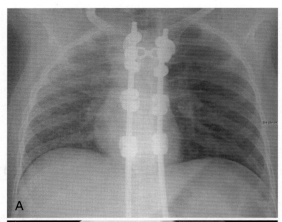

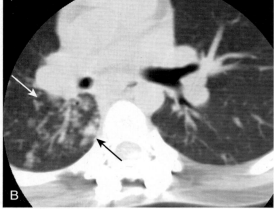

FIGURE 3-36. Aspiration. A, Radiograph in a child suspected of having aspiration shows increased nodular opacities in the right lung. B, High-resolution CT shows multiple nodular opacities (arrows) with tree-in-bud appearance.

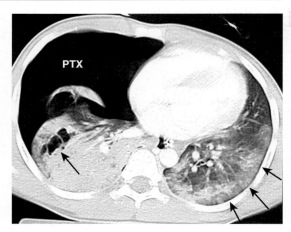

FIGURE 3-37. Lung contusion and laceration after a motor vehicle accident. CT shows characteristic findings of contusion on the left, including posterior location, crescent shape, nonsegmental distribution, and subpleural sparing (arrows). On the right, there is large pneumothorax (PTX) and consolidation of lung with an air-filled cyst (arrow) consistent with lung laceration.

shown to have higher morbidity and mortality rates than those without lung contusions. Although chest CT is not commonly performed to evaluate for lung contusion, the lower lungs are often seen on CT when it is performed to evaluate for abdominal trauma. Characteristic findings in lung contusion on CT include nonsegmental distribution, posterior location, crescent shape, and mixed confluent and nodular characteristics (Fig. 3-37). In children with small lung contusions, the compliance of the chest wall can result in a rim of nonopacified lung between the consolidated contusion and the adjacent ribs seen on CT (see Fig. 3-37). This subpleural sparing can be helpful in differentiating lung contusion from other causes of lung opacification. The CT finding that classifies an opacified area as a lung laceration rather than a lung contusion is the presence of a fluid- or air-filled cyst within the opacified lung

(Fig. 3-38A, B; and see Fig. 3-37). These cystic spaces result from torn lung.

Finally, the sites of rib fracture in children differ from those in adults. Rib fractures in young children in the absence of an obvious traumatic event are highly suspicious for child abuse (Figs. 3-39, 3-40A, B). Pediatric rib fractures are more likely to be posterior than lateral. In child abuse, as a result of squeezing an infant's thorax, the posterior ribs can be excessively levered at the costotransverse process articulation, causing posterior fracture at this site. In the appropriately aged child, these findings are considered pathognomonic for child abuse.

MEDIASTINAL INJURY

The incidence of aortic injury is also much lower in children than in adults. This, in combination with the lower incidence of obesity in children as compared to adults, makes the uncleared mediastinum on a chest radiograph after trauma a much less common scenario in children than in adults. Otherwise, the use of CT and angiography and the imaging findings of aortic injuries are no different from those encountered in adults.

HYDROCARBON INGESTION

The aspiration of the hydrocarbons in gasoline, furniture polish, kerosene, or lighter fluid when young children get into and drink such liquids can cause a combination of chemical

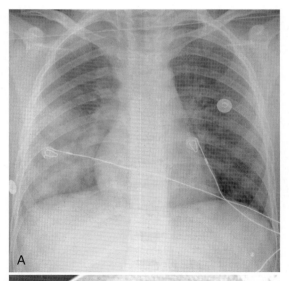

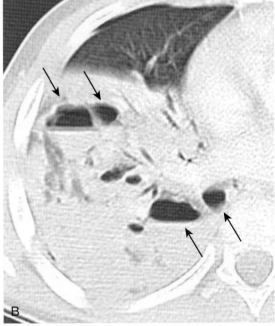

FIGURE 3-38. Lung laceration following motor vehicle accident. **A,** Radiograph shows nonspecific opacification of right lower lobe. **B,** CT shows right lower lobe consolidation with air- and fluid-filled cavities *(arrows)* consistent with lung laceration.

pneumonitis and atelectasis secondary to surfactant destruction. Radiographic findings may not manifest for up to 12 hours after ingestion. However, a normal radiograph at 24 hours after suspected ingestion excludes significant aspiration. The lung opacities tend to be in the lung bases (Fig. 3-41) and may persist for weeks after clinical improvement. Pneumatoceles are not uncommon sequelae.

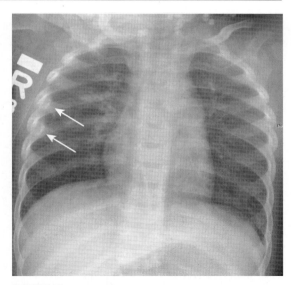

FIGURE 3-39. Child abuse. Radiograph shows healing fractures *(arrows)* of right fourth and fifth ribs.

Mediastinal Masses

The mediastinum is the most common location of primary thoracic masses in children. Also, the majority of mediastinal masses occur in children rather than in adults. As in adults, characterizing the location of the mass as anterior, middle, or posterior mediastinal can focus the differential diagnosis of mediastinal masses (Table 3-4).

ANTERIOR MEDIASTINUM

By far the most commonly encountered issues in the anterior mediastinum are the normal thymus mistaken as a mass and lymphoma. There are a large number of other potential but much less common causes of anterior mediastinal masses in children. They include teratoma (and other germ cell tumors), thymoma, multilocular thymic cysts seen in association with AIDS, and thyroid enlargement and heterogeneity (often with calcifications) in Langerhan cell histiocytosis (in which lung cysts are also present; Fig. 3-42).

TABLE 3-4. **Common Mediastinal Masses by Location**

Anterior	Middle	Posterior
Normal thymus	Lymphadenopathy	Neuroblastoma
Lymphoma	Duplication cyst	
Teratoma		

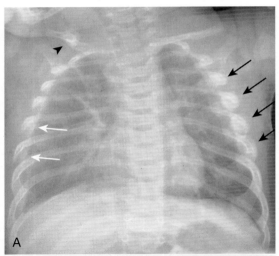

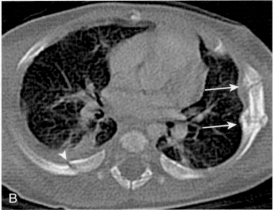

FIGURE 3-40. Child abuse. **A,** Radiograph shows multiple fractures that occurred at different times. There are multiple subacute healing rib fractures *(white arrows)* with callus formation, a subacute healing right clavicle fracture *(arrowhead)*, and multiple acute right-sided rib fractures *(black arrows)* without callus formation. **B,** CT shows callus around healing rib fractures on left *(arrows)* and characteristic acute fracture of the posterior rib *(arrowhead)* on right. A rib fractures against the transverse process when a child is squeezed.

NORMAL THYMUS

One of the most common areas of confusion in the imaging of children is related to differentiating the normal thymus from pathologic processes. This confusion led to thymic radiation therapy in the first half of the 20th century, when children with a normal prominent thymus on chest radiography were radiated because of the erroneous belief that a big thymus compressed the airway and predisposed to death. Distinguishing the normal thymus from disease continues to cause diagnostic problems today, particularly for those who do not often image children.

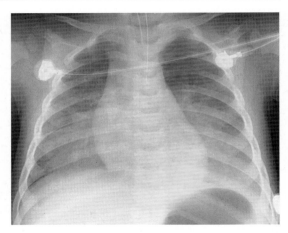

FIGURE 3-41. Hydrocarbon aspiration in a 1-year-old boy who drank gasoline from an orange juice container on the family's garage floor. Chest radiograph shows bibasilar lung consolidation. The patient is intubated.

In children, the thymus has a variable appearance in both size and shape. In children less than 5 years of age, and particularly in infants, the thymus can appear to be very large (Fig. 3-43). Large thymuses are said to be more common in boys. The thymus also has variable configurations. A number of names have become associated with normal variations in the thymus, such as the sail sign (Fig. 3-44), which refers to a triangular extension of the thymus, most commonly to the right, on frontal chest radiography. It resembles a sail. This should not be confused with the spinnaker sail

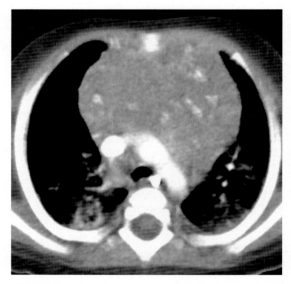

FIGURE 3-42. Enlarged thymus with calcifications in child with Langerhans cell histiocytosis. CT shows prominent thymus with high-attenuation calcifications.

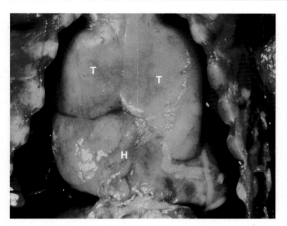

FIGURE 3-43. Normal, prominent size of the thymus. Photograph from autopsy of an infant who died of sudden infant death syndrome shows frontal view of thymus *(T)* after thoracotomy. Note the prominent size of the thymus in relation to the heart *(H)*. The thymus is bilobed. In this patient the left lobe is larger than the right. (Image courtesy Janet L. Strife, MD, Cincinnati, OH.)

sign (Fig. 3-45), which is an indication of pneumomediastinum, in which the abnormally located air lifts the thymus up so it looks like the sail on the front of a racing boat. Between 5 and 10 years of age, the thymus becomes less prominent radiographically because of the disproportionately decreased growth of the thymus in relation to the growth of the rest of the body. During a child's second decade, the thymus should not be visualized as a discrete anterior mediastinal mass on chest radiography.

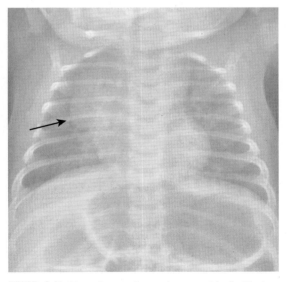

FIGURE 3-44. Normal, prominent thymus with "sail" sign. Radiograph shows prominent but normal thymus with right-ward triangular extension *(arrow)*.

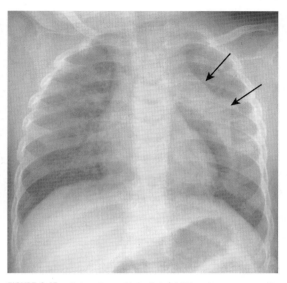

FIGURE 3-45. "Spinnaker sail sign" in child with pneumomediastinum. Radiograph shows thymus *(arrows)* lifted off of mediastinum by air in mediastinum. The uplifted thymus resembles a spinnaker sail.

Abnormality of the thymus (or anterior mediastinum) is suspected when the thymic silhouette has an abnormal shape or an abnormal size in relationship to the patient's age. Displacement or compression of the airway or other structures is suspicious for abnormality. CT, ultrasound, MR imaging, and fluoroscopy can be used to help differentiate the normal thymus from an abnormal mass, but CT is probably used most commonly. When CT is performed to evaluate suspicious cases, the normal thymus should appear homogeneous in attenuation, typically is quadrilateral in shape in young children (Fig. 3-46) and triangular in teenagers (Fig. 3-47A, B), and may have slightly convex margins. Heterogeneity, calcification, and displacement or compression of the airway or vascular structures indicate an abnormality (Fig 3-48A-D; and see Fig. 3-42). True pathologic masses of the thymus are actually quite rare in children.

Thymic rebound is another source of confusion concerning normal thymic tissue. After a patient has ceased receiving chemotherapy for a malignancy, it is normal for the thymus to grow back, as seen in serial CT examinations. Thymic volume has been shown to vary cyclically by as much as 40% during rounds of chemotherapy (see Fig. 3-47). This intervallic increase in soft tissue attenuation in the anterior mediastinum

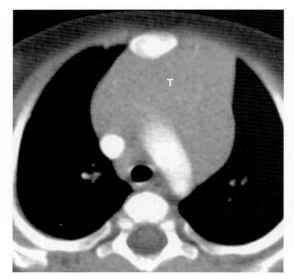

FIGURE 3-46. Normal thymus on cross-sectional imaging. CT in a young child shows thymus *(T)* to be quadrilateral in shape, to have convex margins, and to be of homogeneous attenuation. There is no compression of the trachea or superior vena cava.

should not be considered abnormal when encountered on cross-sectional imaging.

LYMPHOMA

Lymphoma is the third most common tumor in children, exceeded only by leukemia and brain tumors. It is by far the most common abnormal anterior mediastinal mass in children, particularly in older children and teenagers. Therefore, lymphoma is the working diagnosis for newly diagnosed anterior mediastinal masses in children. Age is helpful in differentiating a normal thymus from lymphoma because a normal thymus is most common in small children and lymphoma is most common in teenagers. The most problematic case is the slightly prominent anterior mediastinum in a 10-year-old. One helpful clue in identifying lymphoma is that mediastinal lymphoma is commonly associated with cervical lymphadenopathy.

The most common types of lymphoma that involve the mediastinum include Hodgkin lymphoma and the lymphoblastic type of non-Hodgkin lymphoma. Both lesions can appear as discrete lymph nodes or as a conglomerate mass of lymph nodes, most commonly within the anterior mediastinum (see Fig. 3-48). Lung involvement, when present, is usually contiguous with mediastinal and hilar disease. Calcifications are rare in untreated lymphoma and when present should raise the

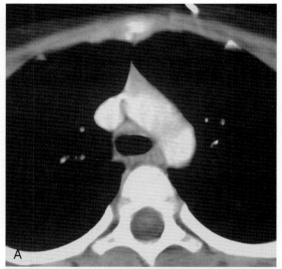

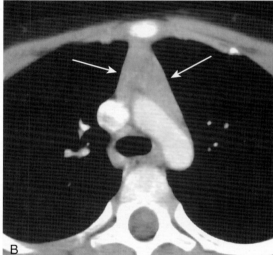

FIGURE 3-47. Thymic rebound in a child on chemotherapy. **A,** CT taken while the child was on chemotherapy shows little thymic tissue. **B,** CT taken 3 months later when child was off chemotherapy shows regrowth of thymus *(arrows)*. Note the typical triangular shape of the thymus as is seen during teenage years.

possibility of other diagnoses such as teratoma (Fig. 3-50).

Most mediastinal masses are initially identified on chest radiography and then further evaluated by CT, which confirms the presence of an anterior mediastinal mass, evaluates the extent of disease, and evaluates for potential complications. The potential complications related to mediastinal lymphoma include airway compression, compressive obstruction of venous structures (superior vena cava, pulmonary veins), and pericardial effusion (see Figs. 3-48, 3-49).

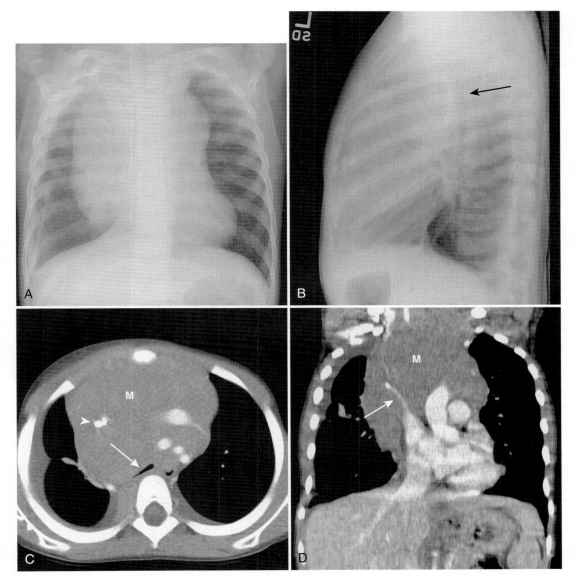

FIGURE 3-48. Lymphoma. **A,** Frontal radiograph shows marked enlargement of superior mediastinum and associated right pleural effusion. **B,** Lateral radiograph shows posterior displacement, compression, and poor visualization of the trachea *(arrow),* further supporting the presence of an abnormal mediastinal mass. **C,** CT shows large anterior mediastinal mass *(M)* with compression and posterior displacement of trachea *(arrow)* and compression of the superior vena cava *(arrowhead).* Note right pleural effusion. **D,** Coronal CT again shows mass *(M)* and compression of superior vena cava *(arrow).*

Airway compression is especially important because it may influence decisions concerning surgical biopsy with general anesthesia versus percutaneous biopsy with local anesthesia. If a patient cannot lie recumbent for CT imaging because of airway compression, the images can usually be obtained with the patient positioned prone because the anterior mediastinal mass falls away from the airway. Compression of the airway by more than 50% from the expected round shape has been shown to be associated with a high risk for complications related to anesthesia. Because of this, some such mediastinal masses are biopsied using ultrasound guidance and local anesthesia.

Middle Mediastinal Masses

Middle mediastinal masses are less common than anterior or posterior mediastinal masses and are usually related to lymphadenopathy or

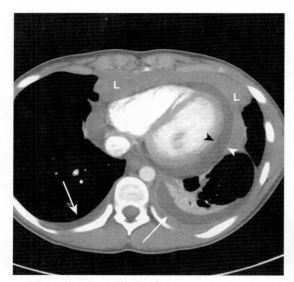

FIGURE 3-49. Lymphoma with pericardial effusion. CT image from level of heart in a child with an anterior mediastinal mass; on more superior images shows extension of lymphoma mass *(L)* inferiorly. Note adjacent pericardial fluid *(arrowheads)* and bilateral pleural fluid *(arrows)*.

duplication cysts. Lymphadenopathy can be inflammatory, most often secondary to granulomatous disease, such as tuberculosis or fungal infection; or to neoplastic growth secondary to metastatic disease or lymphoma. Duplication cysts can be bronchogenic (see Fig. 2-11), enteric, or neurenteric. Duplication cysts are well-defined masses that appear cystic on cross-sectional imaging. Neurenteric cysts, by definition, have

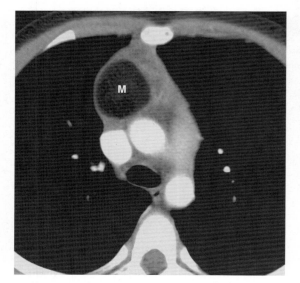

FIGURE 3-50. Teratoma. CT shows anterior mediastinal mass *(M)* that is of fat attenuation.

associated vertebral anomalies. Pathologic processes related to the esophagus can also cause middle mediastinal abnormalities. Chronic foreign bodies can erode through the esophagus and cause a middle mediastinal mass, typically in the cervical esophagus at the level of the thoracic inlet (Fig. 3-51A, B). A dilatated esophagus resulting from achalasia or a hiatal hernia may also appear as a middle mediastinal mass on chest radiography.

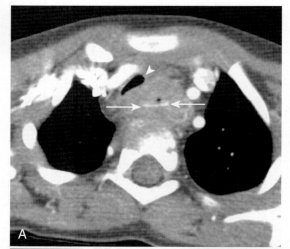

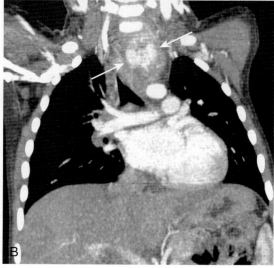

FIGURE 3-51. Chronic esophageal foreign body presenting as dysphagia and stridor in a young child. **A,** Axial CT shows inflammatory mass at thoracic inlet. There is a linear metallic density *(arrows)* suspicious for an eroded, chronic foreign body from the upper esophagus. The trachea is compressed *(arrowhead)*. **B,** Coronal CT shows dense oval structure *(arrows)* in an inflammatory mass. At surgical retrieval, the foreign body was found to be a sequin.

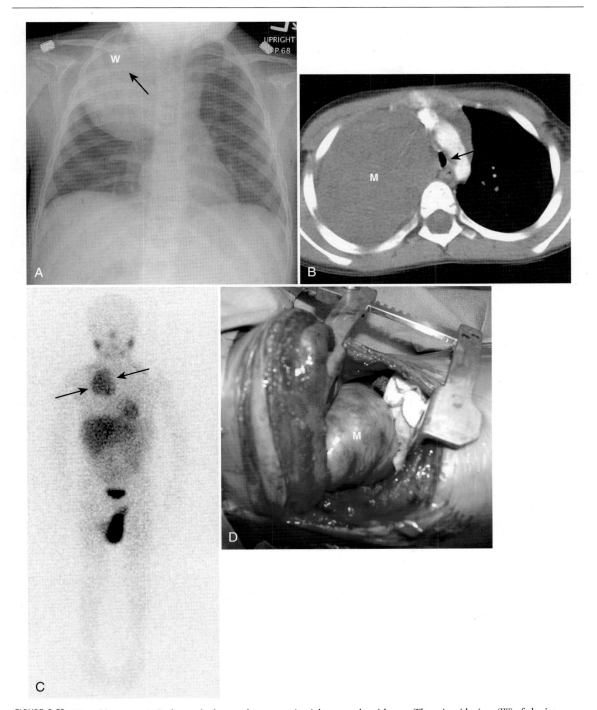

FIGURE 3-52. Neuroblastoma. **A,** Radiograph shows a large mass in right upper hemithorax. There is widening *(W)* of the interspace between the right third and fourth ribs and erosion of the undersurface of the right third rib *(arrow)*. The rib splaying and erosion document chest wall involvement and the posterior nature of the tumor. **B,** CT shows large mass *(M)* with compression of the trachea *(arrow)*. The mass is so large it extends from anterior to posterior chest walls. **C,** MIBG scan shows avid uptake of radiotracer within the mass *(arrows)*, consistent with a neurogenic tumor. **D,** Photograph taken during surgical resection shows a mass *(M)* arising from the posterior chest.

Posterior Mediastinal Masses

There are a number of causes of posterior mediastinal masses in children. They include neural crest tumor, neurofibroma, lateral menigocele, diskitis, hematoma, and extramedullary hematopoiesis. However, just as anterior mediastinal masses in older children are considered to be lymphoma, the working diagnosis for posterior mediastinal masses in young children is neuroblastoma until proven otherwise.

NEUROBLASTOMA

Neurogenic tumors (neuroblastoma, ganglioneuroblastoma, ganglioneuroma) are the most common posterior mediastinal masses in childhood. Neuroblastoma is discussed in detail in the genitourinary section. Approximately 15% of neuroblastomas occur in the posterior mediastinum, most occurring before a child is 2 years of age.

Most neuroblastomas are visible on frontal radiographs of the chest as a posterior opacity. The soft tissue mass is often surprisingly poorly visualized on the lateral view. There is frequently erosion, destruction, or splaying of the adjacent posterior ribs (Fig. 3-52A-D). These findings may be subtle, so whenever a posterior chest opacity is identified an effort should be made to look for rib erosion. The neuroforamina may appear enlarged on the lateral view, secondary to intraspinal extension of the tumor. Calcifications are reported to be visible on chest radiography in as many as 25% of cases, although in my experience it is less than that. Cross-sectional imaging with CT or MR imaging confirms the presence of the tumor and evaluates extent of disease, particularly whether there is intraspinal extension. Thoracic neuroblastomas have better prognosis than abdominal neuroblastomas.

Pediatric Chest Wall Masses

A number of primary malignant processes can arise in the chest walls of children. They include Ewing sarcoma, Askin tumor (primitive neuroectodermal tumor of the chest wall), and other sarcomas (Fig. 3-53). Most of these lesions present with painful enlargement of the chest wall. Metastatic involvement by neuroblastoma, lymphoma, or leukemia is actually more common than are primary tumors. On imaging, all of these malignancies typically appear as

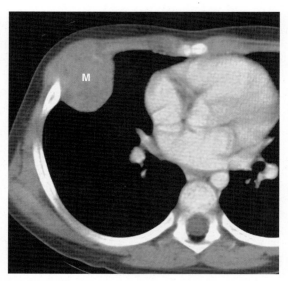

FIGURE 3-53. Undifferentiated sarcoma of the chest wall in a young child. CT shows soft tissue attenuation mass *(M)* involving the anterolateral chest wall on right.

nonspecific aggressive lesions with poorly defined margins that include bony destruction and pleural involvement. However, one must consider that as much as one third of children have variations in the configuration of the anterior chest wall, including asymmetric findings, such as tilted sternum (Fig. 3-54), prominent convexity of anterior rib or costal cartilage, prominent asymmetric costal cartilage, parachondral nodules, or mild degrees of pectus excavatum or carinatum. It is common for these asymmetric variants to be palpated by

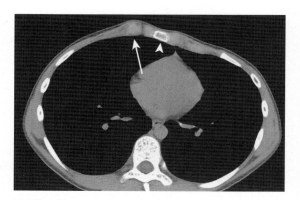

FIGURE 3-54. Tilted sternum with prominent costal cartilage presenting as a palpable mass on physical exam. CT shows the sternum *(arrowhead)* to be tilted with respect to the horizontal right-to-left axis of the body. The right margin of the sternum is more anterior than the right. The associated anterior position of the right costal cartilage *(arrow)*, a normal variant, caused the palpable finding on physical exam.

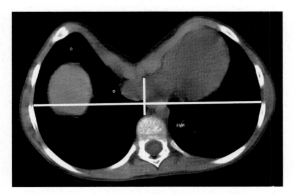

FIGURE 3-55. Pectus excavatum. CT shows severe concavity of anterior chest wall. White lines are the anterior-to-posterior and left-to-right diameters of the chest. These are measured to calculate the Haller index, a quantitative measure of pectus severity.

the Nuss procedure, surgeons commonly request CT examination to document the Haller index, which quantifies the severity of the pectus deformity (Fig. 3-55). To calculate the Haller index, low tube current (mA) images are obtained through the level of the greatest degree of pectus deformity. The Haller index is equal to the transverse left-to-right diameter of the chest, divided by the anterior-to-posterior diameter. The greater the Haller index, the more severe the pectus. A patient with a Haller index greater than 3.2 is considered a surgical candidate.

Suggested Readings

Condon VR: Pneumonia in children, *J Thorac Imaging* 6:31-44, 1991.

Donnelly LF: Maximizing the usefulness of imaging in children with community-acquired pneumonia, *AJR* 172:505-512, 1999.

Donnelly LF, Klosterman LA: Subpleural sparing: a CT finding of lung contusion in children, *Radiology* 204:385-387, 1997.

Donnelly LF, Frush DP: Abnormalities of the chest wall in pediatric patients, *AJR* 173:1595-1601, 1999.

Donnelly LF, Frush DP: Localized lucent chest lesions in neonates: causes and differentiation, *AJR* 172:1651-1658, 1999.

Griscom NT: Respiratory problems of early life now allowing survival into adulthood: concepts for radiologists, *AJR* 158:1-8, 1992.

Griscom NT, Wohl MB, Kirkpatrick JA: Lower respiratory infections: how infants differ from adults, *Radiol Clin North Am* 16:367-387, 1978.

Kunisaki SM, Barnewolt CE, Estroff JA, et al: Large fetal congenital cystic adenomatoid malformations: growth trends and patient survival, *J Pediatr Surg* 42:404-410, 2007.

Merton DF: Diagnostic imaging of mediastinal masses in children, *AJR* 158:825-832, 1992.

Swischuk KE, John SD: Immature lung problems: can our nomenclature be more specific? *AJR* 166:917-918, 1996.

Singleton EB: Radiologic consideration of intensive care in the premature infant, *Radiology* 140:291-300, 1981.

the pediatrician, parent, or patient, and because of the fear of malignancy, cross-sectional imaging is requested. In a previous study that reviewed CT and MR examinations performed to evaluate children with suspected chest wall masses, all of the palpable lesions that were asymptomatic were related to normal anatomic variations. Knowledge that such variations are common should be communicated to referring physicians and parents when imaging is being contemplated in a child with an asymptomatic chest wall "lump."

One of the most common abnormalities in chest wall configuration is pectus excavatum. Although the majority of associated problems due to this deformity are cosmetic, pectus deformities can cause chest pain, fatigue, dyspnea on exertion, palpitations, and restrictive lung disease. When the deformities are severe, surgical repair can be performed. Pectus excavatum is commonly treated by a minimally invasive procedure called a Nuss procedure. Prior to

CHAPTER FOUR

Cardiac

IMAGING MODALITIES IN CONGENITAL HEART DISEASE

Multiple imaging modalities are used to define the morphology, vascular connections, and function of the heart in children with congenital heart disease. Such modalities include radiography, echocardiography, computed tomography (CT), magnetic resonance imaging (MRI), and angiography.

Multiple insults can occur in utero and can lead to congenital heart disease. In many cases, a specific insult results in a single type of anatomic lesion, such as ventricular septal defect (VSD) or coarctation of the aorta. However, insults can result in a variety of anatomic abnormalities, or "complex" congenital heart disease. Historically, chest radiography and clinical symptoms played a large role in limiting the differential diagnosis of the types of congenital heart disease that may be present in a particular patient. With technologic advances and increased use of other imaging modalities, the dependency on chest radiography findings has decreased.

Diagnosing a specific type of congenital heart disease by radiography is difficult. The role of radiography in making the diagnosis of congenital heart disease has probably been overemphasized in education. This is particularly true today because most of the classically described radiographic findings of specific congenital heart disease do not manifest until after the neonatal period, and most patients in developed nations are diagnosed with congenital heart disease and are treated surgically during the neonatal period. However, in some cases the radiologist may be the first person to recognize that the radiographic findings in a newborn suggest that congenital heart disease rather than a pulmonary disorder is the cause of respiratory distress. Therefore, it is important to understand the radiographic findings and the role of radiography in relation to the other imaging modalities in the management of congenital heart disease.

Echocardiography

Echocardiography is the mainstay of congenital heart disease diagnosis. This is particularly true during the fetal and neonatal periods. Most of the highly detailed anatomic and functional information needed for the medical and surgical management of patients with congenital heart disease can be obtained by ultrasound. Color Doppler can be used to identify areas of stenosis or regurgitation. However, there are populations of patients in whom echocardiography is less easily obtained and more prone to inaccuracy. These populations include older children, adults, and postsurgical patients. In these patients, the acoustic window is decreased and echocardiography is more difficult. It is in these circumstances that echocardiography may not provide the necessary information needed for care, so CT and MRI play a role. It is important to keep in perspective the current relatively small role of CT and MRI in cardiac imaging as compared to that of ultrasound.

CT Arteriography

The role of CT in the evaluation of congenital heart disease has rapidly increased as a result of the advent of multidetector CT technology. The rapid speed of acquisition, the ability to acquire volumetric data, and the ability to obtain thin collimation have made CT very useful in patients with congenital heart disease. CT is beneficial in depicting those anatomic structures that are not easily seen on echocardiography, such as the pulmonary arteries, aorta, pulmonary veins, and vascular conduits. CT is often used to depict complex congenital heart disease (Fig. 4-1) and postoperative complications, such as stenosis, occlusions, and pseudoaneurysms. It is useful in evaluating the pulmonary veins such as in suspected anomalous pulmonary venous return. CT is also useful in patients in whom pacemakers preclude the use of MRI. Evaluation of metal stents is often less hampered by artifact in CT than in MRI.

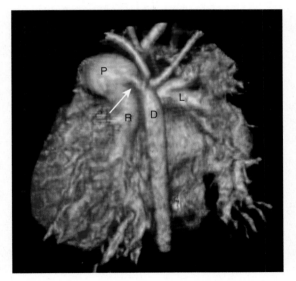

FIGURE 4-1. Hypoplastic left heart syndrome shown on shaded surface rendering of CT arteriogram. CT shows dilatated main pulmonary artery *(P)* supplying descending aorta *(D)* via a PDA *(arrow).* Note left *(L)* and right *(R)* pulmonary arteries. The hypoplastic ascending aorta is not seen.

Magnetic Resonance Imaging

MRI has become a mainstay in the evaluation of certain types of congenital heart disease. MRI studies offer both anatomic and functional information. Cardiac gated spin echo imaging and double inversion recovery imaging, also known as "black-blood" imaging (Fig. 4-2), are the main sequences used to demonstrate anatomic detail and spatial relationships between

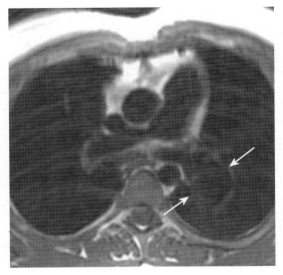

FIGURE 4-2. Dilatated left pulmonary artery *(arrows)* related to poststenotic dilatation from left proximal pulmonary artery stenosis shown on T1-weighted black-blood imaging.

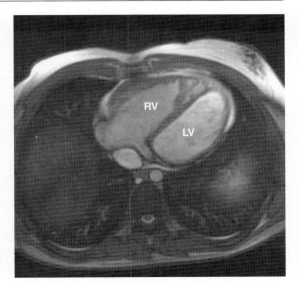

FIGURE 4-3. Gradient echo bright-blood type of image shown through level of left *(LV)* and right *(RV)* ventricles. Such images can be obtained in cine mode and are used to evaluate cardiac motion and functional parameters such as ventricular ejection fraction.

adjacent structures. These sequences allow for precise measurement of anatomic structures.

Cardiac gated cine MRI, or "bright-blood" imaging, is obtained with a number of sequences, such as T2* GRE steady-state sequences (FLASH, SPGR; Fig. 4-3) and steady-state free procession (FIESTA, TRUFISP, balanced fast field echo). Data from these sequences can be processed to provide functional information such as ventricular ejection fractions and can also be used to demonstrate dynamic findings such as turbulent blood flow related to stenosis or regurgitation. MR angiography utilizing gadolinium and maximum projection or shaded surface three-dimensional reconstructions is also useful in demonstrating complex anatomic relationships.

The following are the most common indications for cardiac MRI at our institution: postoperative evaluation of tetralogy of Fallot, evaluation of Duchenne muscular dystrophy, evaluation for possible right ventricular dysplasia, cardiomyopathy, and postoperative evaluation of coarctation.

Computed Tomography versus Magnetic Resonance Imaging

With both CT and MRI becoming increasingly useful in the evaluation of patients with congenital heart disease, there is frequent debate regarding which examination is better for specific clinical indications. Although there are no clear-cut answers, there are advantages and disadvantages of both examinations. The benefits of CT include rapid acquisition time, avoidance of the need for sedation in many cases, greater access to critically ill infants, less artifact resulting from metal stents and other structures, lack of pacemaker safety issues, and visualization of the lungs. The major disadvantage of CT is radiation exposure. Techniques employed in adults, including cardiac gating, thin collimation, overlapping imaging acquisition, and acquisition of multiple sets of images, result in very high radiation doses relative to other CT examinations. Because of the radiosensitivity of children, many of these techniques are not appropriate when imaging children. Other disadvantages of CT include dependence on intravenous contrast bolus and relative lack of functional information. The primary advantages of MRI include lack of ionizing radiation, ability to show more detailed anatomy in some circumstances, and greater depiction of functional information.

Angiography

The use of diagnostic angiography in cases in which percutaneous intervention is not performed is dramatically decreasing because of improvements in noninvasive imaging tools, such as echocardiography, MRI, and CT. At the same time that the role of diagnostic angiography in the evaluation of congenital heart disease is decreasing, percutaneous interventional procedures, such as atrial septal defect (ASD) and VSD closure device deployment, are increasing in number. Diagnostic angiography is commonly performed as part of these interventional procedures to define the anatomy of these abnormalities and to provide procedure guidance.

Approach to the Chest Radiograph in Congenital Heart Disease

It is important to have a basic understanding of the radiographic findings of congenital heart disease because the radiologist may be the first to recognize that respiratory symptoms are secondary to cardiac rather than respiratory disease. Also, understanding the radiographic findings provides a framework for thinking about congenital heart disease. When evaluating a chest radiograph in a patient with potential congenital heart disease, it is important to evaluate pulmonary vascularity, cardiac size, situs, and the position of the aortic arch.

PULMONARY VASCULARITY

The most important radiographic feature for determining the appropriate differential diagnosis in congenital heart disease is the pulmonary vascularity. Unfortunately, it is probably also the most difficult radiographic finding to evaluate. The pulmonary vascularity can be normal or can reflect increased pulmonary arterial flow, increased pulmonary venous flow, or decreased pulmonary flow. In cases of increased pulmonary arterial flow, the pulmonary arteries appear too prominent both in size and in the number of visualized pulmonary arterial structures (Fig. 4-4A, B). A helpful rule is that if the right interlobar pulmonary artery is larger in diameter than the trachea, one should consider increased pulmonary arterial flow to be present. The prominent vascular structures seen in increased pulmonary arterial flow are very distinct and have well-defined borders. In cases with increased pulmonary venous flow, although the pulmonary vascular structures appear prominent in size and distribution, they are very indistinct and poorly defined (Fig. 4-5). Increased pulmonary venous flow is akin to pulmonary venous congestion or mild pulmonary edema. In many cases, such as in left-to-right shunts, there is both increased pulmonary arterial flow resulting from left-to-right shunting as well as increased pulmonary venous flow due to congestive heart failure. If any of the pulmonary arteries in a particular case appear very well defined, it is important to consider at least a component of increased pulmonary arterial flow to be present. In decreased pulmonary arterial flow, there is a paucity of visualized arterial structures throughout the lung (Fig. 4-6). It can at times be difficult to differentiate increased pulmonary arterial flow from the increased peribronchial markings seen with viral pneumonia.

CARDIAC SIZE

Cardiac size may be normal or enlarged. In older children and adults, there may be findings that suggest specific chamber enlargement. However, specific chamber enlargement may be difficult to ascertain in infants because they usually undergo an anteroposterior radiographic technique and have large thymus glands. In these infants, the lateral view commonly offers greater insight into whether cardiomegaly is

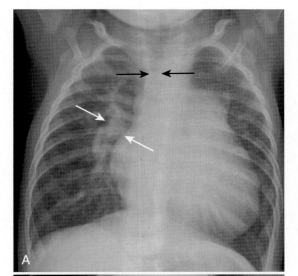

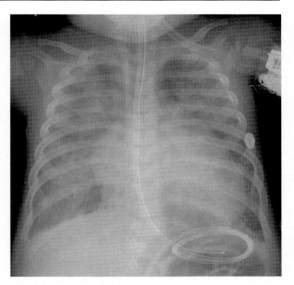

FIGURE 4-5. Increased pulmonary venous flow in neonate with cardiomyopathy. Note the prominent but indistinct pulmonary vascularity.

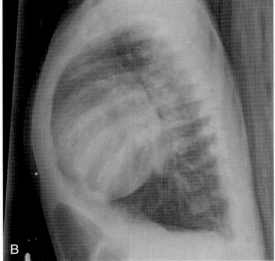

FIGURE 4-4. VSD. **A,** Frontal radiograph shows increased pulmonary arterial flow. Note the prominence of size and number of peripheral pulmonary arterial structures. The diameter of the right interlobar artery *(white arrows)* is wider than the diameter of the trachea *(black arrows),* indicating increased pulmonary arterial flow. Cardiomegaly is present. **B,** Lateral radiograph again shows cardiomegaly and increased pulmonary arterial structures. Note the flattening of hemidiaphragms consistent with hyperinflation, which is often seen in left-to-right shunts.

present than does the frontal view (Figs. 4-7A, B, 4-8A, B, and 4-9A, B). On the lateral view, if the posterior aspect of the cardiac silhouette extends over the vertebral bodies, cardiomegaly should be considered present. *Cardiac axis* is the term given to the configuration of the apex of the heart; it indicates whether the apex points superiorly or inferiorly. If the cardiac apex is oriented superiorly, right-sided cardiac enlargement is suggested (see Fig. 4-6), and if the cardiac axis

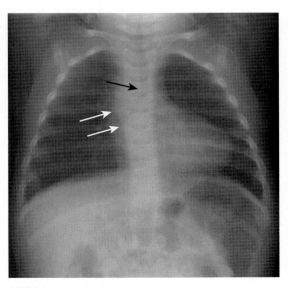

FIGURE 4-6. Tetralogy of Fallot on chest radiography. Note the decrease in identifiable pulmonary markings consistent with decreased pulmonary flow. Also note the upturned cardiac apex and deficient main pulmonary artery area, giving classic boot-shaped appearance of the cardiac silhouette. There is evidence of a right-sided aortic arch, including visualization of a right descending aorta *(white arrows),* indentation on the rightward aspect of the trachea *(black arrow)* from aortic knob, and deviation of the trachea to the left, rather than the typical right deviation.

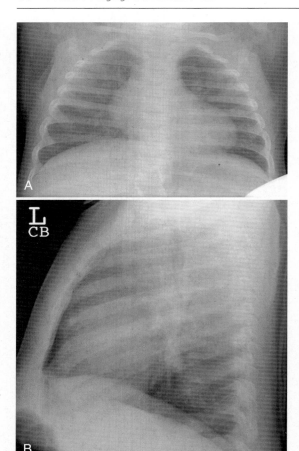

FIGURE 4-7. Exaggerated size of cardiothymic silhouette on anteroposterior frontal radiograph in an infant. **A,** Frontal radiograph demonstrates that the cardiothymic silhouette extends across more than 50% of the thorax. **B,** Lateral radiograph demonstrates the posterior border of the heart to be normally positioned and not to extend posteriorly beyond the spine. No cardiomegaly is present.

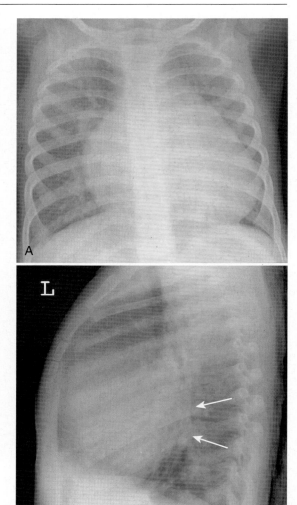

FIGURE 4-8. ASD in an infant demonstrating true cardiac enlargement. **A,** Frontal radiograph demonstrates prominent cardiac silhouette. Also note increased pulmonary arterial flow. **B,** Lateral radiograph better shows cardiomegaly. Note that the posterior aspect of cardiac silhouette *(arrows)* extends beyond the anterior border of the spine.

or apex is oriented inferiorly, left-sided cardiac enlargement is suggested.

SITUS

Situs is defined as the relationship of asymmetric organs to the midline. Identifying disturbances in normal situs (the presence of heterotaxy syndromes) is important because they are associated with the presence of congenital heart disease.

The important structures when evaluating situs on chest radiography are the cardiac apex, the stomach bubble, and the position of the liver. When the cardiac apex and gastric bubble appear on the same side, left or right, there is a much lower incidence of congenital heart disease than in cases in which the cardiac apex is on the opposite side of gastric bubble. When there

is disconcordance between the cardiac apex and the gastric bubble, there is a near 100% incidence of congenital heart disease. Situs solitus is the name given to the normal configuration; it is associated with a 0.6% incidence of congenital heart disease. Situs inversus is the mirror image of normal and is associated with a 3% to 5% incidence of congenital heart disease. With situs ambiguous, there is no clear, straightforward left- or right-sidedness. The major types of situs ambiguous include asplenia (bilateral right-sidedness) and polysplenia (bilateral right-sidedness).

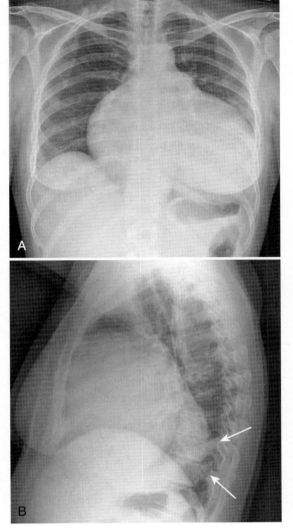

FIGURE 4-9. Epstein anomaly showing marked cardiomegaly. **A,** Frontal radiograph shows marked cardiac enlargement. Note decreased pulmonary flow. **B,** Lateral radiograph shows marked cardiomegaly with posterior aspect of cardiac silhouette *(arrows)* extending well beyond anterior aspect of spine.

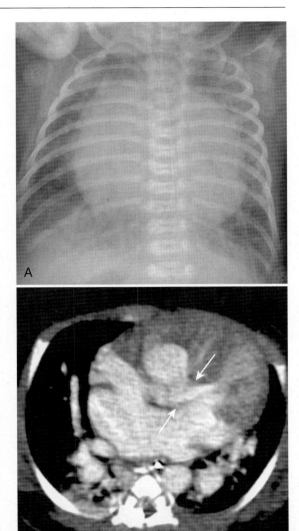

FIGURE 4-10. Asplenia. **A,** Chest radiograph shows marked cardiomegaly and increased pulmonary arterial flow. Note that the stomach bubble is on the right and the cardiac apex is on the left. **B,** CT image shows VSD *(arrows)*. Patient had complex congenital heart disease.

Asplenia (Fig. 4-10A, B) is associated with complex, cyanotic congenital heart disease. Patients are susceptible to infections by encapsulated bacteria because of the lack of a spleen. Other findings include malrotation, microgastria, and midline gallbladder. Radiographic findings include a midline liver, bilateral right-sided-appearing bronchi, decreased pulmonary arterial flow, azygous continuation of the inferior vena cava (IVC), and other findings reflecting the specific type of cyanotic heart disease (see Fig. 4-6).

Polysplenia (Fig. 4-11A, B) is typically associated with less complex acyanotic heart disease,

usually left-to-right shunts. Other associations include azygous continuation of the IVC, bilateral superior vena cava (SVC), malrotation, and absent gallbladder. Radiographic findings include absence of the IVC shadow, prominent azygous vein, midline liver, and increased pulmonary arterial flow.

POSITION OF AORTIC ARCH

The identification of a right-sided aortic arch is also a red flag for the presence of congenital heart disease. When the aortic knob can be identified, as in most cases in adults and older

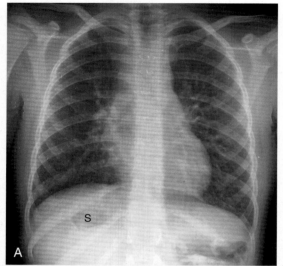

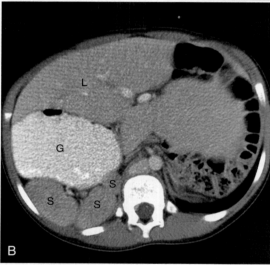

FIGURE 4-11. **Polysplenia. A,** Chest radiograph shows stomach *(S)* on right and cardiac apex on left. **B,** CT shows multiple spleens (S) on the right, a midline liver *(L),* stomach *(G)* on the right, and azygous continuation of the IVC.

trachea, a right-sided aortic arch should be suspected (see Fig. 4-6).

CATEGORIZATION OF CONGENITAL HEART DISEASE

In the traditional classification of congenital heart disease, two of the major features that place the disease into a particular diagnostic category include (1) whether the patient is cyanotic and (2) whether the pulmonary arterial flow is decreased, normal, or increased (Table 4-1). Once these two major features have been identified, other radiographic findings will help to limit the differential diagnosis.

Another important factor to consider is the frequency of occurrence of the various types of congenital heart disease (Table 4-2). Approximately 50% of cases of congenital heart disease are left-to-right shunts. Many of the types of congenital heart disease discussed here are highlighted because of striking anatomic findings but are actually quite rare.

TABLE 4-1. **Categorization of Congenital Heart Disease**

Blue	
	Decreased flow
	Normal heart size
	Tetralogy of Fallot
	Giant heart size
	Ebstein anomaly
	Pulmonary atresia with intact ventricular septum
	Increased flow
	Truncus arteriosus
	Total anomalous pulmonary venous return
	Variable flow
	D-transposition of the great arteries
	Tricuspid atresia
Pink	
	Increased pulmonary arterial flow and left to right shunt (VSD, ASD, AVC, PDA)
	Increased pulmonary venous flow
	CHF in the newborn
	Normal pulmonary flow
	Obstructive lesions
	Coarctation of the aorta
	Aortic stenosis
	Pulmonary artery stenosis
	Postsurgery

children, it is obvious which side the aortic arch is on. However, in infants, the aortic knob is often not identified. In such cases, secondary findings for the presence of the aortic arch must be utilized. Such findings include the position of the descending aorta, tracheal displacement, and tracheal indentation. In a normal left-sided aortic arch, the trachea is displaced slightly toward the right because it moves inferiorly. Also in such cases, there is an indentation on the left aortic border of the trachea as visualized on the frontal view of the chest. If the trachea deviates slightly leftward as it moves inferiorly or if there is a soft tissue indentation on the right aortic border of the

TABLE 4-2. Incidence of More Common Types of Congenital Heart Disease

Diagnosis	% Congenital Heart Disease
Left-to-right shunts (VSD, ASD, atrioventricular canal, persistent PDA)	50 (VSD, 28)
Pulmonic stenosis	9.3
Aortic stenosis/bicuspid aortic valve	7.7
Tetralogy of Fallot	7.5
Coarctation of the aorta	3.8
Single ventricle	2.7
Hypoplastic left heart syndrome	1.8
D-Transposition of the great arteries	1.8
Tricuspid atresia	1.6
Total anomalous pulmonary venous return	1.4
Truncus arteriosus, L-transposition of great arteries, pulmonary atresia, Epstein anomaly	Each ≤1

Blue, Decreased Pulmonary Arterial Flow, Mild Cardiomegaly

The differential diagnosis of patients who are cyanotic and demonstrate decreased pulmonary arterial flow on chest radiograph can be narrowed according to whether the patient has mild or massive cardiomegaly. In the cases in which the heart size is normal or there is only mild cardiomegaly, the differential diagnosis includes tetralogy of Fallot and pulmonary atresia with an associated VSD. These two entities are essentially different spectrums of the same disease.

TETRALOGY OF FALLOT

Tetralogy of Fallot is the most common type of cyanotic congenital heart disease in children. It is usually diagnosed by 3 months of age. There are four classic anatomic components of tetralogy of Fallot: (1) right ventricular outflow tract obstruction, (2) VSD, (3) overriding aorta, and (4) right ventricular hypertrophy. Radiographic features include a normal-sized to slightly enlarged cardiac silhouette with uplifting of the ventricular apex (a superiorly oriented cardiac axis) secondary to right ventricular hypertrophy (see Fig. 4-6). The main pulmonary artery segment is concave because of the small associated pulmonary arteries. The combination of the

deficient main pulmonary artery and the upturned cardiac apex makes the configuration of the cardiac silhouette appear to be boot-shaped. The pulmonary vascularity is decreased. In tetralogy of Fallot the central pulmonary arteries may be confluent or nonconfluent. This is often difficult to evaluate with echocardiography, so MRI can be utilized to evaluate the status of the pulmonary arteries in patients with tetralogy of Fallot (Fig. 4-12A, B). Pulmonary atresia with a VSD is considered to

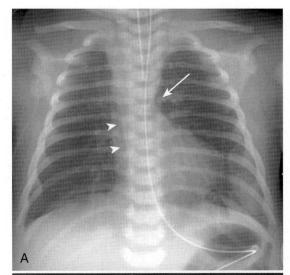

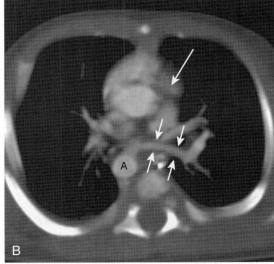

FIGURE 4-12. Tetralogy of Fallot. **A,** Frontal radiograph shows right-sided descending aorta *(arrowheads)*, deficient main pulmonary artery *(arrow)*, decreased pulmonary arterial flow, and upturned cardiac apex. **B,** CT shows deficient main pulmonary artery *(large arrow)* and bronchial collateral artery *(small arrows)* arising from aorta *(A)* and feeding left lung.

be the most severe form of tetralogy of Fallot. It is synonymous with pseudotruncus or truncus arteriosus type 4 because of the larger bronchial arteries arising from the aorta and supplying the lungs.

Blue, Decreased Pulmonary Arterial Flow, Massive Cardiomegaly

In patients who are cyanotic and demonstrate decreased pulmonary flow but have massive cardiomegaly, the first two entities that should be considered are Ebstein anomaly and pulmonary atresia with an intact septum. With these two entities, the degree of cardiomegaly may be the most massive encountered on radiography. The right atrium can dilate to massive size, rather like a balloon; therefore, when massive cardiomegaly is encountered, abnormalities that lead to marked enlargement of the right atrium should be considered.

EBSTEIN ANOMALY

In Ebstein anomaly there is redundancy of the tricuspid valve, which is displaced into the right ventricle causing atrialization of part of the right ventricle. There is functional obstruction at the level of the tricuspid valve that results in massive dilatation of the right atrium and the atrialized portion of the right ventricle. The age of presentation is variable. When the anomaly is severe, infants present with severe cyanosis. On radiography, massive cardiomegaly and decreased pulmonary arterial flow are seen (Fig 4-13A, B; and see Fig. 4-9). Ebstein anomaly is a rare entity.

PULMONARY ATRESIA WITH INTACT VENTRICULAR SEPTUM

Unlike cases of pulmonary atresia with VSD (tetralogy of Fallot), patients with pulmonary atresia and an intact septum have no forward flow from the right heart. This leads to massive dilatation of the right atrium and, to a lesser degree, the right ventricle. Such patients present with marked cyanosis in infancy. The radiographic appearance (Fig. 4-14) may be identical to that of Ebstein anomaly.

Note that there are many other abnormalities that may cause the appearance of a massive cardiopericardial silhouette on the chest radiograph of a newborn. They include cardiac

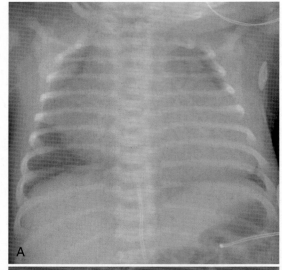

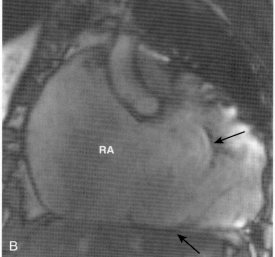

FIGURE 4-13. Ebstein anomaly. **A,** Radiography in a newborn shows massive cardiomegaly and decreased pulmonary arterial flow. **B,** Ebstein anomaly (different patient) shown on coronal-oblique gradient echo bright-blood MRI. There is massive enlargement of the right atrium *(RA).* Note the displaced tricuspid valve *(arrows)* extending into right ventricle.

tumors such as rhabdomyoma (Fig. 4-15A, B), noncardiac mediastinal masses, congenital diaphragmatic hernia prior to aeration of the herniated bowel, and peripheral arterial venous fistulas with associated high output failure. However, when massive cardiomegaly is encountered in the presence of decreased pulmonary flow, Ebstein anomaly and pulmonary atresia with intact septum should be the primary considerations.

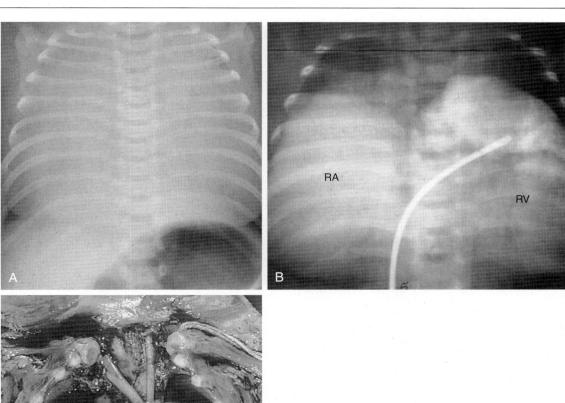

FIGURE 4-14. Pulmonary atresia with intact ventricular septum in a newborn. **A,** Radiograph shows massive cardiomegaly filling the entire chest. **B,** Contrast injection of right ventricle shows massive dilatation of right atrium *(RA)* and right ventricle *(RV).* **C,** Postmortem photograph after thoracotomy shows massively dilatated right atrium. (Donnelly LF and others: The wall-to-wall heart: differential diagnosis for massively large cardiothymic silhouette in newborns, *Applied Radiol* 26:23-28, 1997. Used with permission.)

Blue, Increased Flow

Patients who are cyanotic and have increased pulmonary arterial flow have admixture lesions, in which the systemic and pulmonary circulations are mixed. In infancy, the two entities that should be considered most likely are truncus arteriosus and total anomalous pulmonary venous return (TAPVR).

TRUNCUS ARTERIOSUS

In truncus arteriosus, there is failure of the normal division of the primitive truncus arteriosus into an aorta and a pulmonary artery. Therefore, one single vessel arises from the heart and gives rise to the coronary, systemic, and pulmonary circulations. There is always an associated VSD. The types of truncus arteriosus

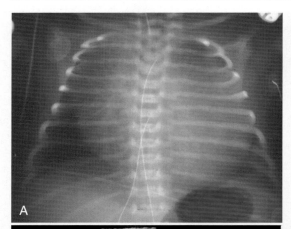

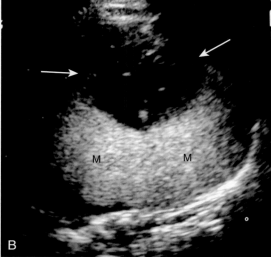

FIGURE 4-15. Cardiac rhabdomyoma with massive cardiomegaly mimicking Ebstein anomaly on radiography. **A,** Frontal radiograph demonstrates massive cardiomegaly. There even appears to be decreased pulmonary arterial flow. **B,** Substernal longitudinal ultrasound demonstrates large infiltrative mass *(M)* arising from and surrounding the heart *(arrows)*. (Donnelly LF and others: The wall-to-wall heart: differential diagnosis for massively large cardiothymic silhouette in newborns, *Applied Radiol* 26:23-28, 1997. Used with permission.)

are classified according to how the pulmonary arteries arise from the primitive truncus. It is an uncommon lesion and usually presents with cyanosis early in infancy.

On chest radiography, there is increased pulmonary arterial flow. A right aortic arch is present in one third of patients. The identification of a right aortic arch in the presence of increased pulmonary arterial flow in a cyanotic child is highly suggestive of the diagnosis (Fig. 4-16). There is usually moderate cardiomegaly as well as superimposed pulmonary venous congestion.

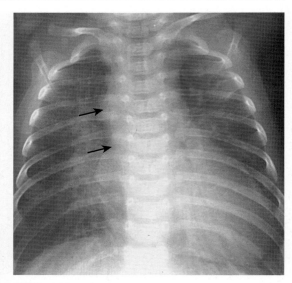

FIGURE 4-16. Truncus arteriosus. Chest radiograph shows increased pulmonary arterial flow, cardiomegaly, and right-sided aortic arch *(arrows)*. Note the indentation on the right wall of the trachea and the straight course of the trachea from superior to inferior, secondary to the right aortic arch.

TOTAL ANOMALOUS PULMONARY VENOUS RETURN

In TAPVR, the pulmonary venous return does not connect to the left atrium but instead connects to systemic venous structures such as the SVC, right atrium, or portal vein. TAPVR can be divided into supracardiac, cardiac, or infracardiac subtypes. Supracardiac is the most common form; in this form the pulmonary veins converge and form a left vertical vein that runs superiorly and connects into the innominate vein. With infracardiac TAPVR, the returning veins penetrate the diaphragm and connect to the IVC below the level of diaphragm. These veins may become obstructed, and the patient may present with a pulmonary edema pattern on chest radiography (Fig. 4-17). If the veins are not obstructed, the lesion may appear with cardiomegaly and increased pulmonary arterial flow, similar to other left-to-right shunts (Fig. 4-18A, B). Supracardiac TAPVR classically demonstrates a "snowman" appearance, in which the dilated left vertical vein and dilated SVC form the superior portion of the snowman, and the cardiac silhouette forms the inferior portion (Fig. 4-19A-D). This classic appearance does not develop until later in life and is not often seen now because these lesions are repaired during infancy.

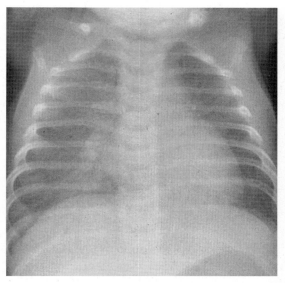

FIGURE 4-17. Total anomalous pulmonary venous return, infra-cardiac type, with venous obstruction in a newborn. Chest radiograph demonstrates diffuse pulmonary opacity with indistinctness of the pulmonary vascularity.

Blue, Variable Pulmonary Arterial Flow

Both D-transposition of the great arteries (D-TGA) and tricuspid atresia can present with variable flow, depending on the anatomy associated with the lesion as well as the age of the patient.

D-TRANSPOSITION OF THE GREAT ARTERIES

D-TGA is the most common congenital heart disease presenting with cyanosis during the first 24 hours of life. With this abnormality, the aorta and pulmonary arteries are transposed. The ascending aorta arises from the right ventricle and the pulmonary artery arises from the left ventricle. Therefore, blood flow runs in two parallel circuits, systemic and pulmonary. Survival depends on communication between these two circles via patent foramen ovale, ASD, VSD, or patent ductus arteriosus (PDA). Historically, D-TGA was categorized as a cardiac lesion associated with increased pulmonary arterial flow. However, in areas with developed health care systems, pulmonary arterial switch procedures are performed during the first week of life; therefore, increased pulmonary flow, which is seen in older children with transposition, is now rarely seen. The most common chest radiographic appearance of a newborn child with D-TGA is normal (Fig. 4-20). Classically described radiographic findings include narrowing of the superior mediastinum due to

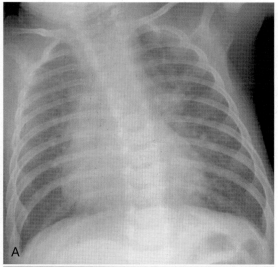

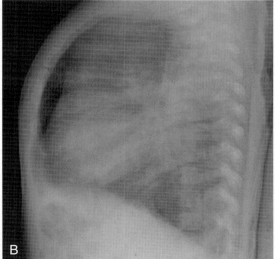

FIGURE 4-18. Total anomalous pulmonary venous return, infracardiac type, without venous obstruction in a newborn. The appearance is typical of a left-to-right shunt. **A,** Frontal chest radiograph shows mild prominence of cardiac silhouette and increased pulmonary arterial flow. **B,** Lateral chest radiograph shows cardiomegaly and hyperinflated lungs, which are commonly seen in left-to-right shunts.

decreased thymic tissue and abnormal relationships of the great vessels and to increased pulmonary arterial flow, as previously mentioned. The appearance of the mediastinum has been likened to that of an egg on a string.

TRICUSPID ATRESIA

In tricuspid atresia, the classic description is that the right atrium is markedly enlarged, causing marked cardiomegaly associated with decreased

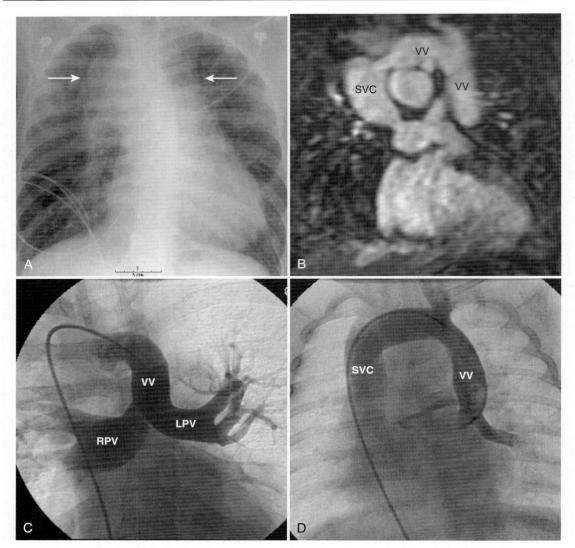

FIGURE 4-19. Total anomalous pulmonary venous return, supracardiac type in an older child. **A,** Chest radiograph shows "snowman" appearance of mediastinum. There is enlargement of the superior mediastinum *(arrows)* secondary to dilatated left vertical vein and SVC. There is also increased pulmonary arterial flow. **B,** MRI coronal gradient echo bright-blood image shows vertical vein *(VV)* draining into superior vena cava *(SVC).* **C,** Venogram with catheter in pulmonary vein shows left *(LPV)* and right *(RPV)* pulmonary veins draining into vertical vein *(VV).* **D,** Later image from venogram shows contrast draining from vertical vein *(VV)* into superior vena cava *(SVC).*

pulmonary flow. However, this classic appearance is seen only in a minority of patients. The radiograph can vary greatly in cases of tricuspid atresia, making radiographic diagnosis a humbling experience (Fig. 4-21).

Pink, Increased Pulmonary Arterial Flow

Children who are acyanotic and demonstrate increased pulmonary arterial flow on chest radiography have left-to-right shunts. Potential shunts include ASD, VSD, PDA (Fig. 4-22), atrioventricular canal, partial anomalous pulmonary venous return, and aortopulmonary window. The particular cardiac chamber enlargement is a clue to which type of shunt is present. In ASD, the right atrium and right ventricle are enlarged. In VSD, the right ventricle, left atrium, and left ventricle are enlarged. In PDA, the left atrium, left ventricle, and aorta are enlarged. However, as previously mentioned, determining chamber enlargement is next to impossible in infants.

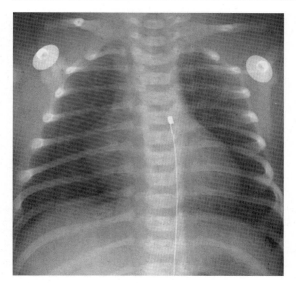

FIGURE 4-20. D-transposition of the great arteries (D-TGA) in a newborn male with a chest radiograph that appears to be relatively normal. Chest radiograph shows normal pulmonary vascularity. The classically described findings of D-TGA, such as increased pulmonary arterial flow and an egg-on-a-string appearance of the mediastinum, are absent.

Perhaps a more practical way of predicting which type of shunt is present is by determining the age at presentation. Patients with very large shunts, such as VSDs or atrioventricular canals, present in infancy. ASDs typically present later in childhood or in early adulthood. PDAs occur most commonly in premature infants. Atrioventricular

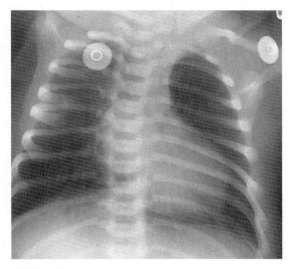

FIGURE 4-21. Tricuspid atresia in a 3-day-old girl with lack of striking findings on radiography. Chest radiograph shows only slightly decreased pulmonary arterial flow.

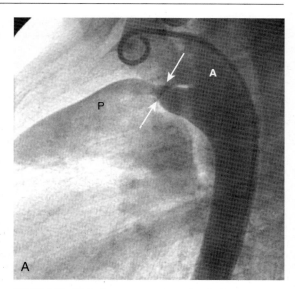

FIGURE 4-22. PDA shown on arteriography. Catheter tip is in ascending aorta (A). Contrast is seen traversing PDA (arrows) and entering into pulmonary artery (P).

canals occur commonly in patients with Down syndrome.

On chest radiography, neonates with left-to-right shunts demonstrate increased pulmonary arterial flow, a variable amount of associated increased pulmonary venous flow (pulmonary edema), and cardiomegaly (see Figs. 4-4, 4-8, and 4-18). It is common for infants with large left-to-right shunts also to have marked hyperinflation on chest radiography (see Figs. 4-4, 4-8, and 4-18). This is thought to be secondary to air trapping due to the peribronchial edema. Therefore, the presence of marked hyperinflation should not dissuade one from the diagnosis of a left-to-right shunt in favor of viral small airway disease.

Pink (or Dusky) With Increased Pulmonary Venous Flow

An acyanotic patient with increased pulmonary venous flow is essentially a patient with congestive heart failure. In the neonate, the differential diagnosis of congestive heart failure is quite extensive and somewhat different from that seen in older children and adults. Residents often have difficulty providing a reasonable differential diagnosis of congestive heart failure in a newborn. An easy way to approach the differential diagnosis is to consider two large

TABLE 4-3. Differential Diagnosis for Congestive Heart Failure in the Newborn

Anatomic	Systemic
Coarctation	Anemia/polycythemia
Aortic stenosis	Hypo- and hyperglycemia
Left ventricular dysfunction and	Hypo- and hyperthyroidism
Anomalous origin of the left coronary artery	Sepsis
Myocarditis	Peripheral arteriovenous malformation
Shock myocardium (birth asphyxia)	Vein of Galen malformation
Glycogen storage disease	Hepatic hemangioendothelioma
Infant of diabetic mother	
Hypoplastic left heart	
Mitral stenosis	
Cor triatriatum	
Pulmonary venous atresia/stenosis	

categories of disease. The first category is that of anatomic left-sided obstruction (Table 4-3). Anything that obstructs the left side of the heart can cause congestive heart failure. If you work your way proximally, starting in the level of the aorta, you won't forget to mention any of the likely candidates. In the aorta, both coarctation of the aorta (Fig. 4-23A, B) and critical aortic stenosis can cause left-sided obstruction. Anything that causes the left ventricle to be dysfunctional also can cause left-sided heart obstruction. The list of possibilities is long and includes cardiomyopathy (see Fig. 4-5), glycogen storage disease, anomalous origin of the left coronary artery with associated cardiac ischemia, birth asphyxia (shock myocardium), infants of diabetic mothers, and hypoplastic left heart syndrome (Fig. 4-24). Within the region of the left atrium, both mitral valve stenosis and cor triatriatum can cause left-sided heart failure. Cor triatriatum is defined as the presence of a membrane dividing the left atrium into two separate chambers. The membrane has a pinlike hole centrally that is the only route for forward blood flow and causes relative obstruction. Pulmonary venous atresia can also cause left-sided heart failure. The most commonly encountered of these abnormalities include hypoplastic left heart syndrome and coarctation of the aorta.

The second large category of entities that can cause left-sided heart failure includes systemic causes of failure, such as anemia and polycythemia, sepsis, or high output failure resulting from a peripheral arteriovenous malformation.

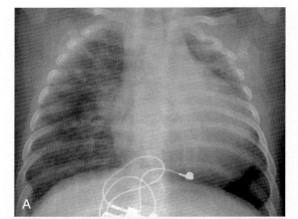

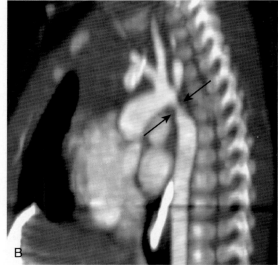

FIGURE 4-23. Coarctation of the aorta associated with congestive heart failure in a newborn. **A,** Chest radiograph shows cardiomegaly and increased and indistinct pulmonary vasculature. **B,** CT arteriography shows coarctation *(arrows)* as narrowing of the aorta in a juxtaductal location.

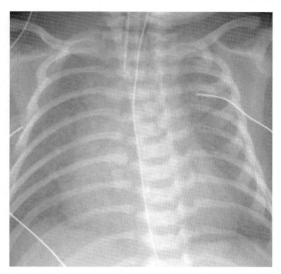

FIGURE 4-24. **Hypoplastic left heart** with associated **congestive heart failure in a newborn.** Radiograph shows **cardiomegaly** and indistinct pulmonary vasculature. Note that patients with hypoplastic left heart do **not** necessarily have hearts that appear to be small.

HYPOPLASTIC LEFT HEART SYNDROME

Hypoplastic left heart syndrome refers to a combination of hypoplasia or aplasia of the ascending aorta, aortic valve, left ventricle, and mitral valve. Children present with congestive heart failure at birth. The lesion is dependent on a PDA. Systemic flow goes from the main pulmonary artery to the descending aorta via the PDA (see Fig. 4-1). Flow to the coronary and cranial areas is retrograde via the hypoplastic ascending aorta. On radiography, there is cardiomegaly and increased pulmonary venous flow (pulmonary edema; see Fig. 4-24). Treatment is the Norwood procedure (Table 4-4).

Pink, Normal Pulmonary Arterial Flow

The three main categories of congenital heart disease that are associated with acyanosis and

TABLE 4-4. **Common Surgical Procedures for Congenital Heart Disease**

Procedure	Indication	Connection
Fontan	Tricuspid atresia Single ventricle Hypoplastic right ventricle Complex congenital heart disease	RA-to-PA conduit or anastomosis
Glenn	Tricuspid atresia Hypoplastic RV Pulmonary atresia	SVC-to-right PA anastomosis (bidirectional provides flow to both pulmonary arteries)
Rastelli	Pulmonary atresia	RV-to-PA conduit
Mustard/Senning (intraatrial baffle)	D-Transposition of the great arteries	Atrial rerouting of venous blood flow
Arterial switch procedure (Jatene)	D-transposition of the great arteries	Switch of aorta and PA with reanastomosis of coronary arteries
Norwood	Hypoplastic left heart syndrome	First stage: use of main PA as ascending aorta, enlargement of aortic arch, systemic shunt to distal PA Second stage: modified Fontan
Blalock-Taussig shunt	Palliative shunt for obstruction of pulmonary blood flow (TOF, pulmonary atresia, tricuspid atresia)	Subclavian artery-to-PA graft
Closure device deployment	Left-to-right shunts (ASD, PDA)	Percutaneous catheter placement of "plugging" closure device across left-to-right shunt
Waterston-Cooley	Palliative shunt for obstruction of pulmonary blood flow	Ascending aorta-to-right PA anastomosis
Potts	Palliative shunt for obstruction of pulmonary blood flow	Descending aorta-to-right PA anastomosis
PA banding	Left-to-right shunting	Band around main PA

PA, pulmonary artery.

normal pulmonary arterial flow include obstructive lesions, extrinsic airway compression, and congenital heart disease with increased or decreased pulmonary arterial flow that has been surgically corrected. (Extrinsic airway compression was discussed in Chapter 2.)

OBSTRUCTIVE LESIONS

Obstructive lesions of the great arteries include aortic stenosis, pulmonic stenosis, and coarctation of the aorta. These lesions can have subtle findings on chest radiography, so when there is a scenario that suggests congenital heart disease but your initial impression is that the chest radiograph is normal, a second glance for subtle mediastinal contour abnormalities may prove fruitful.

AORTIC STENOSIS

Aortic stenosis may occur secondary to a bicuspid aortic valve or previous rheumatic disease. With aortic valvular stenosis, there may be dilatation of the ascending aorta secondary to the "jet" effect through the stenotic valve (Fig. 4-25A-C). The ascending aorta should never be identified in a normal child on frontal radiography. If the rightward border of the ascending aorta is visualized, a dilatated aorta should be suspected (see Fig. 4-25). In addition to aortic stenosis, another cause of a dilatated ascending aorta is an aneurysm secondary to a disorder such as Marfan syndrome. Another supporting sign for aortic stenosis is left ventricular enlargement secondary to hypertrophy. Aortic stenosis can also be supravalvular in

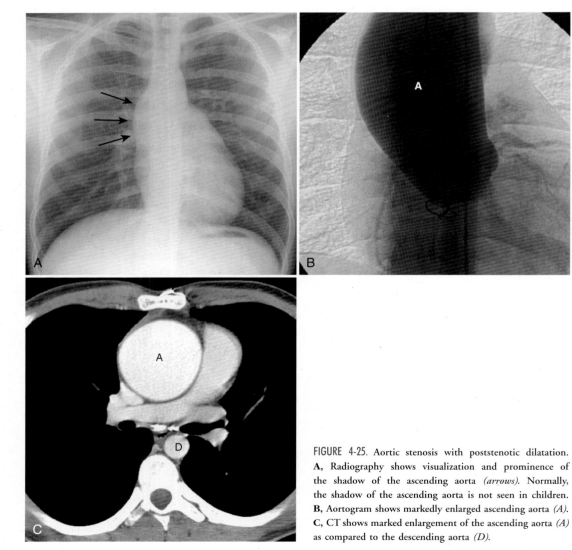

FIGURE 4-25. Aortic stenosis with poststenotic dilatation. A, Radiography shows visualization and prominence of the shadow of the ascending aorta *(arrows)*. Normally, the shadow of the ascending aorta is not seen in children. B, Aortogram shows markedly enlarged ascending aorta *(A)*. C, CT shows marked enlargement of the ascending aorta *(A)* as compared to the descending aorta *(D)*.

location. Williams syndrome is associated with supravalvular stenosis, peripheral pulmonary artery stenosis, and other symptoms, including mental retardation.

PULMONIC STENOSIS

In pulmonary valvular stenosis, there may be dilatation of the main pulmonary artery secondary to the jet effect (Fig. 4-26A, B). On frontal chest radiography this appears as a prominent main pulmonary arterial segment (Fig. 4-27).

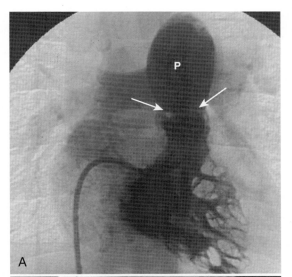

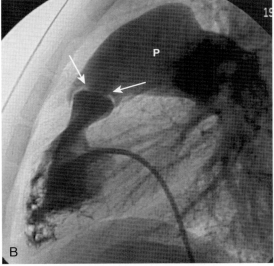

FIGURE 4-26. Pulmonic stenosis in a 3-year-old boy. Arteriogram performed by injection of contrast via the right ventricle. **A,** Frontal projection. **B,** Lateral projection. Both show stenotic valve and jet *(arrows)* and poststenotic dilatation of the main pulmonary artery *(P).*

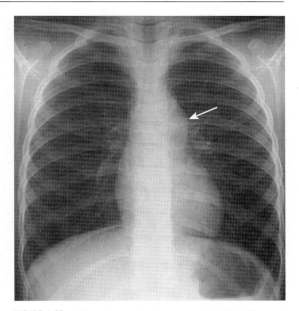

FIGURE 4-27. Pulmonic stenosis in a 7-year-old girl. Radiograph shows slight prominence of the main pulmonary artery *(arrow).*

COARCTATION OF THE AORTA

Coarctation is defined as a congenital narrowing of the aorta. This narrowing can be either diffuse or localized. The localized type, which is more common, is typically located just beyond the left subclavian artery in the vicinity of the level of ductus arteriosus. The clinical presentation is determined by the severity of the narrowing. Severe narrowing presents in infancy with congestive heart failure (see Fig. 4-23). Coarctation can be an isolated lesion or can appear as part of more complex anatomic anomalies (Fig. 4-28A, B). Less severe narrowing may present later in childhood with upper extremity hypertension. On chest radiography, the appearance of the leftward border of the superior mediastinum has been likened to the numeral 3 in coarctation (Fig. 4-29A-C), particularly in older children. The superior portion of the 3 is caused by the prestenotic dilatation of the aorta above the coarctation. The middle or narrow part of the three is caused by the coarctation itself, and the inferior part of the 3 is caused by the poststenotic dilatated portion of the descending aorta. Rib notching may be present secondary to erosion by dilatated intercostal arteries (see Fig. 4-29); it most commonly occurs at the level of the fourth through eighth ribs. In patients with coarctation of the aorta there is increased association with bicuspid aortic valve, which can present later in life with

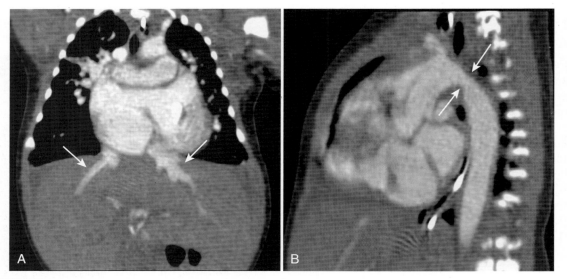

FIGURE 4-28. Coarctation of the aorta associated with asplenia and complex congenital heart disease. **A,** Coronal CT shows midline liver and hepatic veins *(arrows)* draining directly into right atrium. **B,** Sagittal-oblique CT shows narrowing of aorta *(arrows)* in juxtaductal location consistent with coarctation.

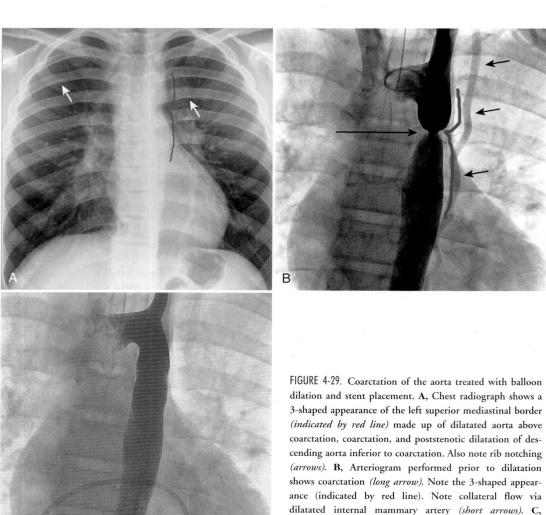

FIGURE 4-29. Coarctation of the aorta treated with balloon dilation and stent placement. **A,** Chest radiograph shows a 3-shaped appearance of the left superior mediastinal border *(indicated by red line)* made up of dilatated aorta above coarctation, coarctation, and poststenotic dilatation of descending aorta inferior to coarctation. Also note rib notching *(arrows).* **B,** Arteriogram performed prior to dilatation shows coarctation *(long arrow).* Note the 3-shaped appearance (indicated by red line). Note collateral flow via dilatated internal mammary artery *(short arrows).* **C,** Postdilation and stent placement, the coarctation has been resolved. Note resolution of flow (nonvisualization on contrast study) of dilatated collateral mammary artery.

resultant aortic stenosis. Treatment involves balloon dilation and stent placement (see Fig. 4-29) or surgical resection. In cases of coarctation, CT and MRI can be used for diagnosis and presurgical planning (site, length, severity, relationship to left subclavian artery, and extent of collateralization; see Fig. 4-25) as well as for postsurgical follow-up in the evaluation of restenosis, aneurysm, or left ventricular hypertrophy.

ABNORMALITIES OF CONOTRUNCAL ROTATION

Several types of congenital heart disease can result from abnormalities of conotruncal rotation. There is often confusion concerning this group of diseases. The primitive truncus is an anterior midline structure during fetal development. Normally, the primitive truncus divides into the aorta and pulmonary artery, which rotate clockwise 150 degrees (Figs. 4-30, 4-31). As a result, the pulmonary artery ends up anterior and to the left of the aorta. Abnormal

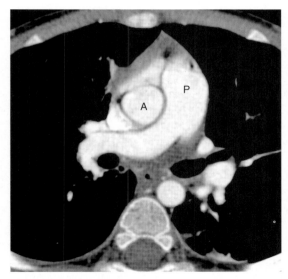

FIGURE 4-31. Normal conotruncal position on axial CT. The pulmonary artery *(P)* is anterior and leftward in relationship to the aorta *(A)*.

division or rotation of this primitive truncus may result in a number of diseases, including L-transposition of the great arteries (L-TGA; Fig. 4-32); D-transposition of the great arteries (D-TGA; Figs. 4-33A, B, 4-34); truncus arteriosus; double-outlet right ventricle; and situs inversus. The anatomic relationship between the aorta and the pulmonary artery as viewed in cross-section at the level of the semilunar valves is characteristic of these abnormalities.

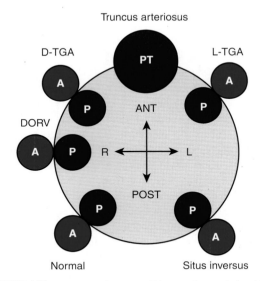

FIGURE 4-30. Conotruncal rotation. Diagram shows relationship of the great arteries at the level of the semilunar valves as depicted by axial cross-sectional MRI. During embryologic development, the primitive truncus is an anterior midline structure. With normal development, the primitive truncus divides into the aorta and the pulmonary artery, which then rotate 150 degrees clockwise. The pulmonary artery then lies anterior to and left of the aorta. Variations in this rotation are characteristic of various conotruncal abnormalities. (A, aorta; DORV, double outlet right ventricle; P, pulmonary artery; PT, primitive truncus; TGA, transposition of the great arteries.)

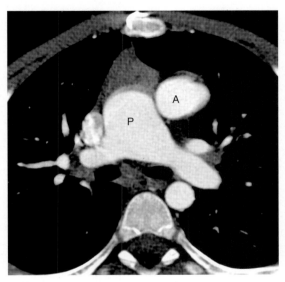

FIGURE 4-32. L-transposition of the great vessels shown on axial CT. The aorta *(A)* is to the left of and anterior to the pulmonary artery *(P)*.

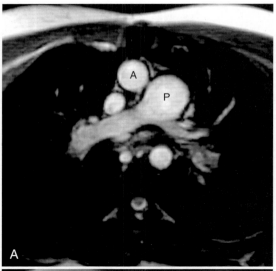

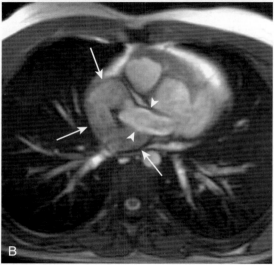

FIGURE 4-33. D-transposition of the great vessels shown on gradient echo bright-blood axial MRI following intraatrial baffle. **A,** The aorta *(A)* is anterior and rightward in relationship to the pulmonary artery *(P)*. **B,** The structures of the intraatrial baffle *(arrows, arrowheads)* are visualized.

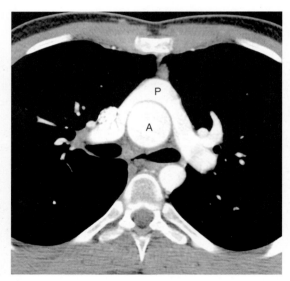

FIGURE 4-34. D-transposition of the great vessels shown following an arterial switch (Jatene) procedure, showing typical post-switch anatomy. The pulmonary artery *(P)* is now anterior to and draped over the more posteriorly positioned aorta *(A)*.

With truncus arteriosus, there is a failure of division of the primitive truncus into a separate aorta and pulmonary artery. Therefore, a single large vessel gives rise to the coronary, systemic, and pulmonary arterial circulation. Truncus arteriosus was discussed in detail previously.

In L-TGA or congenitally corrected transposition of the great arteries, the ventricles and atrioventricular valves are inverted such that there is both atrioventricular and ventriculoarterial discordance. Therefore, the morphologic right ventricle is in the position of and serves as the anatomic left ventricle. L-TGA is often associated with complex congenital heart disease but may occur as an isolated lesion. With L-TGA, there is 30-degree clockwise rotation of the primitive truncus, which causes the aorta to be anterior and leftward as compared to the pulmonary artery (see Figs. 4-30, 4-32).

In contrast, with D-TGA, or complete transposition of the great arteries, there is ventricular-great vessel disconcordance, in which the aorta arises from the right ventricle, and the pulmonary artery arises from the left ventricle. With D-TGA, there is a 30-degree counterclockwise rotation of the primitive truncus, which means that the aorta is rightward and anterior to the pulmonary artery (see Figs. 4-30, 4-33, 4-34).

In the case of a double-outlet right ventricle, more than one half of the origins of the great arteries arise from the morphologic right ventricle. The only outlet for the left ventricle is a VSD. This lesion is commonly associated with other complex congenital heart disease. During development, there is 45-degree counterclockwise rotation of the primitive truncus, which causes the aorta and pulmonary artery to be side by side with the aorta on the right (see Fig. 4-30).

In situs inversus, the rotation of the aorta and pulmonary artery is completely opposite of that which would be considered normal (see Fig. 4-30).

SURGERIES FOR CONGENITAL HEART DISEASE

To understand the imaging appearances on chest radiography and cross-sectional studies of patients who have undergone surgery or interventional procedures for congenital heart disease, knowledge of the types of procedures performed is required. Table 4-4 lists the names, indications, and flow alterations of commonly performed cardiac procedures. The imaging findings related to a number of procedures are also illustrated: balloon angioplasty of coarctation of the aorta (see Fig. 4-29), intraatrial baffle (see Fig. 4-33), arterial switch procedure (see Fig. 4-34), ASD closure device (Fig. 4-35A, B), and Fontan procedure (Fig. 4-36).

Acquired Heart Disease

In addition to congenital heart disease, there are multiple types of acquired heart disease that can occur during childhood. Many of these, such as cardiomyopathy and rheumatic heart disease, have features in common with those found in adult disease. One of the unusual types of acquired heart disease that can occur in children is Kawasaki disease.

KAWASAKI DISEASE

Kawasaki disease (mucocutaneous lymph node syndrome) is an inflammatory disease of unknown cause. Characteristic findings include fever, rash, conjunctivitis, erythema of the lips and oral cavity, and cervical lymphadenopathy. There is an associated generalized vasculitis. Cardiac involvement includes an acute myocarditis, which can lead to congestive heart failure (Fig. 4-37). Delayed cardiac complications include the development of coronary artery aneurysms (Fig. 4-38A-C) as well as coronary artery stenoses. Chest radiographs can show findings of congestive heart failure when the myocarditis is severe. Rarely, the coronary artery aneurysms can calcify (see Fig. 4-38). Gallbladder hydrops, as seen on

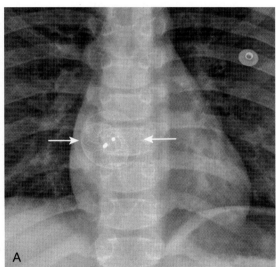
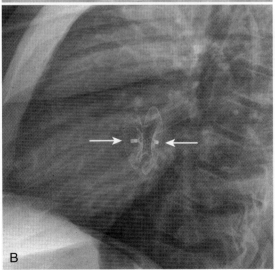

FIGURE 4-35. ASD closure device. **A,** Frontal and **B,** lateral radiographs show ASD closure device *(arrows).* Note the two disk-shaped portions, each one resting on one or the other side of the defect, holding the device in place and blocking flow.

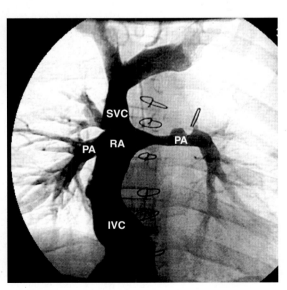

FIGURE 4-36. Fontan procedure. Venogram shows anatomy of Fontan procedure. The SVC and IVC are connected directly to the pulmonary arteries *(PA)* via the right atrium *(RA).*

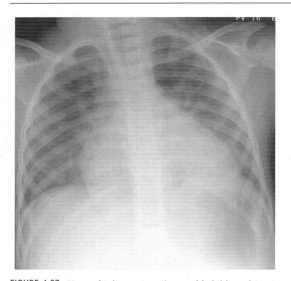

FIGURE 4-37. Kawasaki disease in a 4-year-old child resulting in acute myocarditis. Chest radiograph shows cardiomegaly and indistinct, prominent pulmonary vasculature consistent with venous congestion.

ultrasound, has also been described as a finding. However, this is not included as one of the criteria in making the diagnosis, and ultrasound of the upper abdomen is rarely useful in diagnosing the disease. Treatment with gamma globulin can decrease the severity of the illness and can decrease the likelihood of delayed complications such as coronary aneurysms.

CARDIAC MASSES

There are a number of causes of cardiac masses in children. The majority of them are present during the newborn period. By far, the most common type of congenital heart mass is rhabdomyoma (Fig. 4-39A, B). This lesion is most commonly seen in patients with tuberous sclerosis. Rhabdomyomas typically involute over time and are usually treated conservatively

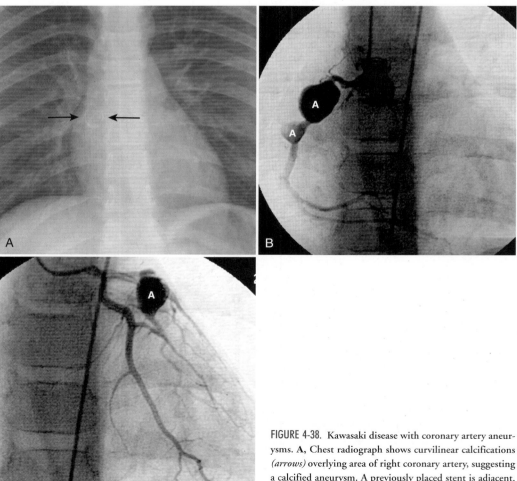

FIGURE 4-38. Kawasaki disease with coronary artery aneurysms. **A,** Chest radiograph shows curvilinear calcifications *(arrows)* overlying area of right coronary artery, suggesting a calcified aneurysm. A previously placed stent is adjacent. **B,** Right coronary arteriogram shows several aneurysms *(A)*. **C,** Left coronary arteriogram shows aneurysm *(A)*.

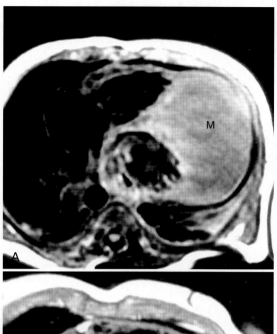

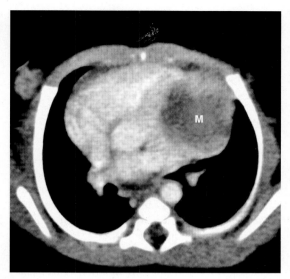

FIGURE 4-40. Cardiac fibroma. CT shows large low attenuation mass *(M)* in left ventricle myocardium.

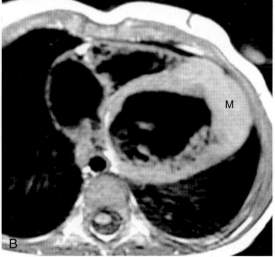

FIGURE 4-39. Rhabdomyoma in a girl with tuberous sclerosis. A, Axial T1-weighted image obtained at 2 days of life shows large mass *(M)* arising from the myocardium of the left and right ventricles, splaying the intraventricular septum. B, Axial T1-weighted image obtained at 2 years of life shows interval decrease in size of mass *(M)*.

often initially diagnosed on in utero or postnatal sonography and then further characterized by MRI.

Suggested Readings

Coussement AM, Gooding CA: Objective radiographic assessment of pulmonary vascularity in children, *Radiology* 109:649-654, 1973.

Donnelly LF, Higgins CB: MR imaging of conotruncal abnormalities, *AJR* 166:925-928, 1996.

Donnelly LF, Gelfand KJ, Schwartz DC, et al: The wall to wall heart: differential diagnosis for massively large cardiothymic silhouette in newborns, *Appl Radiol* 26:23-28, 1997.

Fellows KE, Weinberg PM, Baffa JA, Hoffman EA: Evaluation of congenital heart disease with MR imaging: current and coming attractions, *AJR* 159:925-931, 1992.

Kellenberger CF, Yoo SJ, Valsangiacoma Buchel ER: Cardiovascular MR imaging in neonates and infants with congenital heart disease, *Radiographics* 27:5-18, 2007.

Leschka S, Oechslin E, Husman L, et al: Pre- and postoperative evaluation of congenital heart disease in children and adults with 64-section CT, *Radiographics* 27:829-846, 2007.

Strife JS, Sze RW: Radiographic evaluation of the neonate with congenital heart disease, *Radiol Clin North Am* 37:1093-1107, 1999.

Swischuk LE, Stansberry SD: Pulmonary vascularity in pediatric heart disease, *J Thorac Imaging* 4:1-6, 1989.

Winer-Muram HT, Tonkin IL: The spectrum of heterotaxic syndromes, *Radiol Clin North Am* 27(6):1147-1170, 1989.

(see Fig. 4-39). Other potential cardiac masses include angiosarcoma, fibroma (Fig. 4-40), teratoma, and hemangioma. The most common cause of cardiac tumor associated with pericardial effusion is a hemangioma. These cases are

CHAPTER FIVE

Gastrointestinal

NEONATAL

Necrotizing Enterocolitis

Necrotizing enterocolitis (NEC) is a disease primarily of premature infants in the intensive care unit. It most often occurs 1 to 3 weeks after birth in infants weighing less than 1000 grams but can also occur in older infants under extreme stress, such as after cardiac surgery. The overall mortality rate is 20% to 30%. NEC is an idiopathic enterocolitis that is most likely related to some combination of infection and ischemia. It most commonly affects the ileum and right colon. Symptoms include abdominal distention, feeding intolerance, increased aspirates from nasogastric tube, and sepsis. It is interesting to note that the only parameter associated with decreased incidence of NEC is the use of maternal breast milk. When NEC is suspected, infants are placed in the status of NPO, treated with antibiotics, and monitored by serial abdominal radiographs (anteroposterior supine and a free air view [cross-table lateral or left lateral decubitus]).

Radiographic findings range from normal to suggestive to diagnostic. Suggestive findings include focal dilatation of bowel (especially within the right lower quadrant) or featureless, unfolded-appearing small bowel loops with separation of the loops suggesting bowel wall thickening. An unchanging bowel gas pattern over serial films is worrisome. The most definitive finding of NEC is the presence of pneumatosis (gas in the bowel wall; Figs. 5-1 through 5-4). Pneumatosis appears as multiple bubblelike or curvilinear lucencies overlying the bowel. Its appearance can be similar to that of stool. However, stool is uncommon in sick premature neonates in the intensive care unit. Portal venous gas can also occur (see Figs. 5-2, 5-3). This appears as branching linear lucencies overlying the liver. Free intraperitoneal air is the only radiographic finding seen in NEC that is considered an absolute indication for surgery. Free air may be seen as triangles of anterior lucency on cross-table laterally positioned radiographs (see Fig. 5-2); as overall increased lucency on supine-positioned radiographs (Fig. 5-5); in visualization of both sides of the bowel wall (Rigler sign); or as outlining the intraperitoneal structures such as the falciform ligament (football sign; see Fig. 5-5). In the absence of free air, the decision to perform surgery is made by using a combination of clinical and radiographic findings.

In cases of NEC in which the abdomen is distended but relatively gasless, ultrasound can be helpful. The identification of thickened bowel loops with increased or absent color Doppler flow is suggestive of inflamed or infarcted bowel. A large amount of free fluid is also a poor prognostic finding.

A delayed complication seen in survivors of NEC is bowel stricture (Fig. 5-6). These strictures most commonly involve the left colon.

High Intestinal Obstruction in Neonates

Neonates with suspected intestinal obstruction can be divided into those with upper gastrointestinal obstruction and those with lower intestinal obstruction on the basis of clinical symptoms and radiographic findings. Infants with high intestinal obstruction present predominantly with vomiting. Radiographs may show distension involving the stomach, duodenum, jejunum, or all three, depending on the level of the obstruction. The number of distended small bowel loops is much fewer than that seen with distal bowel obstruction. The most common causes of upper gastrointestinal tract obstruction in neonates include duodenal atresia or stenosis, duodenal web, annular pancreas, midgut volvulus or obstruction by Ladd bands, and jejunal atresia (Table 5-1).

DUODENAL ATRESIA, STENOSIS, WEB, AND ANNULAR PANCREAS

Duodenal atresia, stenosis, web, and annular pancreas are all part of a spectrum of similar abnormalities. All cause either complete or partial duodenal obstruction and usually present at

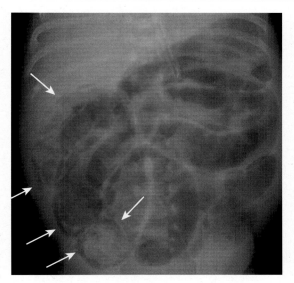

FIGURE 5-1. Necrotizing enterocolitis in a premature infant. Radiography shows multiple dilatated bowel loops with multiple areas of linear lucency *(arrows)* along the bowel wall, consistent with pneumatosis.

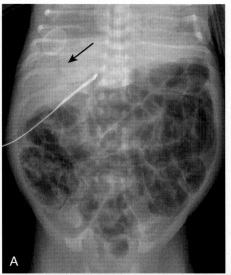

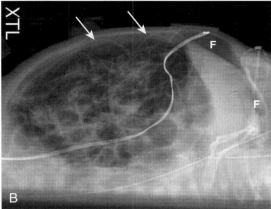

FIGURE 5-2. Necrotizing enterocolitis in a newborn premature infant. **A,** Frontal radiograph shows portal venous gas as branching lucencies *(arrow)* overlying the liver. There are also bubble-like and linear lucencies in the right lower quadrant, worrisome for pneumatosis. Note increased lucency over lateral aspect of right upper quadrant, indicative of free air, which is better seen on a cross-table lateral view. **B,** Cross-table lateral radiograph shows free intraperitoneal air *(F)* adjacent to liver. Note areas where both sides of bowel wall are visible *(arrows)*. Also note how much more striking free air appears on the cross-table lateral as compared to the frontal supine view.

birth or within the first few days of life. Often, components of more than one diagnosis are present. For example, many cases of duodenal atresia have a component of annular pancreas, and annular pancreas almost never occurs without a component of intrinsic duodenal stenosis.

The duodenum is the most common site of intestinal atresia. Duodenal atresia and stenosis almost always occur in the region of the ampulla of Vater. Approximately 30% of cases of duodenal atresia are associated with Down syndrome. Other associations include other intestinal atresias, biliary abnormalities, congenital heart disease, and associations with the complex known as VATER (vertebral defects, imperforate anus, tracheoesophageal fistula, and radial and renal dysplasia). Radiographs of neonates with duodenal atresia typically demonstrate a dilatated stomach and a dilatated proximal duodenum with no gas distal to the proximal duodenum. The two dilatated structures are referred to as a "double-bubble" sign (Fig. 5-7). In the appropriate clinical setting, a double bubble is diagnostic of duodenal atresia, and additional imaging by an upper gastrointestinal series (UGI) is unnecessary. The question that often arises is how do we know that this is not an acute obstruction caused by a midgut volvulus, which is, a surgical emergency? The answer is that dilatation of the duodenal bulb is seen only with chronic causes of obstruction. There is not enough time for the

bulb to become dilated in acute obstruction, such as with midgut volvulus. If it is not clear, a UGI can be performed to document the cause of obstruction. With duodenal stenosis, the double bubble is seen in association with the presence of distal bowel gas.

Duodenal web is another cause of congenital duodenal obstruction. Typically, a web consists of an obstructing membrane; a pin-sized hole in its center is the only lumen. The web

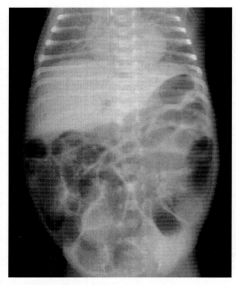

FIGURE 5-3. Necrotizing enterocolitis in a newborn premature infant. Supine radiograph shows linear lucencies over the liver, consistent with portal venous gas; dilatated bowel loops and bubblelike lucencies overlying bowel in right lower quadrant, consistent with pneumatosis.

may stretch downstream, forming a wind-sock configuration seen on UGI (Fig. 5-8). Because the obstruction is not complete, these patients may present later in life than those with atresia. The presence or absence of a component of annular pancreas is not something that can be

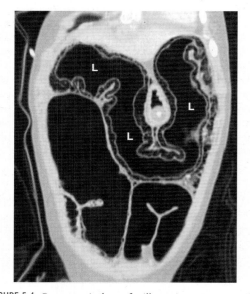

FIGURE 5-4. Pneumatosis shown for illustration purposes on CT in an older child with rotavirus infection. Coronal CT shows linear air extending longitudinally in the bowel wall of the transverse colon. L, lumen of transverse colon.

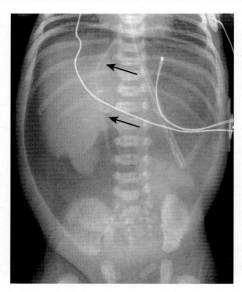

FIGURE 5-5. Free intraperitoneal air in an infant. Radiograph shows marked lucency and distention of abdominal cavity. The falciform ligament *(arrows)* is seen outlined by air (football sign).

determined on UGI in the setting of congenital duodenal obstruction.

MALROTATION AND MIDGUT VOLVULUS

Midgut volvulus is one of the few true emergencies in pediatric gastrointestinal imaging. A delay in the diagnosis of midgut volvulus can result in ischemic necrosis of large portions of the bowel and possibly in death. An understanding of

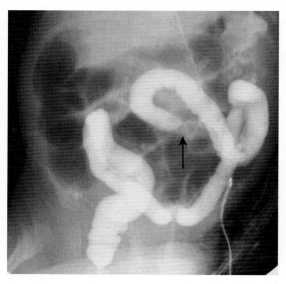

FIGURE 5-6. Colonic stricture resulting from previous necrotizing enterocolitis. Contrast enema shows obstruction of the colon *(arrow)* due to stricture.

TABLE 5-1. Common Causes of Intestinal Obstruction in Neonates

High
Midgut volvulus/malrotation
Duodenal atresia/stenosis
Duodenal web
Annular pancreas
Jejunal atresia

Low
Hirschsprung disease
Meconium plug syndrome (small left colon syndrome)
Ileal atresia
Meconium ileus
Anal atresia/anorectal malformations

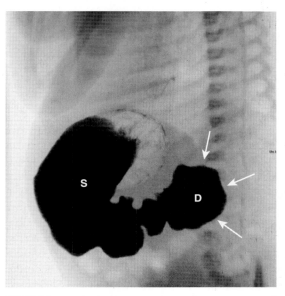

FIGURE 5-8. **Duodenal web in an infant with vomiting. Lateral view from a UGI shows obstruction of the duodenum with a rounded, windsocklike appearance. The duodenal bulb *(D)* is dilatated. There was eventually delayed passage of some contrast into more distal bowel. S, stomach.**

midgut embryogenesis is often emphasized, but an understanding of the end result is more important. With normal embryonic rotation, both the duodenojejunal and ileocolic portions of the bowel rotate 270 degrees about the axis of the superior mesenteric artery. The result is that the duodenojejunal junction (DJJ) is positioned in the left upper quadrant and the cecum is positioned in the right lower quadrant. This results in a long, fixed base that keeps the small bowel mesentery from twisting. If the duodenojejunal and ileocecal junctions are not in their normal positions, the base of the small bowel mesentery may be short and predispose the small bowel to twisting, resulting in a midgut volvulus.

For clarification, note the following definitions:

- Malrotation: abnormal fixation of the small bowel mesentery that results in a short mesenteric base.
- Midgut volvulus: abnormal twisting of the small bowel around the axis of the superior mesenteric artery. Volvulus can result in bowel obstruction, ischemia, or infarction but is not defined by the presence or absence of obstruction or ischemia.
- Ligament of Treitz: also referred to as the DJJ. This is the anatomic location where the duodenum passes through the transverse mesocolon and becomes jejunum. It is also where the bowel changes from retroperitoneal (duodenal) to intraperitoneal (jejunum). This anatomic location is not seen but is inferred on imaging.
- Ladd bands: abnormal fibrous peritoneal bands that can occur in patients with malrotation; they are potential causes of duodenal obstruction, in addition to volvulus.

The diagnosis of malrotation is made on UGI by determining that the DJJ is abnormally positioned. The duodenojejunal junction, the point at which the proximal bowel turns inferiorly on a frontal view, is considered normal

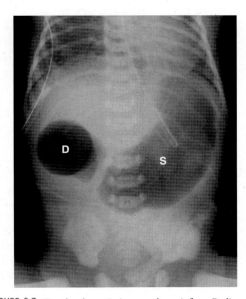

FIGURE 5-7. **Duodenal atresia in a newborn infant. Radiograph shows air-filled, dilatated stomach *(S)* and dilatated duodenal bulb *(D)*, giving the appearance of a double bubble. There is no distal bowel gas.**

when it meets the following two criteria: (1) it is to the left of the spine and (2) it is at the same level as or superior to the duodenal bulb. It is important to evaluate the position of the DJJ during the first pass of contrast through the duodenum and jejunum (see subsequent material; Figs. 5-9A-C, 5-10A-C).

In many cases of malrotation the findings are grossly obvious; the duodenum courses rightward, rather than leftward and never crosses the spine (Fig. 5-11; and see Fig. 5-10). However, when performing UGIs in children, there are many cases that do not quite meet the criteria for normal but are very close. It is probably inappropriate to send all of these cases to the operating room. As you become more experienced in imaging, some things become more and more clear. Others become less clear, and

you realize that many of the rules you were taught should really be thought of more as guidelines. Although germane to the fabric of pediatric radiology, the diagnosis and exclusion of malrotation is not straightforward or easy. In cases with borderline-positioned DJJs (not quite as high as the bulb, not quite to the left of the spine), most pediatric radiologists follow the contrast through the small bowel (see Fig. 5-10). If the jejunum is in the left upper quadrant and the ileum and cecum are in the right lower quadrant, the patient is probably not at risk for midgut volvulus. Also, the DJJ is a mobile structure in children and can "factitiously" be moved into an abnormal position by a space-occupying lesion, such as a mass or distended bowel loops. In addition, the presence of a nasojejunal tube may alter the apparent position of the DJJ.

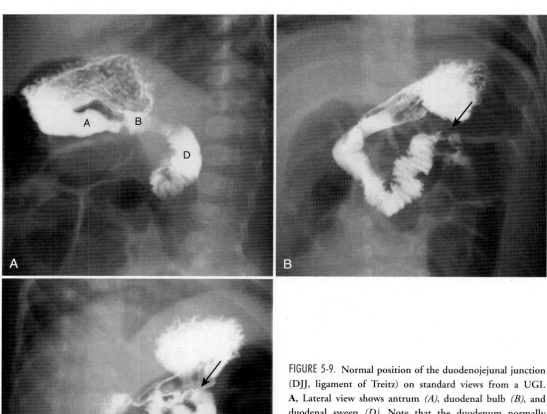

FIGURE 5-9. Normal position of the duodenojejunal junction (DJJ, ligament of Treitz) on standard views from a UGI. **A,** Lateral view shows antrum *(A)*, duodenal bulb *(B)*, and duodenal sweep *(D)*. Note that the duodenum normally extends posteriorly and inferiorly during the retroperitoneal course. **B,** Frontal view obtained during first pass shows the DJJ *(arrow)* identified by the point in the bowel that angles inferiorly. The DJJ is normally to the left of the spine and at the same level (superiorly to inferiorly) as the level of the duodenal bulb. **C,** Oblique view of patient with left side down again shows the level of the DDJ *(arrow)* at the level of duodenal bulb and proximal jejunum in left upper quadrant.

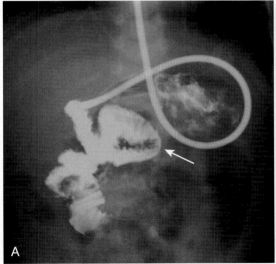
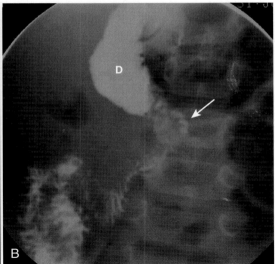
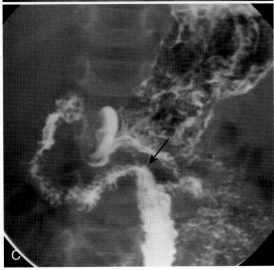

FIGURE 5-10. Abnormal position of the DJJ. **A,** Marked abnormal position of the DJJ. A UGI performed via nasogastric tube shows the DJJ *(arrow)* to be lower than the duodenal bulb and not to the left of the spine. Proximal jejunum is on right of spine. Findings are consistent with malrotation. **B,** Abnormal position of the DJJ associated with dilatation of the proximal duodenum. UGI shows that the DJJ *(arrow)* is not to the left of the spine and is lower than the duodenal bulb. The proximal jejunum is on right of spine. Findings are consistent with malrotation. Dilatation of the proximal duodenum (D) is suspicious for obstruction due to volvulus or Ladd bands. **C,** DJJ that does not quite meet normal criteria. The DJJ *(arrow)* is not quite to the left of the spine and not quite at same level as the bulb. In such cases, most radiologists will follow the contrast through the small bowel. If the cecum is in the right lower quadrant, the small bowel mesentery is most likely long enough not to be at risk for volvulus.

In patients who are malrotated, midgut volvulus may happen at any age; however, more than 90% are present during first 3 months of life. Midgut volvulus can be seen on UGI as a corkscrew appearance of the duodenum and proximal jejunum or as duodenal obstruction (Fig. 5-12A-C). The presence of bilious vomiting and findings of malrotation on UGI, with or without findings of midgut volvulus, is considered a surgical emergency.

Malrotation and midgut volvulus may also be encountered on cross-sectional imaging studies, such as computed tomography (CT) or ultrasound, when these studies are ordered to evaluate abdominal pain or vomiting. This is particularly true in older children in whom malrotation is often not initially suspected as the cause of acute abdominal symptoms. On cross-sectional imaging, the bowel may be seen to form a swirling pattern around the superior mesenteric vessels (Fig. 5-13A, B). In addition, the superior mesenteric vein, which is normally to the right of the superior mesenteric artery, is more often to the left of the superior mesenteric artery in malrotated patients (see Fig. 5-13). However, this is neither sensitive nor specific. The superior mesenteric artery is smaller and rounder than the superior mesenteric vein and is surrounded by fat, giving the artery an echogenic wall, as compared to the vein.

Performing an Upper Gastrointestinal Series in an Infant

There are various ways to accomplish a UGI in an infant, and many pediatric radiologists disagree

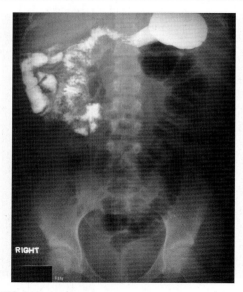

FIGURE 5-11. Malrotation. The duodenum courses rightward and never crosses the spine. The opacified proximal small bowel is in the right upper quadrant. The unopacified colon is in the left abdomen.

about the details. The following is the way I was taught to perform them. I prefer to have the infant secured to an octagon board (an immobilization device). This allows the radiologist to concentrate on the examination (rather than on keeping the child from wiggling or getting hurt), to get images in appropriate positions rapidly, and to minimize the radiation dose. Some think that use of the octagon board is inhumane. The babies do dislike being immobilized and often cry; however, in my experience, if time is taken to explain the procedure and its benefits to the accompanying parent, things usually go well. Some radiologists prefer to administer barium orally and some by nasogastric tube. When the child is willing and able to drink, I administer the contrast orally, usually by bottle. In contrast to adults, in whom many images of the stomach and duodenum are obtained to exclude ulcers and cancer, in normal children, few images are needed. The most important task is to document the position of the DJJ.

I start off with the child feeding in the supine position because they typically are more likely to suck in this position. Once they begin drinking, I obtain an anteroposterior image of the esophagus and then turn them to the lateral position, right side down. I obtain a lateral view of the esophagus and then wait for contrast to pool in the antrum. When the contrast passes through the pylorus and begins to fill

the first and second portions of the duodenum, I obtain a lateral view documenting that the pylorus appears normal and that the duodenum courses posteriorly. This is the crucial point in the examination. The infant is then quickly turned supine and an image is obtained as the contrast courses into the duodenum and proximal jejunum (see Fig. 5-9). If the infant is turned supine too early and not enough contrast is in the duodenum, the contrast will not pass leftward over the spine. You can always put the child back into the right-side-down position and get more contrast in the duodenum. If the child is turned supine too late (the worst-case scenario), the contrast will have passed into more distal loops of the jejunum and will obscure visualization of the position of the DJJ. Appropriate timing comes with experience. The next image that I obtain is an oblique with the left side down, producing an image of the air-filled antrum and bulb. Finally, I obtain either a fluoroscopic spot view or an overhead radiograph once more contrast has passed into the jejunum to document nondilatation of the jejunum and to show that there is no gastroesophageal reflux. Therefore, a normal UGI in an infant should consist of only six images.

Low Intestinal Obstruction in Neonates

It is not uncommon for neonates to fail to pass meconium because of a distal obstructive process. On radiographs of the abdomen, dilatation of multiple loops of bowel is consistent with a distal obstructive process (Fig. 5-14A-C). The only proximal bowel process that may be associated with multiple dilatated loops of bowel is midgut volvulus, when the bowel dilates secondary to ischemia or infarction. These infants, however, are very ill. The neonate who has multiple dilatated loops of bowel on radiographs along with abdominal distention and failure to pass adequate amounts of meconium but is otherwise well on physical exam does not have midgut volvulus as a cause of bowel dilatation and should be evaluated by a contrast enema rather than a UGI. In such a patient without anal atresia on physical examination, the diagnosis is likely to be one of four entities (see Table 5-2). Of these, Hirschprung disease and meconium plug syndrome involve the colon and ileal atresia, and meconium ileus involves the ileum.

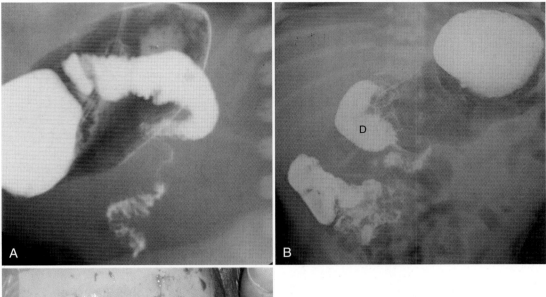

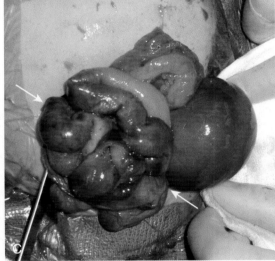

FIGURE 5-12. Midgut volvulus. **A,** Lateral view from UGI shows corkscrew appearance of the duodenum and distention of the proximal duodenum. Findings are consistent with volvulus. **B,** Frontal view from UGI in another patient shows distention of proximal duodenum *(D)* and beaklike area of narrowing. Note that the DJJ is not in the normal position and the proximal small bowel is in the right lower quadrant. Findings are consistent with malrotation and volvulus. **C,** Surgical image from a different patient shows multiple loops of necrotic small bowel secondary to infarction from the volvulus.

Neonatal contrast enemas are typically performed using dilute ionic, water-soluble agents and a non-balloon-tip catheter of appropriate size. Barium is not typically used because it can make the evacuation of meconium plugs or meconium ileus more difficult, whereas water-soluble enemas can be therapeutic.

A microcolon is a narrow-caliber colon secondary to disuse; if it is identified on the enema, the cause is likely to be ileal pathology (Fig. 5-15). If contrast is refluxed into a collapsed terminal ileum and the more proximal non-contrast-filled bowel loops are disproportionately dilatated, the diagnosis is likely to be ileal atresia (Fig. 5-16A, B). If the terminal ileum is distended and has multiple filling defects, the diagnosis is meconium ileus (Fig. 5-17).

Meconium ileus occurs secondary to obstruction of the distal ileum due to accumulation of abnormally tenacious meconium. It occurs exclusively in patients with cystic fibrosis and is the presenting finding of cystic fibrosis in about 10% of cases. It may be complicated by perforation, volvulus of the bowel involved, or meconium peritonitis (Fig. 5-18). Radiographs show findings of distal obstruction, which may be associated with bubblelike lucencies secondary to the accumulated meconium or with calcification when perforation is present. Serial water-soluble enemas are commonly used in an attempt to remove the obstruction nonsurgically. There is debate about the optimal contrast agent to use for such serial therapeutic enemas. Table 5-2 shows a summary of the meconium-related gastrointestinal diseases.

In contrast enemas performed to examine neonatal distal obstruction, if the proximal colon is distended, the cause of distal obstruction

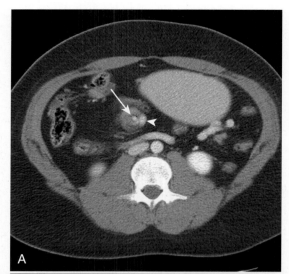

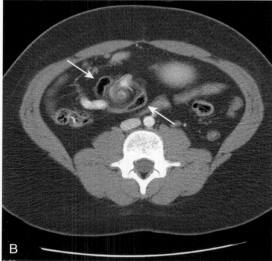

FIGURE 5-13. **Malrotation presenting with intermittent abdominal pain secondary to midgut volvulus in an obese teenager. A,** CT image of the upper abdomen shows inversion of the normal relationship between the superior mesenteric artery *(arrow)* and the vein *(arrowhead),* with the vein situated to the left of the artery. Note swirling vascular structures surrounding the superior mesenteric artery. **B,** A more caudal image shows characteristic swirling pattern of bowel loops *(arrows)* twisting about the axis of the mesenteric vessels, consistent with volvulus.

is likely to be colonic secondary to Hirschprung disease or meconium plug syndrome.

HIRSCHSPRUNG DISEASE

Hirschsprung disease is related to the absence of the ganglion cells that innervate the colon. The denervated colon spasms and causes a functional obstruction. Therefore, the affected portions of colon are small in caliber, and the more proximal, normally innervated colon is dilatated secondary to the obstruction. The rectum and a variable amount of more proximal colon are affected in a contiguous fashion; there are no skip lesions. Most patients with Hirschprung disease (90%) present in the neonatal period with failure to pass meconium (Fig. 5-19; and see Fig. 5-14). However, patients can present later in life with problems related to constipation. Hirschprung disease is much more common in boys (4:1) and is associated with Down syndrome in 5% of cases.

When an enema is being performed to evaluate for possible Hirshprung disease, it is essential to obtain early filling views, collimated to include the rectum and sigmoid colon, in both the lateral and then the frontal position. Findings of Hirschprung disease include a transition zone from an abnormally small rectum and distal colon to a dilatated proximal colon (see Figs. 5-14, 5-19). In a normal patient, the rectum has the largest luminal diameter of the left-sided colon. When the rectum alone is involved by Hirschprung disease, the sigmoid colon is larger than the rectum (see Figs. 5-14, 5-19). This is referred to as an abnormal rectosigmoid ratio. Another, but less common, finding is fasciculations or saw-toothed irregularity of the denervated segment (see Fig. 5-19). If the entire colon is involved by Hirschprung disease (very rare), the entire colon may appear small in caliber and may mimic a microcolon. Patients with Hirschprung disease may present with associated colitis. Therefore, in patients who are suspected to have Hirschprung disease and are ill, contrast enemas should be avoided.

Definitive diagnosis is obtained by rectal biopsy, and patients are treated by surgical resection of the denervated segment. The transition zone depicted on enema does not always accurately predict where the transition from absent to present ganglion cells occurs histiologically.

MECONIUM PLUG SYNDROME

Meconium plug syndrome, also referred to as functional immaturity of the colon or small left colon syndrome, is a common cause of distal neonatal obstruction. It is the most commonly encountered diagnosis in neonates who fail to pass meconium. It is thought to be related to functional immaturity of the ganglion cells. As in Hirschprung disease, the distal colon does not have normal motility, which causes functional obstruction. Unlike Hirschprung disease, it is a temporary phenomenon and resolves. Although most neonates with meconium plug

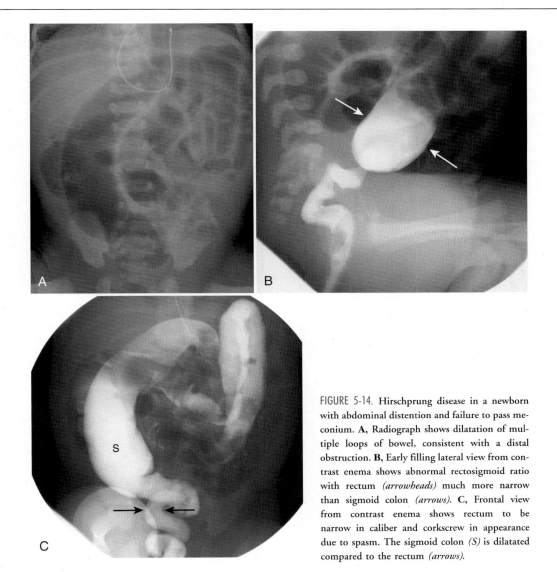

FIGURE 5-14. Hirschprung disease in a newborn with abdominal distention and failure to pass meconium. **A,** Radiograph shows dilatation of multiple loops of bowel, consistent with a distal obstruction. **B,** Early filling lateral view from contrast enema shows abnormal rectosigmoid ratio with rectum *(arrowheads)* much more narrow than sigmoid colon *(arrows)*. **C,** Frontal view from contrast enema shows rectum to be narrow in caliber and corkscrew in appearance due to spasm. The sigmoid colon *(S)* is dilatated compared to the rectum *(arrows)*.

syndrome are otherwise normal and have no abnormal associations, increased incidence occurs in patients who are infants of diabetic mothers or of mothers who have received magnesium sulfate for eclampsia. In neonates with

meconium plug syndrome, there is always concern about underlying Hirschprung disease so at many centers, all neonates who have findings of meconium plug syndrome undergo rectal biopsy. In contrast to meconium ileus, there is

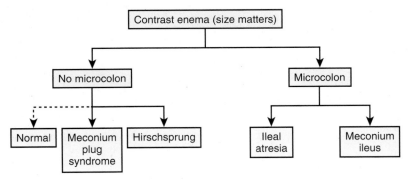

FIGURE 5-15. Schematic for differential diagnosis of contrast enema findings in an infant with failure to pass meconium and distended abdomen. In this scenario, there is a high incidence of pathology, and a normal study is uncommon. If the child has a microcolon, it indicates ileal pathology. If the child does not have a microcolon, the cause is probably colonic.

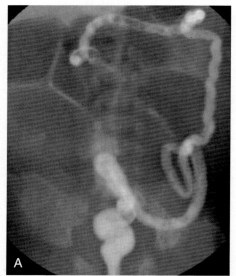

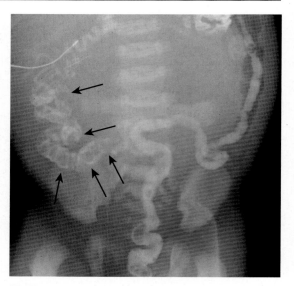

FIGURE 5-17. Meconium ileus in a newborn infant with abdominal distention and failure to pass meconium. The infant was confirmed to have cystic fibrosis. Contrast enema demonstrates a small-caliber microcolon and opacification of the distal ileum, which contains multiple tubular filling defects (arrows), consistent with meconium ileus.

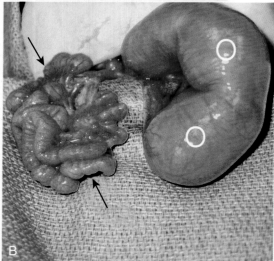

FIGURE 5-16. Bowel atresia. A, Contrast enema shows microcolon. There are multiple very dilatated loops of small bowel. Contrast is not able to be passed into dilatated loops. Findings are consistent with ileal atresia. B, Surgical photograph shows dilatated loops of bowel (O) above the level of obstructive atresia. Distal to the atresia, there are multiple collapsed loops of ileum (arrows).

diameter, as compared to the rectums in infants with Hirschsprung disease. The enema is often therapeutic; plugs of meconium are commonly passed during or shortly after the enema, and symptoms of obstruction often resolve within hours after the enema.

no significant relationship between meconium plug syndrome and cystic fibrosis.

Infants with meconium plug syndrome present with failure to pass meconium. On contrast enema, multiple filling defects (meconium plugs) are seen within the colon (Fig. 5-20). The right and transverse colons maybe more dilatated than the left colon (small left colon syndrome; see Fig. 5-20), although these findings are variable. Microcolon does not occur. The rectum tends to be normal in luminal

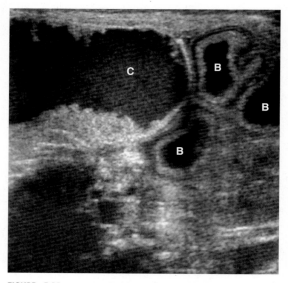

FIGURE 5-18. Meconium peritonitis complicating meconium ileus in a newborn infant with cystic fibrosis. Ultrasound shows large meconium cyst (C) and multiple loops of bowel (B) with bowel wall thickening.

TABLE 5-2. Summary of Meconium-Related Gastrointestinal Diseases

Meconium Ileus
- Occurs only in patients with cystic fibrosis
- Tenacious meconium causes obstruction of distal ileum
- Contrast enema: microcolon, dilatated distal small bowel with filling defects (meconium pellets)

Meconium Plug Syndrome (Small Left Colon Syndrome)
- Not associated with cystic fibrosis
- Immaturity of colon; functional obstruction
- Self-limited, often relieved by contrast enema
- Contrast enema: filling defects (meconium plugs) in colon, small-caliber left colon

Meconium Peritonitis
- Result of in utero perforation of bowel secondary to bowel atresia, in utero volvulus, or meconium ileus
- Imaging: bowel obstruction, peritoneal calcifications, meconium cysts in peritoneal cavity

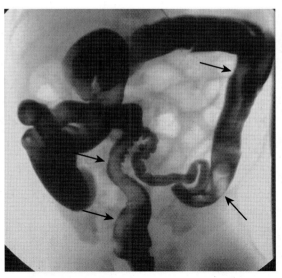

FIGURE 5-20. Meconium plug syndrome (small left colon syndrome) in a newborn infant born of a diabetic mother. Contrast enema demonstrates multiple filling defects *(arrows)* within the colon, consistent with meconium plugs. The left colon is small in caliber. Rectal biopsy, performed to exclude Hirshprung disease, demonstrated normal ganglion cells.

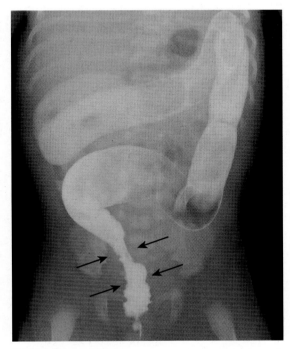

FIGURE 5-19. Hirschprung disease in an infant. Frontal radiograph demonstrates the diameter of the rectum *(arrows)* to be smaller than the diameter of the sigmoid colon, an abnormal rectosigmoid ratio. Note the sawtooth appearance of the abnormal contracted segment.

Esophageal Atresia and Tracheoesophageal Fistula

In esophageal atresia, the esophagus is atretic for a variable length, usually at the junction of the proximal and middle thirds of the esophagus. Esophageal atresia can occur in the presence or absence of a tracheoesophageal fistula. The most common type of esophageal atresia is that with a fistulous communication between the distal esophageal segment and the trachea. Much less commonly, the fistula can connect the proximal or both the proximal and the distal esophageal segments to the trachea. Rarely, tracheoesophageal fistulas can occur in the absence of esophageal atresia; this is called an H-type fistula.

Esophageal atresia presents at birth and is usually encountered by the radiologist after there is failure to pass an orogastric tube. Radiographic findings include a distended air-filled pharyngeal pouch (Fig. 5-21), with or without an indwelling tube. If there is no abdominal bowel gas, a tracheoesophageal fistula is not present; if there is distal bowel gas, there is probably a distal fistula. Further imaging, such as with a UGI, is rarely needed. Because the surgery for esophageal atresia is performed through a thoracotomy contralateral to the

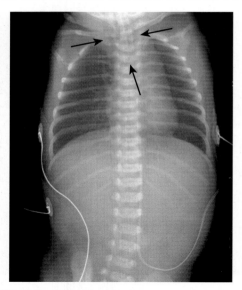

FIGURE 5-21. **Esophageal atresia in a newborn infant. Radiograph shows gasless abdomen and lucent circular area** (arrows) **over upper mediastinum with suction tube in place. This represents the pharyngeal pouch above the atresia.**

aortic arch, it is important to determine on which side the arch is located. Often, echocardiography is used.

Esophageal atresia is usually associated with other congenital anomalies. The acronym VACTERL is used: vertebral anomalies, anal atresia, cardiac anomalies, tracheoesophageal fistula, renal anomalies, and limb (radial array) anomalies. Chest radiographs in such patients should be scrutinized for vertebral and cardiac anomalies.

Children with an H-type fistula present with coughing or choking during feeds or with recurrent pneumonia. Often a UGI is requested to exclude an H-type fistula. Some authors advocate that such an examination should be performed with the patient in the prone position, with a tube positioned in the esophagus, to fully distend the esophagus and maximize potential visualization of the fistula. Others state that this offers no advantage over routine oral administration of contrast via a bottle.

Complications following repair of esophageal atresia include recurrent fistula and esophageal leak during the immediate postoperative period. A large extrapleural fluid collection seen on chest radiography is highly suggestive of a leak. Long-term sequelae include esophageal stricture, esophageal dysmotility, and gastroesophageal reflux.

Abnormalities of Anterior Abdominal Wall

The closure of the anterior abdominal wall occurs during fetal life; failure of proper closure may result in a number of abnormalities, of which the most common are omphalocele, gastroschisis, and cloacal exstrophy. Many of these abnormalities are now diagnosed and evaluated prenatally by ultrasound or fetal magnetic resonance imaging (MRI). Omphalocele results from failure of fusion of the lateral folds. It is a midline defect in which the herniated abdominal contents (bowel or liver) are covered by a sac of peritoneum (Fig. 5-22). As much as two thirds of patients with omphalocele have associated congenital anomalies, most commonly cardiac anomalies.

In contrast, in gastroschisis the defect is lateral to midline, there are typically no associated abnormalities, and the herniated content (usually just bowel) is not covered by a membrane (Fig. 5-23). Because of the lack of a covering membrane, the bowel is exposed to the amniotic fluid, which is toxic to the bowel. These patients often have severe dysmotility problems and present with multiple episodes of pseudoobstruction. Often small-bowel follow-throughs are requested in an effort to differentiate between pseudoobstruction and obstruction related to adhesions. This is a daunting task because these studies can last for days. In this

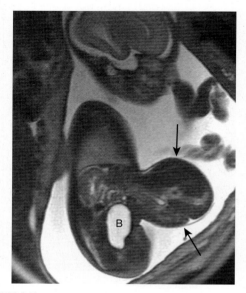

FIGURE 5-22. **Omphalocele demonstrated on fetal MRI. Sagittal image of fetus shows omphalocele** (arrows) **as an anterior pouch containing the liver. Note the smooth appearance of the membrane-covered sac. B, bladder.**

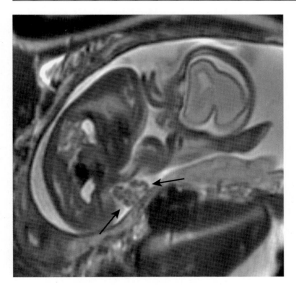

FIGURE 5-23. **Gastroschisis shown on sagittal fetal MRI. There is eviscerated bowel** (arrows) **external to the fetus. Note the irregular margins, consistent with the lack of an enveloping membrane.**

scenario, some have advocated giving the oral contrast and obtaining a film every 24 hours to help minimize radiation exposure.

Cloacal exstrophy is a severe malformation in which there is bladder exstrophy and omphalocele. There is associated diastasis of the pubic bones and spinal dysraphism. Hydrometrocolpos can be associated with cloacal exstrophy and can cause renal failure if not identified because it causes compression and extrinsic obstruction of the distal ureters.

THE VOMITING INFANT

The referral of an infant for an upper GI to rule out reflux is a common event. Typically, such infants are referred to radiology because of excessive "spitting up," or vomiting. There are a number of significant causes of excessive vomiting in infants. They include hypertrophic pyloric stenosis, gastroesophageal reflux, congenital stenosis, lactobezoar, and possibly midgut volvulus. The problem for pediatricians is that spitting up (regurgitation) after feedings is a common and normal event. The degree of such spitting up is also variable. How do pediatricians differentiate prominent but normal regurgitation from vomiting secondary to obstruction or pathologic amounts gastroesophageal reflux? Associated problems such as failure

to gain weight, failure to thrive, or respiratory symptoms suggest pathology. However, this difficult question often results in the performance of a UGI. Although such UGIs are often ordered to rule out reflux, they are actually performed to exclude an anatomic reason for excessive reflux, rather than to exclude reflux itself. Although it is appropriate to document the presence and anatomic extent of gastroesophageal reflux when it occurs, it is not necessary to perform maneuvers to provoke reflux.

Hypertrophic Pyloric Stenosis

Hypertrophic pyloric stenosis is a common idiopathic thickening of the muscle of the pylorus that results in a progressive gastric outlet obstruction. It usually occurs in otherwise healthy infants (between 1 week and 3 months of age) who typically present with projectile, bile-free emesis. It is much more common in males (5:1 ratio). On physical examination, the hypertrophied pylorus can be palpated as an olive-sized mass in the right upper quadrant. It is suggested that palpation of an "olive" in the presence of the appropriate clinical symptoms is diagnostic and that such infants do not need confirmatory imaging studies. However, in practicality, hypertrophic pyloric stenosis is a diagnosis made at imaging, and almost all children have imaging prior to surgery. It should be noted that imaging to confirm or exclude hypertrophic pyloric stenosis is not a medical emergency.

On radiographs, children with hypertrophic pyloric stenosis may show gastric distension, peristaltic waves (caterpillar sign), and mottled retained gastric contents. Both ultrasound and UGI can be used to diagnose hypertrophic pyloric stenosis. Ultrasound allows direct visualization of the pyloric muscle and does not use radiation but is not as reliable in excluding other diagnoses such as midgut volvulus. A UGI does exclude other more serious causes of pathology, but the UGI findings allow the radiologist to infer rather than directly visualize the hypertrophied muscle. The following guidelines may be helpful in making such decisions. If hypertrophic pyloric stenosis is highly suspected on clinical grounds and the purpose of the study is to confirm the diagnosis, ultrasound is probably the test of choice. If the symptoms or patient age are not classic, a UGI may be better both to

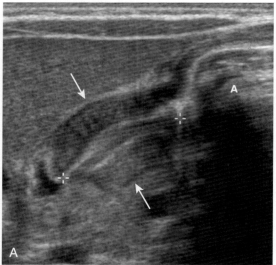

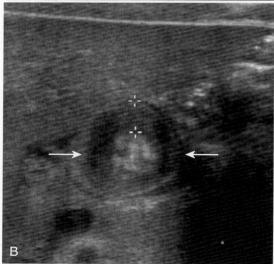

FIGURE 5-24. Hypertrophic pyloric stenosis on ultrasound. **A,** Longitudinal ultrasound image demonstrating findings of hypertrophic pyloric stenosis. The hypertrophied pyloric muscle *(arrows)* is hypoechoic and the mucosa is echogenic. The length of the pylorus is shown between the two cursers. Gastric antrum *(A).* **B,** Transverse ultrasound image shows pyloric muscle with thickness measurement between the two cursors.

evaluate for hypertrophic pyloric stenosis and to exclude other pathology.

On ultrasound, the diagnosis of hypertrophic pyloric stenosis is often obvious and is made on the gestalt of the appearance. The pylorus is anatomically located near the gallbladder, so an easy technique is to find the gallbladder and turn obliquely sagittal to the body in an attempt to visualize the pylorus longitudinally. The hypertrophied muscle is hypoechoic and the central mucosa is hyperechoic (Fig. 5-24A, B). With hypertrophic pyloric stenosis, the pylorus does not open during real-time evaluation. There are measurement criteria that vary slightly from source to source. The pyloric muscle thickness (diameter of a single muscular wall on a transverse image) should normally be less than 3 mm (see Fig. 5-24). The length (longitudinal diameter) should not exceed 15 mm. Another good rule of thumb is that if you send an inexperienced sonographer or resident in to scan the child and they find the pylorus easily, it is probably abnormal. A normal pylorus (Fig. 5-25) is much harder to image than is an abnormal pylorus.

On UGI, there is delayed gastric emptying with hypertrophic pyloric stenosis. When some contrast does pass into the duodenum, the pylorus appears elongated with a narrow pyloric channel (string sign; Fig. 5-26). The lumen may be puckered and have more than one apparent lumen (the double-track sign). The pylorus may indent the contrast-filled antrum (the shoulder sign) or the base of the duodenal bulb (the mushroom sign), and the entrance to the pylorus may be beak-shaped (the beak sign; see Fig. 5-26). After the diagnosis is made, excess barium should be removed from the stomach by nasogastric tube to avoid the risk for aspiration.

INTESTINAL OBSTRUCTION IN CHILDREN

As in adults, the key finding of bowel obstruction on radiography is the presence of disproportionately dilatated proximal small bowel as compared to less dilatated more distal small bowel or colon. In contrast to adults, however, in infants and small children, it may be difficult to differentiate small bowel from colon secondary to a lack of well-defined haustra and valvulae conniventes. The addition of a prone view to the standard two-view abdomen (supine and either upright, cross-table lateral, or left decubitus) can be helpful when differentiation between small and large bowel is difficult. On the prone view, gas moves into the more posterior structures of the colon—the ascending and descending colon and the rectum. On supine views, the colonic gas lies in the more anterior structures, the transverse and sigmoid colon. The position of gas on the combination of these two views is often helpful in identifying

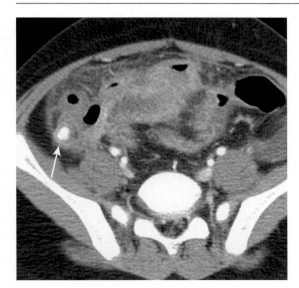

FIGURE 5-30. Perforated appendicitis on CT, which shows a calcified appendicolith *(arrow)* in the right lower quadrant. There is an adjacent inflammatory fluid collection and phlegmonous change.

The value of radiographs in suspected appendicitis is also debated. Radiographs demonstrate an appendicolith in 5% to 10% of patients (Fig. 5-31). Other findings may include air-fluid levels within the right lower quadrant, splinting, and loss of the psoas margin. With perforated appendicitis, there may be findings of small bowel obstruction, right lower quadrant extraluminal gas, and displacement of bowel loops from the right lower quadrant. Free intraperitoneal gas is extremely uncommon secondary to appendicitis.

Intussusception

Intussusception occurs when forward peristalsis results in invagination of the more proximal bowel (the intussusceptum) into the lumen of the more distal bowel (the intussuscipiens) in a telescope-like manner. There are three primary types of intussusception: idiopathic ileocolic intussusception, intussuception secondary to pathologic lead points, and incidentally noted small bowel–small bowel intussusception.

In children, most cases of intussusception (90%) are idiopathic ileocolic (Fig. 5-32). Therefore, when intussusception is referred to in children, this is the type that is generally meant. The idiopathic ileocolic intussusception is thought to be related to lymphoid hypertrophy in the terminal ileum secondary to viral disease. It is more common during the viral months of winter and spring and occurs more commonly in girls than in boys. The typical age for patients to present is between 3 months and 1 year (mean age 8 months), with almost all cases occurring before 3 years of age. If the child is older than 3 years of age, a pathologic lead point should be suspected. Presenting symptoms include crampy abdominal pain, bloody

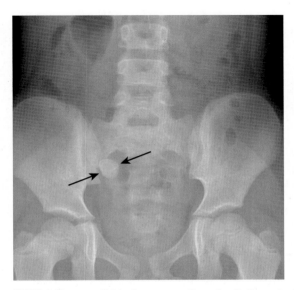

FIGURE 5-31. Appendicitis shown on radiography. Radiograph shows calcified appendicolith *(arrows)* in right lower quadrant, overlying the right sacrum.

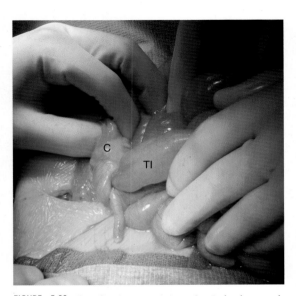

FIGURE 5-32. Ileocolic intussusception. Surgical photograph shows terminal ileum *(TI)* intussuscepted into colon *(C)*.

(currant jelly) stools, vomiting, and palpable right-sided abdominal mass.

Although debated, this is the imaging algorithm often used in the workup of intussusception. Radiographs are commonly the first test obtained. If the radiographs and history are highly suspicious for intussusception, the patient proceeds to reduction enema. If either the radiographic or clinical findings are not highly suspicious, an ultrasound can help to diagnose or exclude intussusception and therefore help to avoid unnecessary reduction enemas. CT plays no role in the workup of suspected intussusception; however, intussusception may be seen on CT when it is obtained for nonspecific abdominal pain, particularly in older children.

Radiographs are rarely completely normal in cases of intussusception. Findings include a paucity of gas within the right abdomen, the absence of an air-filled cecum or ascending colon, the meniscus of a soft tissue mass typically within the ascending or transverse colon (Fig. 5-33), and small bowel obstruction. Because the key to identifying or excluding the diagnosis is related to seeing or not seeing gas in the right colon, left-side-down decubitus- and prone-positioned radiographs are helpful. If air-fluid levels are

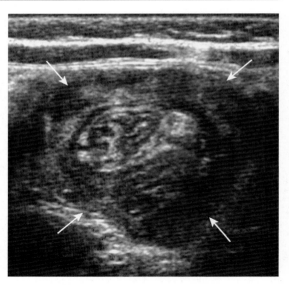

FIGURE 5-34. Appearance of intussusception on ultrasound. Ultrasound shows mass *(arrows)* of alternating hyper- and hypoechogenic rings.

identified within the distal colon, intussusception is unlikely and viral gastroenteritis is a more likely cause of the patient's symptoms. On ultrasound, the intussusception appears as a mass with alternating rings of hyper- and hypoechogenicity (Fig. 5-34). In the transverse plane, the mass has been likened to a donut and in the longitudinal plane to a pseudokidney. When using ultrasound to evaluate for intussusception, it is important to image all four quadrants of the abdomen (Fig. 5-35). The intussusception can travel

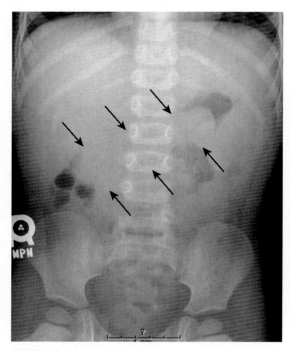

FIGURE 5-33. Intussusception. Radiograph demonstrates nonvisualization of gas in the ascending colon or cecum and a soft tissue mass *(arrows)* overlying the transverse colon, consistent with intussusception.

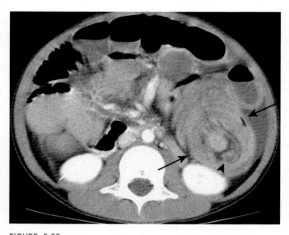

FIGURE 5-35. Intussusception shown on CT, which indicates a mass *(arrows)* of alternating rings of density. Note that intussusception has progressed into the descending colon in the left lower quadrant of the abdomen. This illustrates why it is important to perform ultrasound in all four abdominal quadrants when evaluating for intussusception. Note the lymph node *(arrowhead)* in the intussusception, probably acting as lead point.

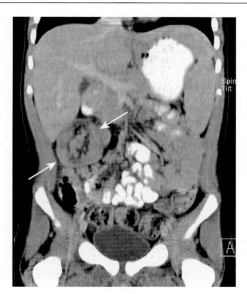

FIGURE 5-36. Intussusception shown on coronal CT image. Note the intussusception *(arrows)* as a mass of alternating high and low attenuation in the region of the hepatic flexure.

the entire route of the colon and therefore may be in any quadrant. If only the right lower quadrant is evaluated, the intussusception may be missed. When encountered on CT, ileocolic intussusception appears as a mass in the cecum or ascending colon with alternating rings of low and high attenuation (Fig. 5-36).

It is being increasingly recognized that small bowel-small bowel intussusceptions are often seen incidentally on ultrasound or CT examinations and that they are a normal, transient phenomenon (Fig. 5-37A-C). However, there are pathologic causes of small bowel-small bowel intussusceptions as well, including lymphoma, Meckel diverticulum, duplication cyst, and Henoch-Schönlein purpura (Fig. 5-38A-C). Findings that help to differentiate incidental from pathologic intussusception include transient presence, lack of associated small bowel obstruction, and length less than 3.5 cm.

Imaging-Guided Reduction of Intussusception

There are several methods of increasing the pressure within the colon in an attempt to invert the intussusception into the normal position by using imaging guidance. They include air insufflation with fluoroscopic guidance, contrast enema with fluoroscopic guidance, and hydrostatic reduction

with ultrasound guidance. Such methods are the primary therapy for intussusception; surgery is reserved for cases in which imaging-guided reduction fails. The choice of reduction method varies with the institution. At our institution, we use air reduction, which is described.

We use the following guidelines in preparing a patient for attempted reduction: adequate hydration with intravenous fluids if needed, a working intravenous port, abdominal examination by an experienced physician, and consultation with the pediatric surgery service. The members of the surgery service must at least know that the reduction is going to be attempted, and it is preferable that they have examined the patient. Contraindications for attempting pressure reduction of an intussusception include peritonitis on physical examination or pneumoperitoneum on radiography. Findings that are not contraindications but are associated with decreased success include small bowel obstruction, long duration of symptoms (>24 hours), and lethargy. In a child with suspected intussusception, lethargy is a sign that the patient is potentially very ill. If a 1-year-old child does not fight you during placement of an enema tip, something is potentially wrong. Members of the surgical team should be present when performing an enema in a lethargic patient.

For air reduction, the patient is immobilized and a Shiels intussusception air-reduction system (Custom Medical Products, Mainville, OH) is utilized. A key to success is generating an adequate rectal seal, so that sufficient colonic pressures can be obtained without leakage of air from the rectum. Pressure generated within the colon should not exceed 120 mmHg when the child is at rest. With air insufflation, the intussusception is encountered as a mass. The reducing intussusception moves retrograde to the level of the ileocecal valve. Criteria for successful reduction include resolution of the soft tissue mass and free reflux of gas into the small bowel (Fig. 5-39A-D). The "mass" often gets stuck at the ileocecal valve. In this case, some radiologists give the child some time to rest and let the edema decrease and then repeat the reduction enema. This is often successful. Overall success rates for reduction enemas are approximately 70% to 90%. The risk for perforation is less than 0.5%. The risk for recurrent intussusception is 5% to 10%, with most occurring within the first 72 hours after the reduction. Recurrence can be treated with repeated reduction enemas up to a recommended three times.

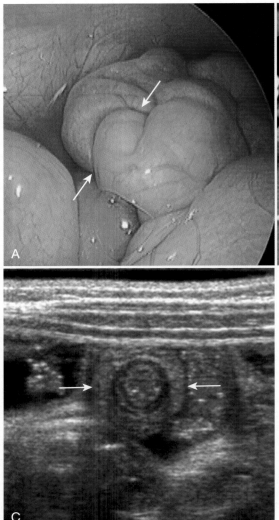

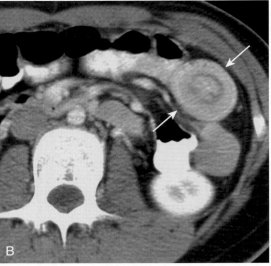

FIGURE 5-37. Incidental small bowel-small bowel intussusceptions in three different children. **A,** Laparoscopic view of small bowel-small bowel intussusception *(arrows)*. **B,** CT examination obtained for trauma shows incidental small bowel-small bowel intussusception *(arrows)* in proximal jejunum. **C,** Ultrasound examination shows small bowel-small bowel intussusception *(arrows)* in a child without abdominal pain. The lesion was shown to be intermittent.

Meckel Diverticulum

The omphalomesenteric duct is a fetal structure that connects the umbilical cord to the portion of the gut that becomes the ileum. Any or all of the structure can abnormally persist into postnatal life, resulting in cysts, sinuses, or fistulae from umbilicus to ileum. Most commonly, the portion adjacent to the ileal end persists and results in what is called a Meckel diverticulum. Meckel diverticula can cause symptoms secondary to bleeding, focal inflammation, perforation, or intussusception (Fig. 5-40A-D). Bleeding is the most common complication and occurs secondary to the presence of ectopic gastric mucosa. Although most Meckel diverticula do not contain gastric mucosa, almost all of those associated with bleeding do. Therefore, the imaging modality of choice to detect bleeding Meckel diverticula is nuclear scintigraphy with Tc 99m pertechnetate, which accumulates in gastric mucosa. Such studies demonstrate foci of increased activity within the right lower quadrant of the abdomen (see Fig. 5-40). Meckel diverticula are difficult to visualize on other studies such as CT and small bowel follow-through. However, in a patient with CT findings of right lower quadrant inflammation that do not fit appendicitis, Meckel diverticula should be considered.

Gastrointestinal Duplication Cysts

Gastrointestinal duplication cysts are congenital lesions that are typically round, attached to the

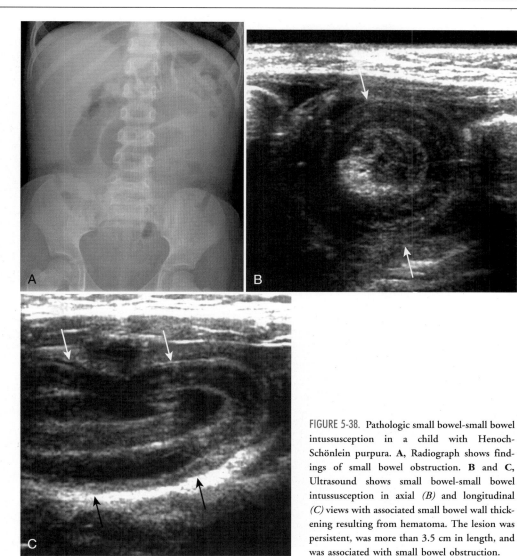

FIGURE 5-38. Pathologic small bowel-small bowel intussusception in a child with Henoch-Schönlein purpura. **A,** Radiograph shows findings of small bowel obstruction. **B** and **C,** Ultrasound shows small bowel-small bowel intussusception in axial *(B)* and longitudinal *(C)* views with associated small bowel wall thickening resulting from hematoma. The lesion was persistent, was more than 3.5 cm in length, and was associated with small bowel obstruction.

gastrointestinal tract, and do not communicate with the gastrointestinal lumen. The most common locations are the terminal ileum and the distal esophagus. These cysts may present because of a palpable mass, compression of adjacent anatomic structures, bowel obstruction, or ulceration and perforation. They are most likely to be present during the first year of life. Duplication cysts have a typical ultrasound appearance. They appear as a cystic mass with a "bowel wall signature" on ultrasound. The cyst wall demonstrates alternating hypoechoic and hyperechoic layers that correlate with the mucosa (hyperechoic) and the muscular layers (hypoechoic) (Fig. 5-41). Much less commonly, duplications can appear tubular rather than round and can communicate with the gastrointestinal lumen.

SWALLOWED FOREIGN BODIES

The majority of foreign bodies swallowed by children pass through the gastrointestinal tract without complication. If the initial series of radiographs demonstrates that the foreign body lies within the stomach or more distally in the gastrointestinal tract, follow-up films are not indicated unless the child develops obstructive symptoms or peritonitis. However, foreign bodies may lodge within the esophagus. The most common site of esophageal foreign bodies, and also the least likely area from which foreign bodies will spontaneously pass, is the proximal esophagus at the thoracic inlet. Because most infants with esophageal foreign bodies are initially asymptomatic, radiographs

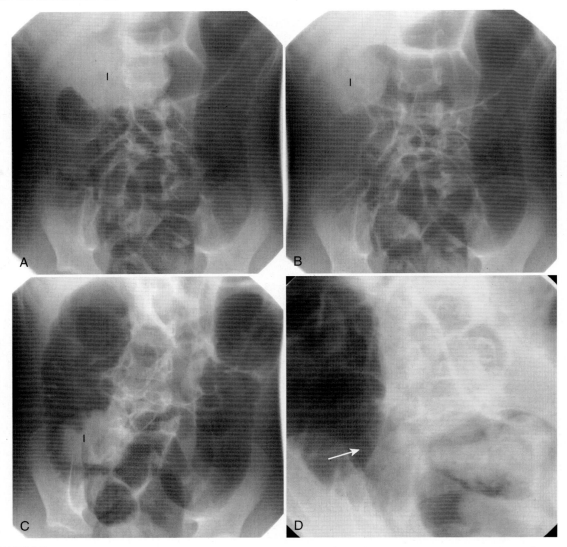

FIGURE 5-39. Air-reduction of intussusception. A, Upon onset of performance of air-reduction enema, intussusception *(I)* is in the region of the transverse colon. B, Intussusception *(I)* moving retrograde, now in the hepatic flexure. C, Intussusception *(I)* now in the region of the ileocecal valve. D, The region of previously seen soft tissue mass *(arrow)* is now resolved, and there is reflux of gas into the terminal ileum, consistent with resolved intussusception.

should be obtained when ingestions are witnessed, regardless of whether symptoms are present, to confirm that the foreign body has passed into the stomach. The most common foreign body to lodge in the esophagus is a coin (Fig. 5-42). Coins may be removed from the esophagus by using a Foley balloon catheter and fluoroscopic guidance. The catheter is inserted via the nose and the balloon is blown up in the esophagus beyond the level of the coin. The catheter is pulled retrograde, moving the coin into the oral pharynx. Chronic esophageal foreign bodies may result in complications such as a tracheoesophageal fistula. They may

also cause an inflammatory mass that leads to compression of the trachea. Such foreign bodies may present with respiratory rather than gastrointestinal symptoms.

Lodged esophageal foreign bodies may also be a sign of underlying pathology, such as a stricture or vascular ring that did not allow the foreign body to pass. Esophageal strictures can occur secondary to a number of causes in children, including corrosive ingestion, previous esophageal atresia repair, epidermolysis bullosa, and gastroesophageal reflux. Such strictures are often dilated utilizing balloon catheters and fluoroscopic guidance.

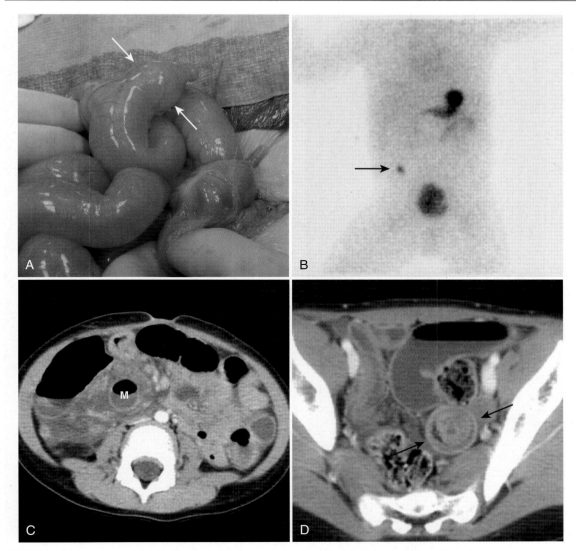

FIGURE 5-40. **Meckel diverticulum. Various types of presentations are illustrated in different children. A, Surgical photograph showing Meckel diverticulum** *(arrows)* **arising from the ileum. B, 99m technetium pertechnetate image demonstrates abnormal increased activity** *(arrow)* **within the anterior right lower quadrant. Normal activity is seen within the stomach, proximal bowel, and bladder. C, Meckel diverticulitis. CT shows round structure** *(M)* **in right abdomen with surrounding inflammatory change. D, Intussusception secondary to Meckel lead point. CT shows bowel** *(arrows)* **with alternating high and low attenuation consistent with small bowel-small bowel intussusception.**

There are several circumstances and types of foreign bodies that deserve special mention: zinc pennies, multiple magnets, and button batteries.

- Zinc pennies: Post-1982 U.S. pennies are zinc-based (rather than the pre-1982 copper-based pennies) and if retained in the stomach, the zinc-based coins can corrode and react with the hydrochloric acid in the stomach to create gastric ulceration. Radiography of such coins commonly shows irregular coin margins and developing radiolucent holes in the coins.

If a penny is retained in the stomach and the patient is symptomatic, the coin should be removed endoscopically.

- Multiple magnets: Recent reports have shown that small colorful pieces of certain toys that contain magnets can be swallowed by children. When multiple magnets are swallowed, they can become attracted to each other across the thin walls of the small bowel, and this may lead to ischemia, necrosis, obstruction, and perforation (Fig. 5-43). It should be considered a surgical emergency when identified.

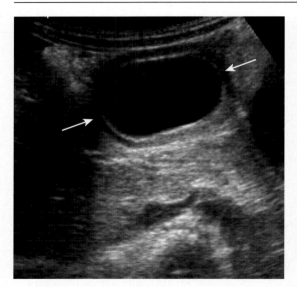

FIGURE 5-41. Gastric duplication cyst demonstrated on ultrasound. The structure appears as a cystic lesion *(arrows)* with bowel wall signature of alternating hyper- and hypoechoic rings.

- Button batteries: Button batteries are the disk-shaped batteries such as those used in cameras, watches, and hearing aids. When swallowed by children, these batteries can cause caustic injury to the mucosa, particularly when lodged in the esophagus. The shape of these batteries is slightly different from that of a coin (Fig. 5-44A, B). On a lateral view, the front edge of the battery is beveled with a central protrusion. In other words, the central portion is thicker than the peripheral portion. On a frontal view of a coin, the periphery may appear to have two circular edges. These batteries may also develop corrosive holes if they are present for some time. The potential presence of a button battery should be communicated to the care givers immediately to allow for expedited removal.

ABNORMALITIES OF THE PEDIATRIC MESENTERY

The mesentery does not have easily recognizable boundaries on imaging. Therefore, localization of an abnormality to the mesentery can be difficult. The relative paucity of mesenteric fat seen in the pediatric population can make detection and localization of processes in the mesentery even more difficult than in adults, in whom fat is typically abundant. The following criteria are helpful in localizing a process to the

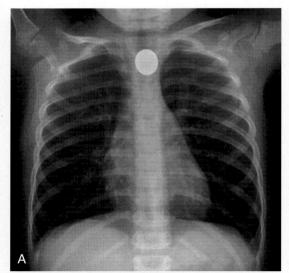

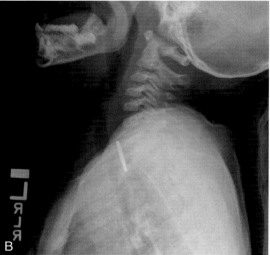

FIGURE 5-42. Coin lodged within the esophagus at the thoracic inlet. **A,** Frontal radiograph shows coin at region of upper esophagus. **B,** Lateral view shows coin in esophagus posterior to airway. Note that there is no soft tissue thickening between the coin and the airway to suggest chronic inflammation.

mesentery in children: (1) partial or complete envelopment of the superior mesenteric artery or vein, (2) peripheral displacement of jejunal or ileal bowel loops, or (3) extension of the process from superocentral to inferoperipheral in a conelike manner. Mesenteric disorders are divided into the specific patterns of involvement that can readily be identified by imaging: developmental abnormalities of mesenteric rotation, diffuse mesenteric processes, focal mesenteric masses, and multifocal mesenteric masses. Abnormalities of mesenteric rotation have been discussed.

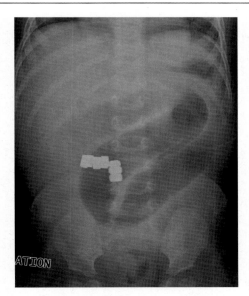

FIGURE 5-43. Multiple magnets. Radiograph shows multiple radiodense structures adjacent to each other, consistent with many swallowed magnets. There is an associated small bowel obstruction.

Processes that can involve the mesentery diffusely include edema, hemorrhage, and inflammation. Diffuse mesenteric processes characteristically demonstrate replacement of mesenteric fat by soft tissue attenuation with resultant loss of vascular definition. Focal masses within the mesentery in the pediatric population can be secondary to lymphoma, mesenteric cysts, desmoids, teratomas, and lipomas. Mesenteric cysts, also known as lymphatic malformations, are developmental anomalies in which focal lymphatic channels fail to establish connections with the central lymphatic system. Lymphatic malformations are often multiseptated and quite large (Fig. 5-45A, B).

Multifocal mesenteric masses most commonly represent lymphadenopathy. On imaging studies such as CT, mesenteric lymph nodes are considered abnormal if they are greater than 5 mm in diameter. Mesenteric lymphadenopathy can be a manifestation of either a malignant neoplastic or an inflammatory process. Malignant entities include lymphoma, lymphoproliferative disorder, and metastatic disease. Lymphomatous involvement of the mesentery most often occurs in association with non-Hodgkin disease and usually involves both the mesentery and the retroperitoneum. Most cases of non-Hodgkin lymphoma that involve the abdomen demonstrate lymphadenopathy rather than parenchymal masses. Mesenteric lymphadenopathy can also be caused by infectious disorders such as

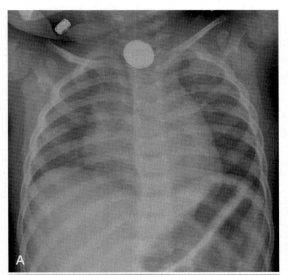

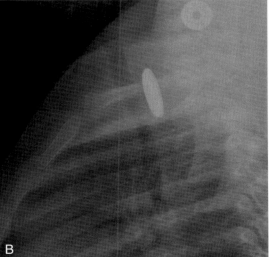

FIGURE 5-44. Button battery in proximal esophagus. **A,** Frontal view shows radiopaque round structure at the thoracic inlet. On close inspection, the edge of the circle is beveled and also has some peripheral erosions. **B,** On the lateral view, the edge is again seen to be beveled, with the central portion thicker than the peripheral portion. These findings are suspicious for a button battery, rather than a coin.

tuberculosis, cat scratch disease, or fungal infection. Central low attenuation with peripheral enhancement favors an inflammatory over a neoplastic cause. Central low attenuation of lymph nodes has been described as characteristic of tuberculosis and is present in as many as 60% of cases. With tuberculosis, it has been suggested that the mesenteric adenopathy is often more pronounced relative to the degree of retroperitoneal adenopathy. Note that visualization of prominent but smaller than 5-mm lymph

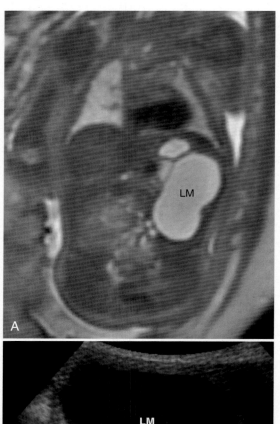

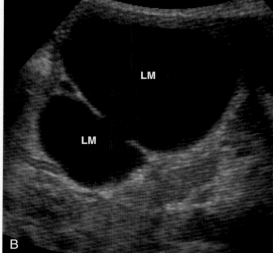

FIGURE 5-45. Mesenteric lymphatic malformation (mesenteric cyst). **A,** Fetal MRI in coronal plane shows multicystic mass *(LM)*. **B,** Postnatal ultrasound shows multicystic nature of large mass *(LM)*.

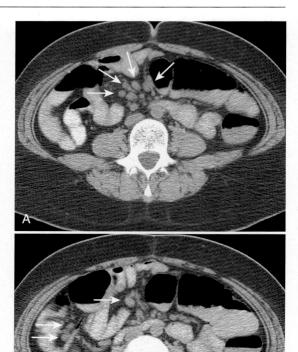

FIGURE 5-46. Mesenteric adenitis in an obese teenage boy with right lower quadrant pain. **A,** CT shows a cluster of lymph nodes in the mesentery *(arrows)*, centrally located in relationship to adjacent bowel. **B,** A more inferior CT image shows right lower quadrant lymph nodes *(arrows)* as well as more mesenteric lymph nodes.

nodes in the inferior mesentery and right lower quadrant is common in children and has no clinical significance.

Mesenteric Adenitis

Mesenteric adenitis is a clinical entity that is related to benign inflammation of the mesenteric lymph nodes, sometimes associated with enteritis. Patients present with nausea, vomiting, diarrhea, right lower quadrant abdominal pain and tenderness, fever, and leukocytosis. Because of the marked overlap in clinical symptomatology, differentiation between appendicitis and mesenteric adenitis can be extremely difficult, if not impossible, on a clinical basis. The diagnosis is often made at laparotomy and nontherapeutic appendectomy. CT findings include enlarged and clustered lymphadenopathy in the bowel mesentery just anterior to the right psoas muscle (78%) or in the small bowel mesentery (56%) or ileal wall thickening (33%) and inflammatory changes in the mesentery (Fig. 5-46A, B). The presence of diffuse mesenteric lymph nodes and the absence of findings of appendicitis suggest mesenteric adenitis as the cause of right lower quadrant pain. When the diagnosis is made at imaging, unnecessary surgical exploration may be avoided.

NEONATAL JAUNDICE

Some degree of "physiologic jaundice," or hyper-bilirubinemia, is common in neonates and is related to physiologic destruction of red blood cells in the polycythemic newborn. Jaundice that persists beyond 4 weeks of age is due to biliary atresia or neonatal hepatitis in 90% of cases.

Biliary Atresia Versus Neonatal Hepatitis

It is important to identify children with biliary atresia because they can benefit from early surgical intervention (prior to 3 months of age). In contradistinction, it is essential to avoid unnecessary laparotomies in patients with neonatal hepatitis. Because the two entities have similar clinical, laboratory, and pathologic findings, diagnostic imaging plays an important role in differentiating them. In biliary atresia, there is congenital obstruction of the biliary system with bile duct proliferation intrahepatically and focal or total absence of the extrahepatic bile ducts. Cirrhosis ultimately develops unless there is corrective surgery. There is an association with the abdominal heterotaxy syndromes such as polysplenia and with trisomy 18.

Ultrasound is the initial imaging procedure in neonates with jaundice. It can exclude the presence of choledochal cysts and dilatation of the bile duct system due to other causes of obstruction. Absence of a visualized gallbladder is suggestive of biliary atresia, although 20% of normal patients have small or barely visible gall bladders. The finding of a normal or enlarged gall bladder is supportive of the diagnosis of neonatal hepatitis. Visualization of a triangular echogenic structure adjacent to the main portal vein is referred to as the triangular cord sign and is thought to be the remnant of the common bile duct in biliary atresia. The hepatic parenchyma and intrahepatic bile ducts usually appear normal in patients with neonatal hepatitis and biliary atresia.

Hepatobiliary scintigraphy with 99m technetium-IDA derivatives can be one of the most reliable ways to differentiate between neonatal hepatitis and biliary atresia. The radiopharmaceutical is usually administered after pretreatment with oral phenobarbital. Normally, radiopharmaceutical uptake and clearance by hepatocytes exceeds cardiac blood pool tracer activity and radio tracer can be visualized within

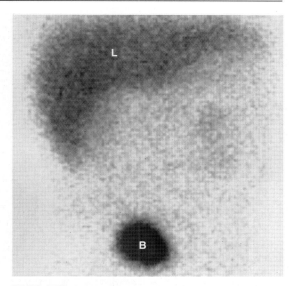

FIGURE 5-47. Biliary atresia in a newborn with persistent jaundice. Radionuclide hepatobiliary image obtained at 4 hours shows prompt uptake in liver *(L)* and faint activity in kidneys. No activity is present in the gastrointestinal tract. Radioactivity is seen in the urinary bladder *(B)*.

the biliary tree and intestines 15 minutes after administration. Classically described scintigraphic appearance of neonatal hepatitis includes delayed uptake of radio tracer by hepatocytes, slow clearance of blood pool radio tracer, but eventual radio-tracer excretion in the intestines. In biliary atresia, radio-tracer uptake and clearance by hepatocytes are adequate, with prominent low activity identified, but the tracer never reaches the gastrointestinal tract, even on 24-hour delayed imaging (Fig. 5-47).

Choledochal Cyst

Choledochal cyst is defined as a local dilatation of the biliary ductal system and is categorized into types based on the anatomic distribution of dilatation. These types include localized dilatation of the common bile duct below the cystic duct, dilatation of the common bile and hepatic ducts, localized cystic diverticulum of the common bile duct, dilatation of the distal intramedullary portion of the common bile duct (choledochocele), and multiple cystic dilatations involving both the intra- and extrahepatic bile duct radicals (Caroli disease). Choledochal cysts are uncommon and the cause is unknown. They most commonly present early in life with

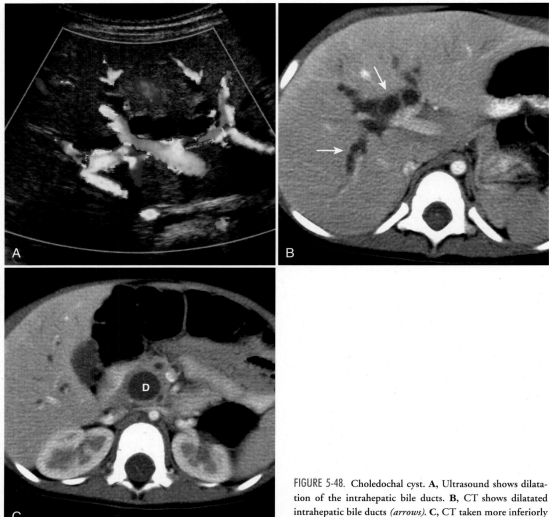

FIGURE 5-48. Choledochal cyst. **A,** Ultrasound shows dilatation of the intrahepatic bile ducts. **B,** CT shows dilatated intrahepatic bile ducts *(arrows)*. **C,** CT taken more inferiorly shows the common bile duct *(D)* is markedly dilatated.

jaundice (80%), abdominal mass (50%), or abdominal pain (50%). Ultrasound demonstrates a cystic mass in the region of the porta hepatis that is separate from an identifiable gall bladder (Fig. 5-48A-C). The presence of a dilatated common bile duct or cystic duct or visualization of the hepatic duct directly emptying into the cystic mass confirms the diagnosis. In cases in which there is a nonspecific cyst in the region of the porta hepatis, hepatobiliary scintigraphy can be used to demonstrate radio-tracer accumulation within the cyst, confirming the diagnosis.

LIVER MASSES

Hepatic masses constitute only 5% to 6% of all intraabdominal masses in children, and primary hepatic neoplasms constitute only 0.5% to 2% of all pediatric malignancies. Primary hepatic neoplasms are the third most common abdominal malignancy in childhood, after Wilms tumor and neuroblastoma and are by far the most common primary malignancy of the gastrointestinal tract.

Most children with benign or malignant liver masses present with a palpable mass on physical examination. Other presenting symptoms include pain, anorexia, jaundice, paraneoplastic syndromes, hemorrhage, and congestive heart failure. Although it is commonly obvious that these children have an upper abdominal mass, the organ of origin may not be clear without imaging. Whether CT or MRI is the modality of choice for definitive imaging of liver masses is a controversial issue. There are no pathognomonic imaging features for hepatic malignancies. The major role of imaging is to define accurately the extent of the lesion in relation to hepatic lobar anatomy and vascular and biliary structures for preoperative planning and to monitor tumor response to chemotherapy or radiation. For most hepatic malignancies, complete tumor resection or liver transplantation is essential for cure. The types of liver resection performed include left lobectomy, left lateral segmentectomy, right lobectomy, or trisegmentectomy (right lobe and medial segment of the left lobe). Therefore, a mass must be confined to the left or right lobe or the right lobe plus the medial segment of the left lobe to be considered resectable. If a lesion does not meet anatomic requirements for resectability at initial imaging, the child is often initially treated with chemotherapy, with or without radiation, and then reimaged.

The differential diagnosis for liver masses in children includes benign and malignant neoplasms such as hepatoblastoma, hemangioendothelioma, mesenchymal hamartoma, hepatocellular carcinoma, hemangiomas, lymphoproliferative disorder, lymphoma, hepatic adenomas, metastatic disease, and uncommon sarcomas, such as undifferentiated embryonal sarcoma and angiosarcoma. Nonneoplastic causes of liver masses include abscesses (fungal, bacterial, or granulomatous) and hematomas. Several factors help to focus the differential diagnosis, including the age of the child, the presentation, the alpha-fetoprotein level, and whether the lesion is solitary or multiple (Table 5-4). The differential diagnosis of liver

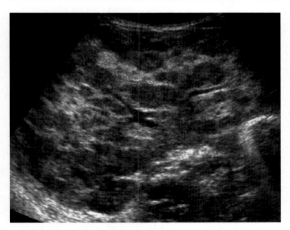

FIGURE 5-49. Liver metastasis from neuroblastoma. Ultrasound shows heterogeneous liver with multiple liver masses.

tumors is different in younger and older children. The most common hepatic tumors in children younger than 5 years of age include hepatoblastoma, hemangioendothelioma, mesenchymal hamartoma, and metastatic disease resulting from neuroblastoma or Wilms tumor. In children older than 5 years of age, the previously mentioned lesions are uncommon; the most common tumors include hepatocellular carcinoma, undifferentiated sarcoma, hepatic adenoma, hemangioma, and metastatic disease. Liver tumors that are associated with elevated serum alpha-fetoprotein levels include hepatoblastoma and hepatocellular carcinoma. Hemangioendothelioma can show elevated serum alpha-fetoprotein levels in a minority (less than 3%) of lesions. Other liver masses are not associated with an elevated serum alpha-fetoprotein. The presence of multiple liver lesions favors metastatic disease (Fig. 5-49), abscesses, cat scratch disease, lymphoproliferative disorder, or hepatic adenomas associated with a predisposing syndrome (Fanconi anemia, Gaucher disease).

TABLE 5-4. Causes of Pediatric Hepatic Masses

Age Less Than 5 Years
Hepatoblastoma (+ AFP)
Hemangioendothelioma
Mesenchymal hamartoma
Metastatic disease (Wilms, neuroblastoma)

Age Greater Than 5 Years
Hepatocellular carcinoma (+ alpha-fetoprotein level)
Undifferentiated embryonal sarcoma
Hepatic adenoma
Hemangioma
Metastatic disease

Immunocompromised state
Lymphoproliferative disorder
Fungal infection

Hepatoblastoma

Hepatoblastoma is the most common primary liver tumor of childhood, composing 43% of total liver masses. Hepatoblastoma is usually seen in infants and young children and occurs primarily in those less than 3 years of age. Predisposing conditions include Beckwith-Wiedemann syndrome, hemihypertrophy, familial polyposis coli, Gardner syndrome, Wilms tumor, and biliary atresia. However, most hepatoblastomas are seen in patients without associated conditions. The most common presentation

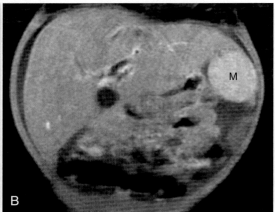

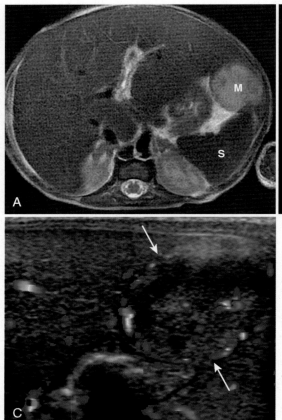

FIGURE 5-50. Hepatoblastoma in a 4-day-old infant. A, Axial T2-weighted image shows well-defined mass (M) arising from the very leftward aspect of the left lobe of the liver to be heterogeneously high in the T2-weighted signal. Note the dark signal within the spleen (S), which is normal in neonates. The spleen does not take on the typical high T2-signal appearance until after the white pulp develops at several weeks of age. B, Coronal MR image after contrast shows homogeneous enhancement of mass (M). C, Transverse sonogram shows a well-defined, heterogeneous mass (arrows) to be slightly hyperechoic to liver and shows some internal flow on color Doppler images.

is a painless mass. There is usually not a history of underlying liver disease. Serum alpha-fetoprotein levels are elevated in more than 90% of patients. Therefore, a liver mass presenting in a child younger than 3 years of age with an elevated alpha-fetoprotein level is almost always hepatoblastoma. On imaging, the lesions are most commonly well defined and have a tendency to displace rather than invade adjacent structures such as the falciform ligament (Fig. 5-50A-C). The lesions may be heterogeneous secondary to necrosis or hemorrhage. Overall survival rate for hepatoblastoma is 63% to 67%.

Infantile Hemangioendothelioma

Infantile hemangioendothelioma is the most common symptomatic vascular lesion of infancy. The lesions most commonly present in young infants as abdominal masses associated with either high-output congestive heart failure, consumptive coagulopathy (thrombocytopenia), or hemorrhage. Approximately 85% of the lesions present by 6 months of age. They can be well-defined or diffuse. The imaging appearance is variable; however, the lesions are most often heterogeneous and typically enhance with contrast. There may be prominent vessels within the lesions (Fig. 5-51A-C). On all imaging modalities, the descending aorta superior to the level of the hepatic branches of the celiac artery may appear abnormally enlarged as compared to the infrahepatic aorta because of differential flow.

The differentiation between hemangioendothelioma and multiple liver hemangiomas is not completely clear on the basis of either imaging or histology. Hemangioendotheliomas tend to spontaneously involute without therapy over a course of months to years. Sequential ultrasounds are often used to follow lesions and most often demonstrate a progressive decrease in size and an increase in degree of calcification.

Mesenchymal Hamartoma of the Liver

Mesenchymal hamartoma of the liver is a very rare, benign, predominately cystic liver mass

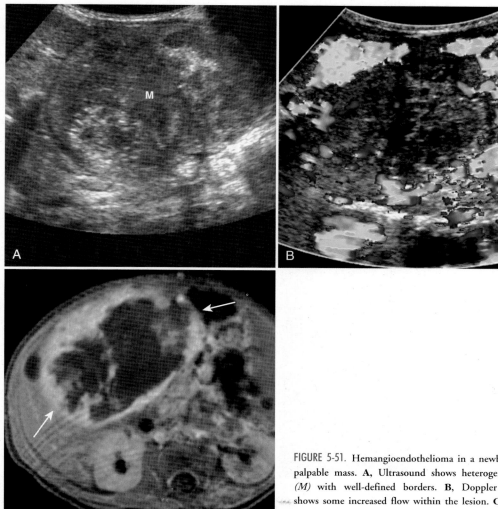

FIGURE 5-51. Hemangioendothelioma in a newborn with a palpable mass. **A,** Ultrasound shows heterogeneous mass *(M)* with well-defined borders. **B,** Doppler evaluation shows some increased flow within the lesion. **C,** Contrast-enhanced axial MRI shows peripheral enhancement of lesion *(arrows).*

that most commonly presents in infancy, almost always before 2 years of age. The lesion is considered a developmental anomaly rather than a true neoplasm. Patients usually present with a large painless abdominal mass and a normal serum alpha-fetoprotein level. At imaging, lesions appear as large, multilocular, cystic masses with thin internal septations (Fig. 5-52A-C). Occasionally, the solid component of the lesion can be more predominant, with multiple smaller cysts giving the lesion the appearance of Swiss cheese.

BLUNT ABDOMINAL TRAUMA

Blunt abdominal trauma is a common indication for CT of the abdomen and pelvis in children. In children, the most common cause of blunt abdominal trauma is motor vehicle accidents. Other causes include a direct blow resulting from abuse or from a handlebar when falling off a bike. Many aspects of the imaging of pediatric trauma, such as the appearance of parenchymal lacerations, are similar in children and adults and are not discussed in detail here. However, there are several significant differences that are emphasized.

Focused abdominal ultrasound for trauma has been advocated as a way of triaging patients with potential blunt abdominal trauma. It consists of a rapid ultrasound search for free fluid in all four quadrants. However, it has been shown that many significant parenchymal injuries can occur without associated free fluid. For these reasons, at our institution we use CT as the primary imaging modality to evaluate for blunt abdominal trauma.

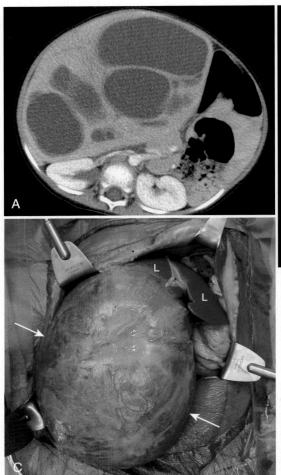

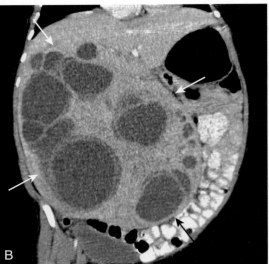

FIGURE 5-52. Mesenchymal hamartoma of the liver in a 3-week-old girl with an asymptomatic abdominal mass. **A,** Axial CT shows multicystic mass within liver. **B,** Coronal CT shows the multicystic mass *(arrows)* to be pedunculated off the inferior aspect of the liver. **C,** Operative photograph shows large pedunculated mass *(arrows)* extending off of the inferior aspect of the liver *(L).*

Parenchymal Organ Injuries

The order of frequency of parenchymal organ injuries in children is liver (36%), spleen (34%), kidney (22%), adrenal gland (11%), and pancreas (6%). Injury to multiple organs occurs in up to 21% of trauma cases. Most solid organ injuries are treated conservatively; operation is reserved for cases that are hemodynamically unstable. The size and appearance of a parenchymal organ injury have been shown to be inaccurate predictors of which patients with solid organ injury will need surgery. However, the visualization of active extravasation of contrast from a lacerated organ (density as high as the enhancing aorta seen within the peritoneum) strongly predicts the need for operation (Fig. 5-53).

Artifactual areas of low attenuation can be seen within the spleen; this is known as transient splenic heterogeneity, which is a normal flow phenomenon commonly seen during the arterial phase of

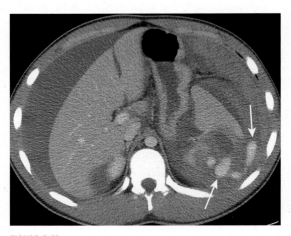

FIGURE 5-53. Active arterial extravasation resulting from splenic rupture in a 13-year-old who was hit in the abdomen playing American football. CT shows rupture of the spleen with arterial extravasation *(arrows)* shown as high-attenuation material exuding from the spleen. There is also a large amount of hemoperitoneum.

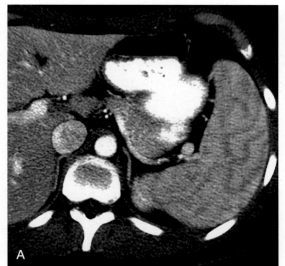

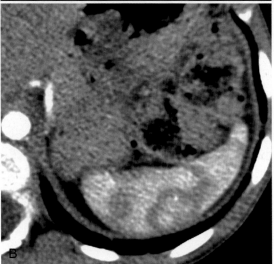

FIGURE 5-54. Heterogeneous splenic enhancement related to imaging during the arterial phase of enhancement. **A** and **B,** Examples in two children. They should not be mistaken for splenic injury.

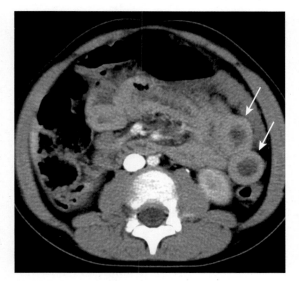

FIGURE 5-55. Bowel injury. CT shows focal bowel wall thickening *(arrows)* involving several jejunal loops. There is also edema in the base of the mesentery.

contrast enhancement. These artifacts should not be mistaken for splenic injury. Patterns of splenic heterogeneity included archiform (alternating bands of low and high attenuation (Fig. 5-54A, B), focal, and diffuse heterogeneity.

Bowel Injury

Injury to the bowel represents approximately 8% of abdominal injuries after trauma. Bowel injury is more common in children who have had lap-belt-type injuries. The most commonly

encountered CT findings include focal bowel wall thickening (Fig. 5-55), associated prominent bowel wall enhancement, mesenteric soft tissue stranding, and unexplained free peritoneal fluid (fluid in the absence of solid organ injury). When subtle, these findings may be suggestive but not diagnostic of a bowel injury. It is inappropriate to send all of such patients to the operating room. More often, the findings are communicated to the surgical team and kept in mind in case the patient develops increasingly severe abdominal symptoms. More specific findings of bowel injury are less common and include free intraperitoneal air, extraluminal bubbles of gas in the vicinity of the injury and, much less commonly, active extravasation of enteric contrast.

A patient who receives a focal, direct blow to the upper abdomen, most commonly caused by either a bicycle handle when falling or by abuse, is at increased risk for having a duodenal hematoma/laceration or pancreatitis (Figs. 5-56, 5-57). On CT, duodenal hematomas appear as high- or low-attenuation masses or as wall thickening in the third portion of the duodenum. Fluid seen between the splenic vein and the pancreas is said to be the most sensitive finding of pancreatic trauma. Lacerations of the pancreas are seen as hypoattenuating linear structures through the pancreas.

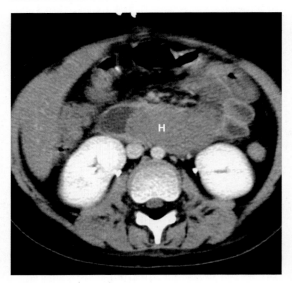

FIGURE 5-56. Duodenal hematoma. CT scan shows increased attenuation mass *(H)* within the portion of the duodenum that crosses the spine. This is the portion of the duodenum most commonly injured by blunt trauma.

Hypoperfusion Complex

It has been suggested that the clinical findings of hypovolemic shock can be masked for a longer time in children than in adults because of more pronounced peripheral vasospasm

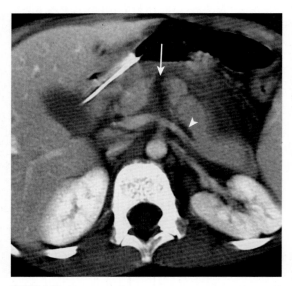

FIGURE 5-57. Traumatic pancreatic transection in an 11-year-old girl after a handlebar injury. CT shows low-attenuation cleft *(arrow)* traversing the pancreas and soft tissue stranding in the peripancreatic portion of the anterior pararenal space. There is also fluid *(arrowhead)* between the pancreas and splenic vein, a sensitive finding of pancreatic injury.

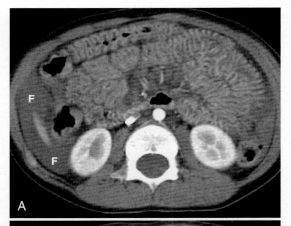

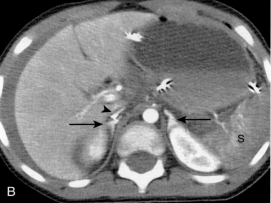

FIGURE 5-58. Hypoperfusion complex secondary to volume loss resulting from trauma. **A,** CT shows diffuse abnormal bowel enhancement and free intraperitoneal fluid *(F)*. **B,** A more superior CT image shows splenic rupture *(S)*, intense enhancement of the adrenal glands *(arrows)*, and small-caliber inferior vena cava *(arrowhead)*.

and tachycardia. The CT appearance of such children has been referred to as the hypoperfusion complex or as "shock bowel." CT findings include abnormal intense enhancement of the bowel wall, mesentery, adrenal glands, liver, kidneys, and pancreas, intense enhancement and decreased caliber of the inferior vena cava and aorta, and diffusely dilatated, fluid-filled bowel loops (Fig. 5-58A, B). This appearance on CT may be identified prior to clinical findings of shock and is associated with the potential development of hemodynamic instability. The bowel findings (bowel wall enhancement and dilatation over a diffuse distribution) should not be confused with the focal dilatation and bowel wall thickening or enhancement more typical of bowel injury. In cases in which the cause of the bowel findings is unclear, identifying other findings of the hypoperfusion complex is helpful.

THE IMMUNOCOMPROMISED CHILD

The population of immunocompromised children has greatly increased. Children can be immunocompromised because of therapy for malignancy, bone marrow transplantation, solid organ transplantation, primary immunodeficiency, and AIDS. These patients can have many different types of problems, including those related to immunodeficiency (infection, lack of neoplasm surveillance); thrombocytopenia (bleeding); other therapy-related complications, including mucositis, radiation injury, and the development of secondary neoplasm; recurrence of the primary neoplasm; and normal childhood illnesses that are unrelated to the patients' oncologic problems. The gastrointestinal tract is commonly involved with such processes. These patients commonly present with nonspecific symptoms, and imaging, usually with CT, is requested. Immunocompromised children are often referred for abdominal CT imaging to rule out abscess. However, drainable focal intraabdominal fluid collections are uncommon in immunocompromised children. More often, the abdominal source of sepsis is related to bowel wall compromise secondary to a variety of types of enterocolitis. Common bowel diseases in immunocompromised children are listed in Table 5-5. Most of these enterocolitides are managed medically unless there is evidence of perforation (extraluminal gas, fluid collection). When intraabdominal abscesses are present, they are often related to systemic fungal infection with such organisms as *Candida albicans* or *Aspergillus* species. These abscesses appear as multiple small, low-attenuation lesions within the liver, spleen, or kidneys.

TABLE 5-5. **CT Findings Helpful in Differentiating Bowel Diseases in Immunocompromised Children**

Entity	Typical Distribution	Imaging Features
Pseudomembranous colitis	Pancolitis	Marked bowel wall thickening Nonprominent pericolonic inflammatory changes
Neutropenic colitis	Cecum, right colon, terminal ileum	Bowel wall thickening Pericolonic inflammatory changes
Cytomegalovirus (CMV) colitis	Cecum, right colon, terminal ileum	Bowel wall thickening Pericolonic inflammatory changes
Mucositis	Small and large bowel	Fluid-filled, dilatated small and large bowel Thin but enhancing bowel wall Absent bowel wall thickening or adjacent inflammatory changes
Graft-vs-host disease	Diffuse small and large bowel	Mucosal enhancement Fluid-filled dilatated bowel Mild wall thickening, isolated to small bowel Prominent mesenteric inflammatory changes
Lymphoproliferative disorder	Focal involvement, typically small bowel	Marked focal bowel wall thickening Aneurysmal dilatation of bowel lumen Parenchymal (liver) masses Lymphadenopathy/mesenteric masses
Gastrointestinal bleeding	Anywhere	High-attenuation fluid or heterogeneous mass (solid thrombus) within lumen Associated underlying enterocolitis

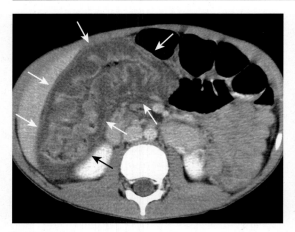

FIGURE 5-59. Pseudomembranous colitis. CT shows marked thickening of the colon *(arrows)*, shown here in the hepatic flexure. There is mucosal enhancement, low-attenuation bowel wall thickening, and disproportionately little pericolonic inflammatory change as compared to the degree of bowel wall thickening.

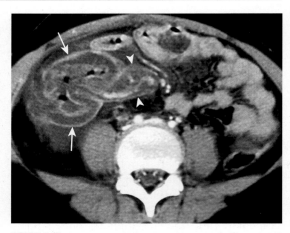

FIGURE 5-60. Neutropenic colitis. CT shows marked bowel-wall thickening, adventitial enhancement, low-attenuation of the central bowel wall, and pericolonic inflammatory change involving both the cecum *(arrows)* and terminal ileum *(arrowheads)*. The descending colon and the remainder of the small bowel appear to be normal.

Pseudomembranous Colitis

Because immunocompromised patients commonly receive antibiotics, they are at risk for developing pseudomembranous colitis, which is related to the overgrowth of and toxin production by *Clostridium difficile*, usually after the use of antibiotics. On gross inspection of the colon, there are discrete yellow plaques (pseudomembranes) involving the mucosal surface. The plaques are usually separated by normal-appearing mucosa. The CT findings, although nonspecific, are often highly suggestive of pseudomembranous colitis (Fig. 5-59). In the majority of cases, there is diffuse colonic involvement (pancolitis). There is marked colonic wall thickening (average 15 mm), greater in degree than that seen in most other types of colitis. It is common for contrast material to insinuate between the pseudomembranes and swollen haustra creating an accordion sign, which is highly suggestive of the diagnosis. Because pseudomembranous colitis involves predominantly the mucosa and submucosa, the degree of inflammatory change in the pericolonic fat is often disproportionately subtle compared to the degree of colonic wall thickening (see Fig. 5-59).

Neutropenic Colitis

Neutropenic colitis (typhlitis, necrosing enteropathy) is a life-threatening right-sided colitis associated with severe neutropenia. Pathologically, there is necrosing inflammation of the cecum and ascending colon with associated ischemia and secondary bacterial invasion. CT shows bowel wall thickening, pericolonic fluid, and inflammation of the pericolonic fat, usually isolated to the cecum and ascending colon (Fig. 5-60). The adjacent terminal ileum may also appear abnormal, but involvement of other portions of the small bowel or left colon is unusual.

Graft-Versus-Host Disease

Acute graft-versus-host disease is a process specific to bone marrow transplant recipients, in which donor T lymphocytes cause selected epithelial damage of recipient target organs. Histopathologically, there is extensive crypt cell necrosis and, in severe cases, diffuse destruction of the mucosa throughout both the large and small bowel and replacement with a thin layer of highly vascular granulation tissue. CT findings include diffuse enterocolitis from the duodenum to the rectum. Compared with the previously discussed causes of enterocolitis, bowel wall thickening may be mild, isolated to the small bowel, or absent. More characteristically, there is abnormal bowel wall enhancement in a central, mucosal location corresponding pathologically with the thin layer of vascular granulation tissue replacing the destroyed mucosa (Fig. 5-61). Both the small and large

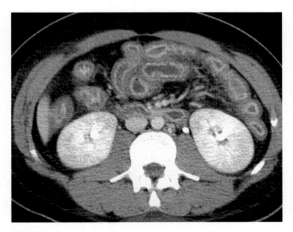

FIGURE 5-61. Acute graft-versus-host disease. CT shows abnormal mucosal enhancement and mild diffuse wall thickening in all visualized bowel loops.

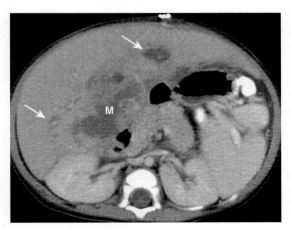

FIGURE 5-62. Lymphoproliferative disorder in a liver transplant recipient. CT shows heterogeneous, poorly defined mass *(M)* in central liver. There are also varying degrees of periportal low-attenuation masses surrounding the portal vein branches *(arrows)*.

bowel are usually filled with fluid and dilatated. There is often prominent infiltration of the mesenteric fat and soft tissue attenuation.

Mucositis

Gut toxicity has been described in association with multiple chemotherapeutic agents. The damage to the mucosa, the impaired ability of the bowel to regenerate its protective cell lining (mucosa), and the resultant inflammation are often referred to as mucositis. Patients present with nonspecific abdominal complaints, including nausea, vomiting, and abdominal pain, and they demonstrate an ileus pattern on abdominal radiographs. The symptoms may be severe and difficult to separate clinically from the previously discussed processes. On CT, the predominant finding of mucositis is dilatated, fluid-filled loops of small and large bowel. There may be mild associated small bowel wall enhancement. Marked bowel wall thickening, predominance of colonic involvement, and marked abdominal inflammatory changes suggest other diagnoses. Treatment for mucositis is supportive.

Lymphoproliferative Disorder

Lymphoproliferative disorders are lymphoma-like diseases related to an uncontrolled proliferation of cells infected by the Ebstein-Barr virus in an immunocompromised host. Although they can occur in any immunocompromised individual, they are most commonly encountered in patients after solid organ transplantation. Similar to the variable appearances of lymphoma, there are a spectrum of imaging findings of abdominal involvement in lymphoproliferative disorders, including focal parenchymal mass (Fig. 5-62), diffuse lymphadenopathy, mesenteric mass, bowel wall thickening, and associated aneurysmal dilatation of the small bowel lumen. In contrast to typical non-Hodgkin lymphoma, which manifests more commonly as abdominal lymphadenothy, lymphoproliferative disorder is more often associated with parenchymal organ involvement, most commonly the liver. In solid organ transplant recipients, the distribution of disease tends to occur in the vicinity of the transplant organ. Therefore, liver transplant recipients are more likely to have abdominal disease than are heart transplant recipients. Therapeutic options include reduction of immunosuppressive therapy, when possible, and chemotherapy.

COMPLICATIONS RELATED TO CYSTIC FIBROSIS

Newborn infants with cystic fibrosis presenting with meconium ileus have already been discussed. Older children and adults can present with a similar syndrome, distal intestinal obstruction syndrome, also known as meconium ileus equivalent. These children develop obstruction secondary to inspissated, tenacious intestinal contents lodging within the bowel lumen. On radiographs, there is abundant stool within the right colon and distal small bowel and findings

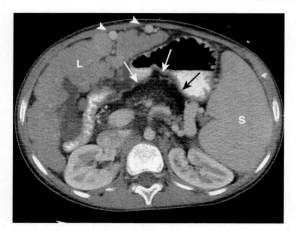

FIGURE 5-63. Abdominal complications of cystic fibrosis. CT shows irregular liver *(L)* consistent with cirrhosis. There are findings consistent with portal hypertension, including spleno-megaly *(S)* and multiple varices *(arrowheads)*. Note atrophy and fatty replacement of pancreas *(arrows)*.

of obstruction. When other therapies fail to resolve the obstruction, contrast enemas with gastrografin (meglumine diatrizoate) may be effective. However, it should be noted that patients with cystic fibrosis who develop pseu-domembranous colitis can develop abdominal pain and bloating, much like those with distal intestinal obstruction syndrome, and often do not have the diarrhea typically seen with pseu-domembranous colitis. If colonic wall thickening is identified on imaging studies such as CT or contrast enemas, the possibility of pseudomem-branous colitis should be raised. In these cases, enemas are definitely not indicated.

Another cause of bowel pathology in cystic fibrosis is the development of colonic thickening

or stricture resulting from iatrogenic damage caused by pancreatic enzyme replacement ther-apy. Other gastrointestinal problems associated with cystic fibrosis include cirrhosis, portal hypertension and varices, gallstones, and pan-creatic atrophy (Fig. 5-63). Patients with cystic fibrosis may have striking atrophy and fatty replacement of the pancreas on imaging studies such as CT, sonography, and MRI.

Suggested Readings

Zarewych ZM, Donnelly LF, Frush DP, Bisset JS III: Imaging of pediatric mesenteric abnormalities, *Pediatr Radiol* 29:711-719, 1999.

Buonomo C: Neonatal gastrointestinal emergencies, *Radiol Clin North Am* 35:845-864, 1997.

Long FR, Kramer SS, Markowitz RI, et al: Intestinal obstruc-tion in children: tutorial on radiographic diagnosis in dif-ficult cases, *Radiology* 198:775-780, 1996.

Berdon WE, Baker DH, Santulli TV, et al: Microcolon in new-born infants with intestinal obstruction: its correlation with the level and time of onset of obstruction, *Radiology* 90:878-885, 1968.

Kliegman RM, Fanaroff AA: Necrotizing enterocolitis, *N Engl J Med* 310:1093-1103, 1984.

Teele RL, Smith EH: Ultrasound in the diagnosis of idiopathic hypertrophic pyloric stenosis, *N Engl J Med* 296: 1149-1150, 1977.

Kirks DR: Air intussusception reduction: "the winds of change", *Pediatr Radiol* 25:89-91, 1995.

Frush DP, Donnelly LF: State of the art: spiral CT: technical considerations and applications in children, *Radiology* 209:37-48, 1998.

Sivit CJ, Taylor JA, Bulas DI, et al: Posttraumatic shock in children: CT findings associated with hemodynamic insta-bility, *Radiology* 182:723-726, 1992.

Donnelly LF, Bisset GS III: Pediatric liver imaging, *Radiol Clin North Am* 36:413-427, 1998.

Donnelly LF: CT imaging of immunocompromised children with acute abdominal symptoms, *Am J Roentgenol* 167:909-913, 1996.

CHAPTER SIX

Genitourinary

URINARY TRACT INFECTIONS

Urinary tract infection (UTI) is the most common problem of the genitourinary system encountered in children. The urinary tract is the second most common site of infection in children overall, with the upper respiratory tract being the first. The incidence of UTI is higher in girls than in boys, probably because of the short length of the female urethra. There is some current controversy concerning when children with UTIs should be imaged. Most physicians would agree that boys should be studied after the first UTI and that girls should be studied after the second UTI. However, there are some physicians who advocate that all children should be imaged after the first UTI. The immediate goals of imaging children with UTIs include identifying underlying congenital anomalies that predispose the child to UTI, identifying vesicoureteral reflux, identifying and documenting any renal cortical damage, providing a baseline renal size for subsequent evaluation of renal growth, and establishing prognostic factors. The long-term goal is to eliminate the chance of renal damage leading to chronic renal disease and hypertension.

The workup of a child with a UTI typically involves both a renal ultrasound and a voiding cystourethrogram. Voiding cystourethrograms can be performed using fluoroscopy or nuclear medicine. There is some debate about the indications for one or the other of the two studies. The advantage of the fluoroscopic cystourethrogram is that it demonstrates better anatomic detail. The advantage of the nuclear cystogram is that the patient is exposed to less radiation. However, in modern fluoroscopic units with pulse fluoroscopy, the difference in radiation dose between the two techniques is minimal. Because of the need for sharp anatomic detail in all boys and in girls with anatomic abnormalities demonstrated on ultrasound, most would advocate fluoroscopic cystograms for those patients. Nuclear cystograms are adequate for girls with normal ultrasound examinations.

Renal Ultrasound

At Cincinnati Children's Hospital Medical Center, renal ultrasounds are performed with the patient both in the supine and the prone positions. Transverse and longitudinal images are obtained of the kidney and bladder. Renal lengths are measured in both the prone and supine positions but are often more accurate with the patient in the prone position. In every case, it is important to compare the patient's renal length with tables that plot normal renal length against age. Also, the left and right kidneys should normally be within 1 cm of each other. If there is a discrepancy of more than 1 cm, an underlying abnormality should be suspected. A size discrepancy may result from a disorder that causes one of the kidneys to be too small, such as global scarring, or from a process that causes one of the kidneys to be too large, such as acute pyelonephritis or renal duplication.

The kidneys of infants have several characteristics that are different from those of older children and adults. They commonly have a prominent undulating contour. This is a normal appearance secondary to fetal lobulation (Fig. 6-1). In addition, infants' kidneys can demonstrate prominent hypoechoic renal pyramids (see Fig. 6-1) in contrast to the more echogenic renal cortex. These findings should not be mistaken for hydronephrosis.

Fluoroscopic Voiding Cystourethrogram

The most common indication for a fluoroscopic voiding cystourethrogram (VCUG) is the evaluation of UTI. Other indications include voiding dysfunction, enuresis, and the workup for hydronephrosis. The VCUG demonstrates the presence or absence of vesicoureteral reflux and also documents anatomic abnormalities of the bladder and urethra. Because catheterization is used for the procedure, there can be a great deal of anxiety for both the patient and the parents. Education of the parents and patient prior to

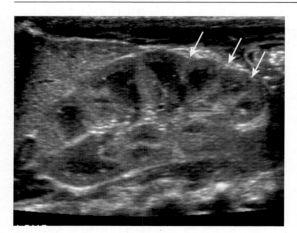

FIGURE 6-1. Normal ultrasound appearance of neonatal kidney. Longitudinal ultrasound shows prominent hypoechoic renal pyramids. This normal finding should not be confused with hydronephrosis. Also note fetal lobulation as focal indentations *(arrows)* located between medullary pyramids.

the examination is crucial to optimizing the patient's experience. VCUGs are performed under fluoroscopy with the patient awake. The patient is catheterized under sterile conditions on the fluoroscopy table, typically using an 8F catheter. A precontrast scout view of the abdomen is usually obtained to evaluate for calcifications, to document the bowel pattern so that it is not later mistaken for vesicoureteral reflux, and to document the catheter position within the bladder. Contrast is then instilled into the bladder. An early filling view of the bladder should be obtained to exclude a ureterocele. A ureterocele appears as a round, well-defined filling defect on early filling views. On later full views of the bladder, a ureterocele can be compressed and obscured. Once the patient's bladder is full, bilateral oblique views are obtained to visualize the regions of the ureteral vesicular junctions. These views are typically obtained with the collimators open from top to bottom, with the bladder positioned at the inferior aspect of the screen and the expected path of the ureter included on the film. During voiding, the male urethra is optimally imaged with the patient in the oblique projection. The female urethra is best seen on the anteroposterior view. It is critical to obtain an image of the urethra during voiding, particularly in males. In order to ensure that a view of the urethra is obtained, an image should be obtained during urination with the catheter in place and then a second view can be obtained after the catheter has been removed. After the patient has completed

voiding, images are obtained of the pelvis and over the kidneys, documenting the presence or absence of vesicoureteral reflux and evaluating the extent of postvoid residual contrast within the bladder. The use of fluoroscopy should be brief and intermittent during bladder filling. Fluoroscopic last-image hold images can often substitute for true exposures in order to further decrease radiation dose.

Sometimes, particularly in older children, it may be difficult to get the child to void on the table. Almost all children will eventually void and a great deal of patience is required during such prolonged examinations. There are several maneuvers that may help the child to void. They include placing warm water on the patient's perineum or toes; placing a warm, wet washcloth on the patient's lower abdomen; tilting the table so that the head is up; letting the patient hear the sound of running water in the sink; and dimming the lights.

The expected bladder capacity of small children can be calculated by adding 2 to the patient's age in years and multiplying that number by 30. This yields the bladder capacity in milliliters. Obviously, this formula works only up to a certain age.

Acute Pyelonephritis

There is some confusion concerning the terminology used for infections of the urinary tract in children. The definition of UTI is the presence of bacteria in the urine, but the term typically refers to infections of the lower urinary tract. Acute pyelonephritis is defined as urinary tract infection that involves the kidney. Young children may present with nonspecific symptoms, such as fever, irritability, and vague abdominal pain. In older children, the findings may be more specific, such as fever associated with flank pain. In patients in whom the diagnosis is straightforward, no imaging is needed during the acute infection, but the patients are imaged later as the standard workup for UTI. In patients in whom there is clinical difficulty in distinguishing an upper from a lower UTI, cortical scintigraphy using dimercaptosuccinic acid (DMSA) has been advocated as being the most sensitive test. In the case of pyelonephritis, this study demonstrates single or multiple areas of lack of renal uptake of the radiotracer. These areas tend to be triangular and peripheral (Fig. 6-2). Other imaging studies

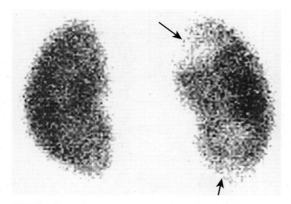

FIGURE 6-2. Acute pyelonephritis. Nuclear scintigraphy with dimercaptosuccinic acid (DMSA) shows areas of decreased uptake *(arrows)* in the upper and lower poles of the right kidney, consistent with pyelonephritis in a child with known reflux and flank pain.

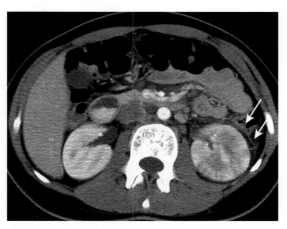

FIGURE 6-4. Acute pyelonephritis on CT obtained for abdominal pain. Pyelonephritis appears as asymmetric increased volume of left kidney, striated low attenuation within peripheral aspect of left kidney, and perinephric stranding with thickening of Gerota fascia *(arrows)*.

that have also been advocated to detect acute pyelonephritis include color Doppler ultrasound and contrast-enhanced helical computed tomography (CT). These studies typically demonstrate lack of color flow or contrast enhancement of triangular, peripheral portions of the kidney (Fig. 6-3). CT may show a striated nephrogram (Fig. 6-4). Also, pyelonephritis can be very focal and can mimic a mass on all of these studies (Fig. 6-5A, B). Ultrasound and CT may also demonstrate disproportionate enlargement and swelling of the affected kidney as compared to the contralateral side. Sometimes the findings of pyelonephritis will be encountered on these imaging studies when the studies were obtained for other suspected causes of abdominal pain such as appendicitis.

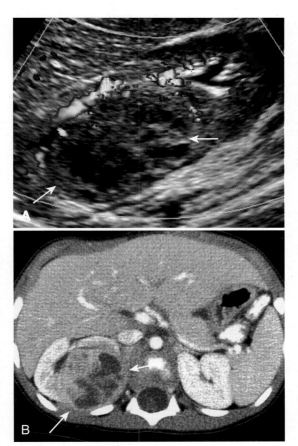

FIGURE 6-5. Acute, focal pyelonephritis presenting as a mass. **A,** Longitudinal ultrasound shows a heterogeneous mass *(arrows)* with areas of low echogenicity. **B,** CT shows heterogeneous mass *(arrows)* with low attenuation.

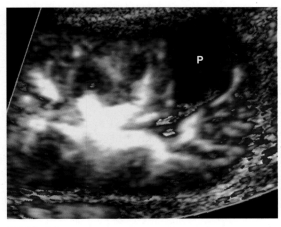

FIGURE 6-3. Acute pyelonephritis on Doppler ultrasound. Longitudinal ultrasound shows lesion (P) as peripheral area of absent color flow.

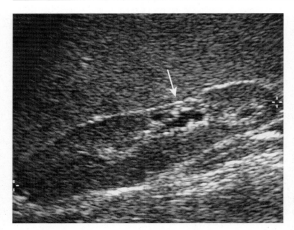

FIGURE 6-6. Global renal scarring shown on longitudinal ultrasound of the left kidney. There is diffuse thinning of the renal parenchyma, most striking in the lower pole *(arrow)*, where the renal surface is in close approximation to the collecting system.

Chronic Pyelonephritis

Chronic pyelonephritis is defined as the loss of renal parenchyma resulting from previous bacterial infection. It is synonymous with renal scarring. Normally, the renal cortical thickness should be symmetric and equal within the upper, mid, and lower poles of the kidneys. The loss of renal cortical substance as seen by ultrasound, most commonly at one of the renal poles, is suggestive of the diagnosis (Fig. 6-6). This should not be confused with fetal lobulation (also known as an interrenicular septum; Fig. 6-7A, B), a normal variant. In pyelonephrotic scarring, the indentations of the renal contour tend to overlie the renal calyces, whereas in fetal lobulation, the indentations are between renal calyces (see Fig. 6-7).

EVALUATION OF PRENATALLY DIAGNOSED HYDRONEPHROSIS

As a result of the increasing use of prenatal ultrasound, pediatric radiologists are more frequently having to perform postnatal workups of prenatally diagnosed hydronephrosis. The evaluation of such patients typically includes both ultrasound and VCUG. The controversy revolves around the timing of the ultrasound evaluation. In neonates, there is a relative state of dehydration that occurs after the first 24 hours of life. Reports have shown that this relative state of dehydration can lead to underestimation or nondetection of hydronephrosis by ultrasound.

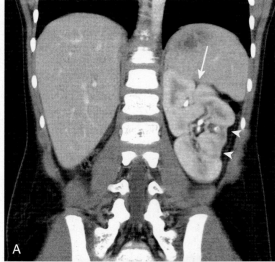

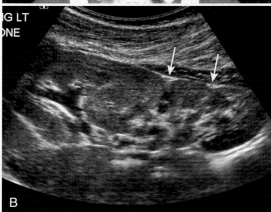

FIGURE 6-7. Differentiation between fetal lobulation and focal scarring; both are demonstrated in the same patient with a solitary left kidney. **A,** Coronal CT shows solitary left kidney. There are indentations of the renal cortex directly over the medullary pyramids *(arrowheads)*. These areas represent focal scarring. There is also an indentation in the renal cortex between the medullary pyramids *(arrow)*. This is consistent with fetal lobulation. **B,** Longitudinal ultrasound in same patient again shows indentations of the renal cortex directly over the medullary pyramids *(arrows)*, which is consistent with focal scarring.

Therefore, it is recommended that the postnatal evaluation of prenatally diagnosed hydronephrosis be performed during the first 24 hours of life or after 1 week of age. The disadvantage of doing the ultrasound during the first 24 hours of life is the interruption of mother-child bonding, whereas the disadvantage of performing the examination at 7 days of life is the potential of parental noncompliance and losing the patient for follow-up.

Congenital Anomalies

Congenital anomalies of the genitourinary tract are commonly encountered during workups for UTIs or other abnormalities.

Vesicoureteral Reflux

Vesicoureteral reflux (VUR) is defined as retrograde flow of urine from the bladder into the ureter. It is thought to be a primary abnormality related to immaturity or maldevelopment of the ureterovesicular junction. Normally, the ureter enters the ureterovesicular junction in an oblique manner such that the intramural ureter traverses the bladder wall for an adequate length to create a passive antireflux valve. When the angle of entrance of the ureter is abnormal, vesicoureteral reflux results. VUR occurs in less than 0.5% of asymptomatic children but is present in as much as 50% of children with UTIs. There is an increased incidence of VUR in siblings of children with VUR, in children of parents who had VUR, and in non-blacks as compared to blacks. The importance of VUR is its association with renal parenchymal scarring. VUR is present in almost all children with severe renal scarring. Also, a direct correlation between the grade of VUR and the prevalence of scarring has been demonstrated. Other complications associated with

VUR include acute pyelonephritis, interference with the normal growth of the kidney, and development of hypertension. The degree of VUR is graded on the basis of several characteristics (Fig. 6-8): the level to which the reflux occurs (ureteral vs. ureteral and collecting system); the degree of dilatation; the calyceal blunting; and papillary impressions. Grade 1 reflux is confined to the ureter. Grade 2 reflux fills the ureter and collecting system, but there is no dilatation of the collecting system. Grade 3 reflux is associated with blunting of the calyces. In deciding whether a calyx is dilatated or not, I was taught that if it looks like you could pick your teeth with a calyx, it is not dilatated (Fig. 6-9). Grade 4 reflux is identified by progressive, tortuous dilatation of the renal collecting system. Grade 5 reflux is defined by the presence of a very tortuous dilatated ureter. Both grade 4 and grade 5 reflux can be associated with intrarenal reflux. It is surprising, but significant VUR can be present in spite of a normal renal ultrasound. Lack of dilatation on ultrasound in no way excludes the presence of VUR. Dilatation of the ureter or collecting systems can sometimes be seen intermittently when VUR is present.

Most low-grade VUR resolves spontaneously by the age of 5 to 6 years unless there is an underlying anatomic abnormality. In children without anatomic reasons that prohibit spontaneous resolution of reflux, most are

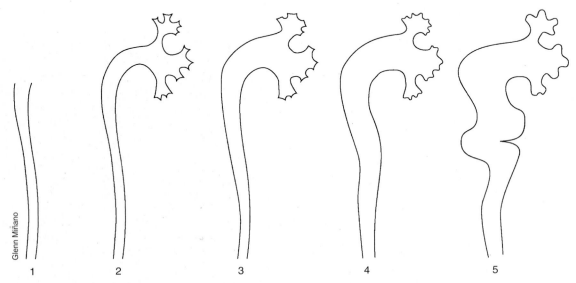

FIGURE 6-8. Grading system for vesicoureteral reflux. Grade 1 Reflux is confined to the ureter. Grade 2: Reflux fills the ureter and collecting system without dilatation of the collecting system. Grade 3: Reflux is associated with blunting of the calyces. Grade 4: Reflux results in progressive, tortuous dilatation of the renal collecting system. Grade 5: Reflux is defined by the presence of a very tortuous, dilatated ureter.

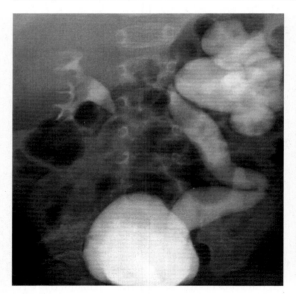

FIGURE 6-9. Vesicoureteral reflux shown on voiding cystoure-throgram: right, grade 2, and left, grade 5. Image shows reflux of contrast filling a nondilatated right renal collecting system. Note that the calyces are sharp in appearance and are not blunted. On the left, there is reflux of contrast filling a markedly dilated ureter and collecting system. The calyces are markedly blunted. The ureter is tortuous.

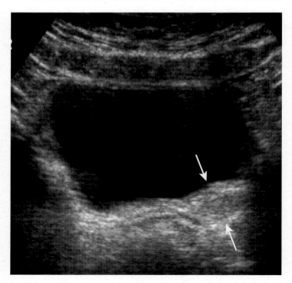

FIGURE 6-10. Ultrasound appearance following minimally inva-sive endoscopic treatment of VUR using periureteral injection of Deflux. Ultrasound shows echogenic mound (arrows) at base of bladder in region of left ureterovesicular junction.

treated with prophylactic antibiotics alone. Antibiotic therapy is discontinued when the reflux has resolved. Surgical reimplantation of the ureter or periureteral injection (minimally in-vasive endoscopic treatment) is considered when the degree of VUR is severe, if there is evidence of renal scarring, if the VUR has not resolved over a reasonable time, or if break-through infections occur frequently. After peri-ureteral injection, ultrasound will show an echo-genic mound in the bladder wall in the region of the treated ureteral orifice (Fig. 6-10).

Ureteropelvic Junction Obstruction

Ureteropelvic junction (UPJ) obstruction is defined as an obstruction of the flow of urine from the renal pelvis into the proximal ureter. It is the most common congenital obstruction of the urinary tract. There is an increased inci-dence of other congenital anomalies of the uri-nary tract in patients with UPJ obstruction. They include vesicoureteral reflux, renal duplication, and ureterovesicular junction obstruction. In addition, UPJ obstruction may be present bilat-erally but the severity may be asymmetric. The cause of most UPJ obstructions is intrinsic

narrowing at the UPJ. However, extrinsic com-pression secondary to anomalous vessels is also occasionally identified. On ultrasound, there is dilatation of the renal collecting system without dilatation of the ureter (Fig. 6-11). The degree of dilatation may be severe. Renal scintigraphy using 99m technetium-MAG3 with diuretic (fur-osemide) challenge is often used to evaluate the severity of the UPJ obstruction. Children with

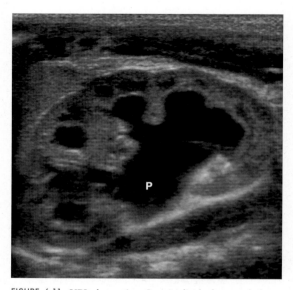

FIGURE 6-11. UPJ obstruction. Longitudinal ultrasound shows dilatation of renal collecting system, which connects to central, dilatated renal pelvis (P). The ureter was not dilatated.

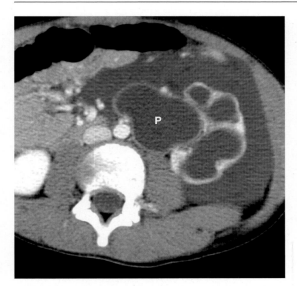

FIGURE 6-12. **Renal injury to child with UPJ obstruction follow-ing minor trauma. CT shows findings of UPJ obstruction with dilatation of the renal collecting system and central, dilatated renal pelvis *(P).* There is a large amount of perinephric fluid secondary to injury to the dilatated collecting system.**

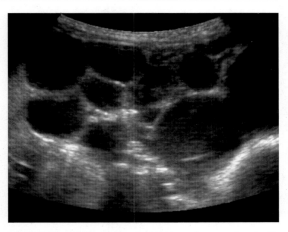

FIGURE 6-13. **Multicystic dysplastic kidney shown on longitudi-nal ultrasound as cluster of anechoic cysts without dominant central cyst. Scintigraphy showed no renal activity.**

UPJ obstruction and other congenital anomalies are predisposed to renal injury even by minor abdominal trauma (Fig. 6-12). Mild to moderate UPJ obstructions are sometimes treated conser-vatively, but most urologists treat severe UPJ obstruction surgically.

Multicystic Dysplastic Kidney

Multicystic dysplastic kidney (MCDK) is thought to be related to severe obstruction of the renal collecting system during fetal development. The site of the obstruction determines the imaging appearance. The most common appearance of MCDK is that of a grapelike collection of variably sized cysts that do not appear to communicate (Fig. 6-13). The absence of a central dominant cyst differentiates MCDK from severe hydrone-phrosis. However, if the level of the fetal obstruc-tion is within the proximal ureter, the "hydronephrotic" form of MCDK can occur; in this there is a central pelvis surrounded by dila-tated cysts. In such cases, renal scintigraphy can be useful in differentiating severe UPJ obstruction from MCDK. In MCDK, no trace or accumulation is seen within the renal pelvis on 4-hour images. In patients with MCDK, it is important to exclude other associated congenital anomalies of the contralateral kidney. UPJ obstruction is

commonly identified. Rarely, MCDK can be iso-lated to an upper or lower pole.

Most MCDKs slowly decrease in size over time. Often the remaining residual dysplastic renal tissue will no longer be visualized by imag-ing techniques. Although in the past, nephrectomy was the usual treatment for MCDK, most patients are currently treated nonoperatively. They are, however, followed by ultrasound because there is some controversy as to whether there may be an increased risk for developing malignancy in an MCDK. MCDK can also predispose patients to hypertension, and if hypertension develops, nephrectomy is usually performed.

Ureteropelvic Duplications

The term *ureteropelvic duplication* refers to a broad range of anatomic variations ranging in severity from incomplete to complete. The incom-plete form of duplication is more common than the complete form. With incomplete duplication, there can be a bifid renal pelvis, two ureters super-iorly that join in midureter, or duplicated ureters that join just prior to insertion into the bladder wall. With complete duplication there are two completely separate ureters that have separate ori-fices into the bladder. Ureteropelvic duplication is thought to occur secondary to premature division or duplication of the ureteral bud. Such duplica-tions are five times more common unilaterally than bilaterally. On ultrasound, incomplete renal duplication may appear as an area of echogenicity similar to the renal cortex separating the echogen-ic central renal fat into superior and inferior

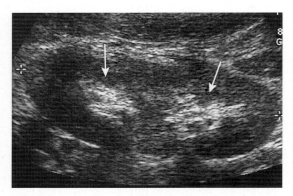

FIGURE 6-14. Intrarenal duplication shown on longitudinal ultrasound as an area of echogenicity similar to that of the renal cortex separating the central pelvicalyceal fat into separate superior and inferior components *(arrows)*.

components (Fig. 6-14). Noncomplicated, incomplete renal duplications have little significance and should be thought of as a normal variation. Children with incomplete duplication are not at increased risk for urinary tract disease as compared to children without duplications.

In patients with complete ureteropelvic duplication, there is a higher incidence of urinary tract infection, obstruction, vesicoureteral reflux, and parenchymal scarring. In these patients the ureteral orifice of the upper pole moiety inserts more medially and more inferiorly than the orifice of the lower pole ureter. This is known as the Weigert-Meyer rule. The lower pole system is more prone to vesicoureteral reflux and UPJ obstruction. The upper pole system is more prone to obstruction secondary to ureterocele (Figs. 6-15A-C, 6-16A, B).

URETEROCELE

A ureterocele is defined as dilatation of the distal ureter. The dilatated portion of the ureter lies between the mucosal and muscular layers of the bladder. The ureteral orifice is usually stenotic or obstructed. Ureteroceles are defined as simple when they are positioned at the expected orifice of the ureter at the lateral aspect of the trigone; they are defined as ectopic when they are associated with an ectopic insertion of the ureter. Ectopic ureteroceles can be quite large

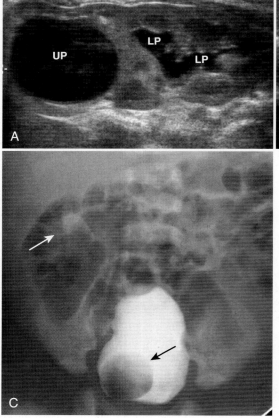

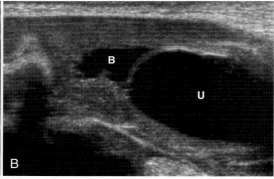

FIGURE 6-15. Duplicated right renal collecting system with lower pole reflux and a ureterocele causing obstruction of the upper pole. **A,** Longitudinal ultrasound of right kidney shows a markedly dilatated upper pole collecting system *(UP)*, secondary to an obstructing ureterocele, and a mild dilatation of lower pole collecting system *(LP)*, secondary to VUR. **B,** Longitudinal ultrasound, right paramidline, of pelvis shows a ureterocele *(U)* as a thin-walled cystic structure within the bladder *(B)*. **C,** Image from VCUG shows a ureterocele *(black arrow)* as a round filling defect within the bladder. Note reflux into the lower pole collecting system *(white arrow)*. Also note that the opacified lower pole collecting system is displaced inferiorly by the dilatated, nonopacified, obstructed upper pole collecting system. This is called the "drooping lily" sign.

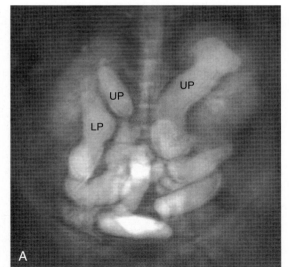

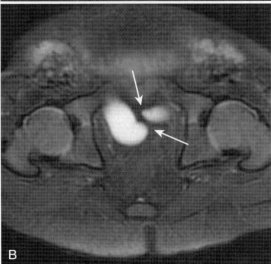

FIGURE 6-16. Complex bilateral duplication shown on an MRI urogram. **A,** MRI urogram shows marked dilatation of the upper pole collecting systems and ureters *(UP)* bilaterally, secondary to obstruction by ectopic ureter insertion. The right lower pole collecting system and ureter *(LP)* is also dilatated secondary to VUR. **B,** Axial T2-weighted MR image shows ectopic low-inserting bilateral ureters *(arrows)*. Both ureters insert into the urethra below the bladder base.

and are almost always associated with a duplicated collecting system (see Figs. 6-15, 6-16). The ureter from the upper pole moiety is associated with the ureterocele. There can be marked associated dilatation of that ureter and the upper pole moiety collecting system. On VCUGs, ureteroceles appear as round, well-defined filling defects, best visualized on early filling views (see Fig. 6-15). Ureteroceles may be compressed and not visualized when the

bladder is distended by contrast. Sometimes the ureteroceles can invert and appear as diverticula. On ultrasound, typically a dilatated ureter is seen to terminate in a round, anechoic intravesicular cystic structure (see Fig. 6-15). Usually there is associated dilatation of the upper pole moiety.

Renal Ectopia and Fusion

Renal ectopia is defined as abnormal position of the kidney. It results from abnormal migration of the kidney from its fetal position within the pelvis to its expected position in the renal fossa. Most ectopic kidneys lie within the pelvis and are malrotated. Renal fusion is defined as a connection between the two kidneys. It results from failure of separation of the primitive nephrogenic cell masses into two separate left and right blastemas. With ectopia, the ectopic kidney most commonly lies within the pelvis. Most ectopic kidneys are also malrotated. With cross-fused renal ectopia, both kidneys lie on the same side of the abdomen and are fused (Fig. 6-17). The ureter from the ectopic kidney crosses the midline and enters the bladder in the expected location of the contralateral ureterovesical junction. The most common type of renal fusion is horseshoe kidney, which occurs in approximately 1 in 600 births. With horseshoe kidney, there is fusion of the lower

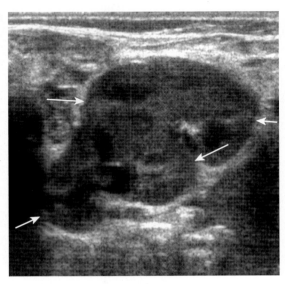

FIGURE 6-17. Crossed-fused renal ectopia is demonstrated as fusion of the "left" and right kidneys to the right of the midline on ultrasound. The *arrows* point to the upper and lower poles of the two kidney units.

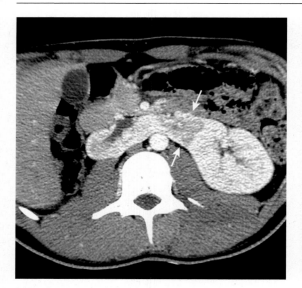

FIGURE 6-18. CT of horseshoe kidney with contusion due to a minor injury. There is an area of low attenuation *(arrows)* within the horseshoe kidney, consistent with a contusion.

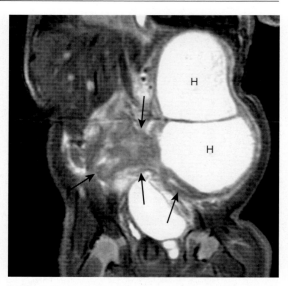

FIGURE 6-19. Horseshoe kidney with associated left hydronephrosis. Coronal T2-weighted MRI shows horseshoe kidney *(arrows)* with a parenchymal connection of the kidneys across the midline. Note hydronephrosis *(H)* of the left renal moiety.

pole of the two kidneys across the midline. The connecting isthmus may consist of functional renal tissue or fibrous tissue and cross the midline anterior to the aorta and inferior vena cava. Most horseshoe kidneys are located more inferiorly than normal. The number of ureters arising from a horseshoe kidney is variable and they exit the kidney ventrally rather than ventromedially. Horseshoe kidneys and other types of renal fusions are at increased risk for infection, injury from mild traumatic events (Fig. 6-18), renal vascular hypertension, stone formation, and hydronephrosis (Fig. 6-19); there is also a slight increase in incidence of Wilms tumor and adenocarcinoma. On ultrasound, horseshoe kidney may be difficult to diagnose on the standard longitudinal and axial planes. It may also be difficult to obtain accurate measurements of the kidneys in the longitudinal plane because of the poorly defined inferior pole. If the ultrasound probe is moved posterolaterally and the patient is scanned in the coronal plane, the two kidneys and connecting isthmus can be visualized on a single image (Fig. 6-20A-C). Such images are most easily obtained in infants. Horseshoe kidneys are readily visualized on CT scanning (see Fig. 6-20).

Primary Megaureter

Primary megaureter can be thought of as the ureteral equivalent of Hirschsprung disease.

With primary megaureter, there is an aperistaltic segment of the distal ureter that results in a relative obstruction (Fig. 6-21). The normal more proximal ureter dilates as a consequence of the relative obstruction. It is more common on the left and in boys. Children affected with primary megaureter may present with infection or be diagnosed prenatally. Ultrasound demonstrates hydronephrosis and enlargement of the ureter above the aperistaltic segment.

Posterior Urethral Valves

Posterior urethral valves are the most common cause of urethral obstruction in male infants. They are identified most commonly in infancy but can be diagnosed in older children. The high back pressure and associated reflux can damage the kidneys and result in renal failure. Affected children can be diagnosed prenatally and present with renal failure or with urinary tract infection.

Typical ultrasound features include a thick-walled bladder with associated bilateral dilatation of the renal collecting systems and ureters (Figs. 6-22A-D, 6-23A-C). Occasionally, a dilatated posterior urethra can be identified inferior to the bladder. On VCUG, the posterior urethra appears very dilatated (see Figs. 6-22, 6-23). The actual valve itself may be difficult to visualize but can appear as a membranelike obstruction

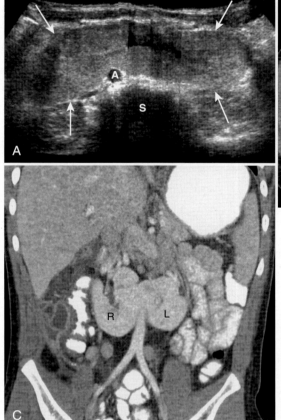

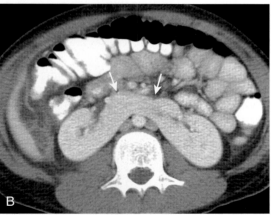

FIGURE 6-20. Horseshoe kidney in two children. **A,** Horseshoe kidney shown on axial ultrasound of an infant. The right and left kidneys *(arrows)* are connected by a parenchymal isthmus. A, aorta; S, spine. **B,** Axial CT of a different child shows right and left kidneys joined by a parenchymal bridge *(arrows)*. **C,** Coronal CT again shows right *(R)* and left *(L)* kidneys connected by a parenchymal bridge.

(see Fig. 6-22). The bladder is trabeculated. Vesicoureteral reflux is present in approximately 50% of patients with posterior urethral valves.

Anything that relieves the increased pressure within the urinary system of patients with posterior urethral valves protects the patients from developing renal failure and is associated with a better prognosis. Such entities include unilateral vesicoureteral reflux (with protection of the kidney contralateral to the reflux; see Fig. 6-23), large bladder or calyceal diverticuli, or development of intrauterine ascites. It is the potential of posterior urethral valves that makes obtaining an image of the urethra during voiding a vital part of every VCUG performed on boys.

Urachal Abnormalities

The urachus is an embryologic structure that communicates between the apex of the bladder and the umbilicus. Normally, it closes by birth.

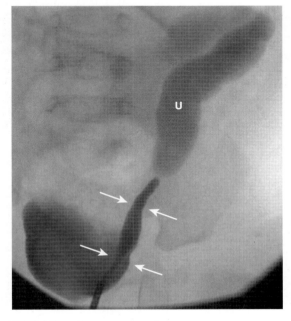

FIGURE 6-21. Primary megaureter. Retrograde contrast injection of ureter shows narrowed distal ureter *(arrows)* with dilatation of the more proximal ureter *(U)*, secondary to relative obstruction.

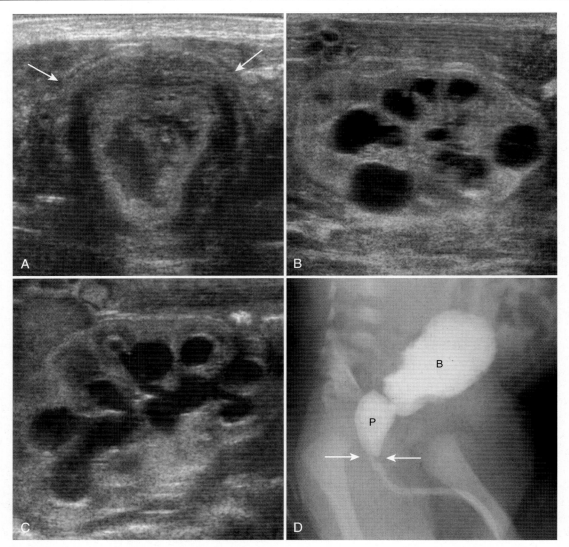

FIGURE 6-22. Posterior urethral valves in a newborn with renal failure. **A,** Axial ultrasound shows markedly thick-walled bladder *(arrows).* The bladder is empty. **B,** Longitudinal ultrasound of the left kidney shows hydronephrosis and echogenic renal parenchyma. **C,** Longitudinal ultrasound of the right kidney shows hydronephrosis and echogenic renal parenchyma. **D,** VCUG shows trabeculated, thick-walled bladder *(B),* dilatated posterior urethra *(P),* and visible posterior urethral valve *(arrows).*

If any portion of this embryologic structure remains patent, a urachal abnormality results. The type of the urachal anomaly present is determined by which portion of the urachus remains patent (Figs. 6-24, 6-25A-C). If the urachus remains patent in its entirety from the umbilicus to the bladder, it is a patent urachus (see Fig. 6-25). A neonate with a patent urachus will have urine draining from the umbilicus. Patent urachus can be demonstrated by VCUG, fistula tract injection, or ultrasound.

If the urachus remains patent only at the bladder end of the urachus, a urachal diverticulum is present. On ultrasound or VCUG, a

diverticulum of variable size is demonstrated arising from the anterosuperior aspect of the dome on the bladder (see Fig. 6-25). Ultrasound may also demonstrate a fibrous tract extending from the diverticulum to the umbilicus.

If the urachus remains patent only at the umbilical end, a urachal sinus is present. If the urachus remains patent only at its midportion and is closed at both its umbilical and its bladder ends, a urachal cyst is present. Urachal cysts may present as palpable masses but more commonly present with inflammatory changes after becoming infected. Ultrasound or CT will show a cystic mass anterior and superior to the bladder dome in the midline (see Fig. 6-25). Urachal carcinoma is rare in adults and extraordinarily rare in children.

Prune Belly Syndrome

Prune belly syndrome, or Eagle-Barrett syndrome, is the name given to the rare condition in which there is a triad of hypoplasia of the abdominal muscles, cryptorchidism, and abnormalities of the urinary tract system. Potential urinary tract abnormalities include severe bilateral hydronephrosis, a trabeculated and hypertrophied bladder, urachal diverticulum, and hydroureter. Radiographic manifestations include bulging flanks secondary to abdominal wall hypoplasia and the previously described renal manifestations (Fig. 6-26A, B). There are multiple associated congenital anomalies. Even more rarely, the syndrome can be incomplete (pseudo prune belly syndrome) in girls, who obviously cannot have cryptorchidism, and it can occur unilaterally.

Hydrometrocolpos

Genital outflow tract obstructions may lead to hydrometrocolpos or hematometrocolpos. *Hydrometrocolpos* is the term given to a rare condition in which the vagina and uterus dilate when fluid accumulates in the reproductive tract; this occurs in response to hormonal stimulation, so it occurs during infancy, secondary to maternal hormones, or during puberty. Hematometrocolpos is the accumulation of blood in a dilatated vagina and uterus that occurs after menarche in patients with a genital outflow tract obstruction. In both hydrometrocolpos and hematometrocolpos, a fixed midline mass may be palpable; the mass can become large enough to cause ureteral obstruction and result in hydronephrosis. Radiography or ultrasound can demonstrate the midline abdominal mass. On ultrasound, the mass appears tubular or elliptical and at the midline. In hematometrocolpos there is heterogeneous echogenicity secondary to the underlying hemorrhage (Fig. 6-27A, B). Because the vagina is more elastic, it becomes markedly dilatated and composes the bulk of the mass. The uterus may also be dilatated but cannot expand to the degree that the vagina can. Often the uterus can be identified as a small C-shaped cavity arising from the

anterosuperior aspect of the distended vagina on ultrasound (see Fig. 6-27). Ultrasound also can reveal the degree of obstructive hydronephrosis. In problematic cases, MRI can be helpful in confirming the cause and the anatomy of the lesion (see Fig. 6-27).

Renal Cystic Disease

In children, renal cysts can occur secondary to polycystic kidney disease; can be associated with a variety of syndromes; can occur secondary to cystic neoplasms; or can be related to other cystic processes such as multicystic dysplastic kidney (Table 6-1). The categorization of and nomenclature for renal cystic disease in children can sometimes be confusing. In addition, it is important to note that although much less common than in adults, solitary simple renal cysts are not uncommonly identified in children. When such unilocular, solitary cysts are encountered during the workup for a urinary tract infection or hematuria, they are usually of no clinical significance and do not necessarily suggest an underlying developing polycystic kidney disease. As in adults, the ultrasound criteria for diagnosing a simple renal cyst include an anechoic, well-defined, round lesion; an imperceptible wall; and increased through-transmission. No central echoes or vascular flow is present within the lesion or within its walls.

AUTOSOMAL RECESSIVE POLYCYSTIC KIDNEY DISEASE

Autosomal recessive polycystic kidney disease, also known as infantile polycystic kidney disease, encompasses a range of recessive diseases that are associated with varying amounts of cystic disease in the kidneys as well as with hepatic fibrosis. It is a very rare condition. When the renal findings (severe renal tubular ectasia) predominate, the disease most commonly presents on in utero imaging or during infancy and is termed infantile polycystic kidney disease. When the liver disease (severe fibrosis) predominates and there is minimal renal disease, the disease usually presents later in childhood and is referred to as juvenile polycystic kidney disease. In the infantile form, the kidneys are markedly enlarged and replaced by numerous small, 1- to 2-mm cysts throughout the cortex and medulla. On ultrasound, the kidneys are grossly enlarged and demonstrate

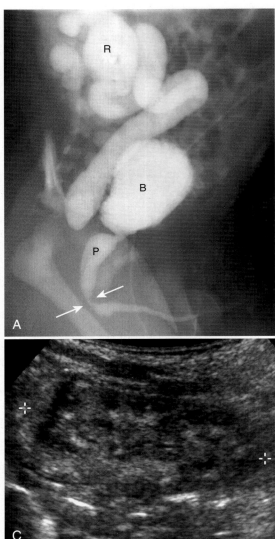

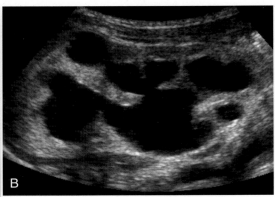

FIGURE 6-23. Posterior urethral valves and unilateral vesicoureteral reflux serving as a protective mechanism for the contralateral kidney. **A,** VCUG shows trabeculated, thick-walled bladder *(B)*, dilatated posterior urethra *(P)*, and narrowing *(arrows)* of the urethra without the valves being directly visualized. There is unilateral right, grade 5 vesicoureteral reflux *(R)*. **B,** Longitudinal ultrasound of right kidney shows marked dilatation of the renal collecting system and cortical thinning. **C,** Longitudinal ultrasound of protected left kidney shows a normal kidney.

diffuse increased echogenicity (Fig. 6-28A, B). Discrete cystic structures are sometimes not identified because of the small size of the cysts. In the juvenile form, patients usually present with hepatosplenomegaly and portal hypertension. The kidneys may demonstrate enlargement and cysts of varying sizes but may also appear normal. The liver usually shows increased echogenicity related to the diffuse hepatic fibrosis.

AUTOSOMAL DOMINANT POLYCYSTIC KIDNEY DISEASE

Autosomal dominant polycystic kidney disease, also known as adult polycystic kidney disease, is a dominantly inherited disease with variable penetrance. It is relatively common. Usually, the diagnosis is first encountered in early adulthood, when the patient presents with hypertension, hematuria, or renal failure. However, the cysts can be encountered during childhood. Some patients even present during the neonatal period. During childhood several cysts of varying sizes may be identified in both the cortex and medulla. The intervening renal parenchyma appears normal. The cysts gradually progress in size and number with time, and the normal renal parenchyma can be compressed and destroyed. Cysts may also be found in other organs, most commonly in the liver or pancreas. There is an association between the disease and the presence of intracranial berry aneurysms (10% of cases).

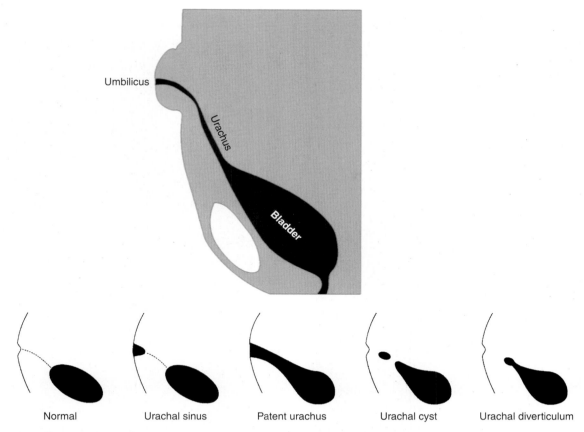

Umbilicus

Urachus

Bladder

Normal   Urachal sinus   Patent urachus   Urachal cyst   Urachal diverticulum

FIGURE 6-24. Urachal abnormalities. The superior image demonstrates the urachus as a patent connection between the umbilicus and bladder during fetal life. The inferior row of images demonstrates the potential urachal anomalies that occur when a portion or all of the urachus remains patent after birth. The type of urachal abnormality present depends upon which portion of the urachus remains patent.

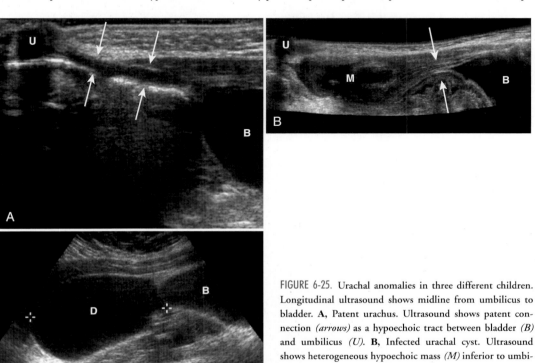

FIGURE 6-25. Urachal anomalies in three different children. Longitudinal ultrasound shows midline from umbilicus to bladder. **A,** Patent urachus. Ultrasound shows patent connection *(arrows)* as a hypoechoic tract between bladder *(B)* and umbilicus *(U)*. **B,** Infected urachal cyst. Ultrasound shows heterogeneous hypoechoic mass *(M)* inferior to umbilicus *(U)*, with associated tract *(arrows)* to bladder *(B)*. **C,** Urachal diverticulum. Ultrasound demonstrates diverticulum *(D)* extending from superior aspect of bladder *(B)*.

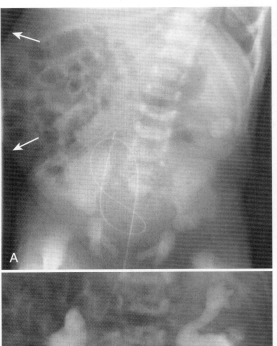

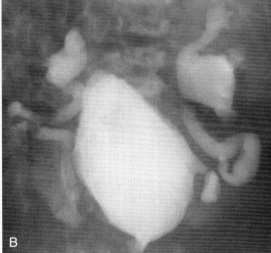

FIGURE 6-26. Prune belly syndrome. **A,** Radiograph shows bulging flanks *(arrows)*. **B,** VCUG shows bilateral grade 5 VUR and trabeculated bladder.

RENAL TUMORS

Wilms Tumor

Wilms tumor is the most common renal malignancy in children. It accounts for approximately 8% of all childhood malignant tumors. Also referred to as nephroblastoma, Wilms tumor is a malignant embryonal neoplasm. Its peak incidence occurs at approximately 3 years of age, with about 80% of cases detected between 1 and 5 years of age. Wilms tumor presents most commonly as an asymptomatic abdominal mass but may present with abdominal pain, particularly when there is intratumoral hemorrhage (Fig. 6-29A-C). Although most cases of Wilms tumor occur in otherwise normal children,

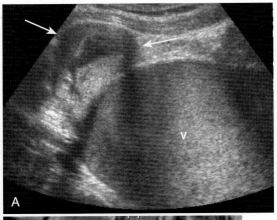

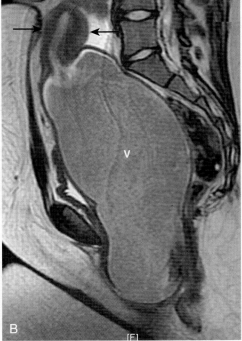

FIGURE 6-27. Hematometrocolpos shown in two different girls. **A,** Longitudinal midline ultrasound shows elliptical echogenic mass *(V)*, which represents the vaginal cavity markedly distended with blood products. The uterus *(arrows)* extends from the superior aspect of the mass. The uterine cavity is slightly dilatated but not nearly as much as the vaginal cavity. **B,** Sagittal T1-weighted MRI of a different girl shows massively dilatated vaginal cavity *(V)*. The uterus *(arrows)* extends from the superior aspect of the mass. The uterine cavity is slightly dilatated but not nearly as much as the vaginal cavity.

Wilm's tumor: Beckworth Wiademan

there is an association between the development of Wilms tumor and overgrowth disorders (congenital hemihypertrophy, Beckwith-Wiedemann syndrome), sporadic aniridia, and other malformations. Wilms tumor can be bilateral in approximately 5% of cases. Invasion of the renal vein and extension into the renal vein into the inferior

TABLE 6-1. Renal Cyst Disease in Children

Solitary simple cyst
Autosomal recessive polycystic renal disease
Autosomal dominant polycystic renal disease
Multicystic dysplastic kidney
Syndromes
    Tuberous sclerosis
    von Hippel-Lindau
    Meckel-Gruber
Cystic neoplasms
    Wilms tumor
    Multilocular cystic nephroma
Calyceal diverticulum

Wilm's ——→ lungs.

vena cava occurs commonly in Wilms tumor. Lung metastatic disease occurs in as many as 20% of cases.

On ultrasound, Wilms tumors typically appear as large, well-defined masses arising from the kidney (see Fig. 6-29). The masses are typically of increased echogenicity and may show heterogeneity related to areas of intratumoral hemorrhage, necrosis, or calcification. Doppler ultrasound is excellent in detecting extension of the tumor into the renal vein or inferior vena cava. It is especially important to document extension of the tumor thrombus into the right atrium because in such cases cardiothoracic surgery usually also becomes involved.

Confirmation of the lesion and evaluation of the anatomic extent of disease is usually performed using CT or MRI (Fig. 6-30A, B; and see Fig. 6-29). When evaluating a suspected Wilms tumor with either modality, it is important to document the following features: lymph node involvement, liver and lung metastases, involvement of the contralateral kidney by a synchronous Wilms tumor, the anatomic distribution of the intrarenal tumor, involvement of the renal vein or inferior vena cava, and the path of the ureters in relation to the mass. Identification of the ureter as anterior or posterior to the mass is important so that the ureters are not inadvertently injured when the mass is removed.

One of the most important issues when evaluating a mass in the region of the suprarenal fossa is determining whether the mass arises from the kidney and is therefore most likely a Wilms tumor or whether it arises from the suprarenal region and is a neuroblastoma. Differential features between these two lesions are described in Table 6-2. In the case of a Wilms tumor, the mass usually

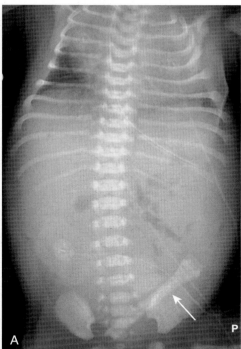

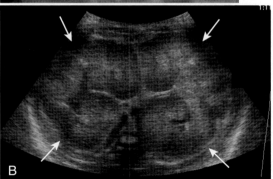

FIGURE 6-28. **Recessive polycystic kidney disease in an infant. A,** Radiography shows prominence of soft tissue in expected region of kidneys bilaterally. Incidentally, note the shadow caused by the umbilical clamp *(arrow)*, a common overlying artifact seen on radiographs of newborn infants. **B,** Axial ultrasound shows massive enlargement of bilateral kidneys *(arrows)*, which fill the majority of the abdominal cavity. The kidneys are of diffusely increased echogenicity, and no discrete cysts are identified.

appears as a well-defined, large, round mass on CT and MRI. The mass tends to grow in a ball, displacing blood vessels rather than engulfing them, as does neuroblastoma. As Wilms tumor arises in the kidney, the renal parenchyma often surrounds a portion of the mass, resulting in the "claw sign." When the mass crosses the midline, the lesion usually passes anterior to the aorta, as compared to neuroblastoma, which can surround the aorta posteriorly and raise it anteriorly, away

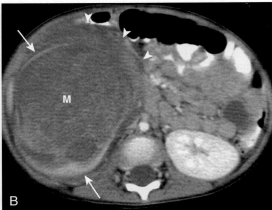

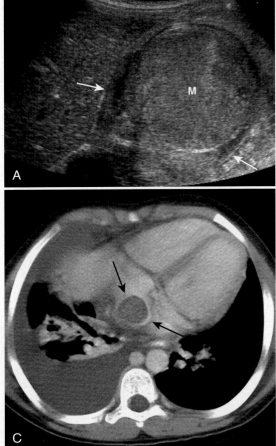

FIGURE 6-29. Wilms tumor in a 3-year-old presenting with acute pain secondary to intratumoral hemorrhage. **A,** Longitudinal ultrasound shows heterogeneously echogenic mass *(M)* arising from right kidney *(arrows)*. Note that the mass is round and ball-like. **B,** CT shows heterogeneous mass *(M)* arising from right kidney *(arrows)*. The parenchyma of the right kidney forms a claw sign, indicating that the mass is truly arising from the right kidney and is not a suprarenal mass. Note the crescent of heterogeneous attenuation *(arrowheads)* around the anterior aspect of the mass, consistent with hemorrhage. **C,** CT shows tumor thrombosis *(arrows)* as a filling defect extending along the inferior vena cava and into the right atrium. Note the right pleural effusion.

from the spine. Wilms tumors commonly appear to be solid, but larger lesions may have areas of heterogeneity or cystic components due to previous hemorrhage or necrosis.

the more nonenhancing nephrogenic rests. Typically, cases of Wilms tumor associated with syndromes are the ones that develop from nephroblastomatosis.

Nephroblastomatosis

Nephroblastomatosis is a rare entity that is related to the persistence of nephrogenic rests within the renal parenchyma. These nephrogenic rests are precursors of Wilms tumors. Most patients with nephroblastomatosis are monitored by ultrasound, MRI, or CT for the development of Wilms tumors. On imaging, nephrogenic rests appear as plaquelike peripheral renal lesions and may be confluent (Fig. 6-31). The development of a Wilms tumor is suggested when a lesion appearing spherical demonstrates an increase in size compared to previous studies or demonstrates progressively increasing inhomogeneous enhancement as compared to

Multilocular Cystic Nephroma

Multilocular cystic nephroma is a rare type of cystic mass that contains multiple septa. The lesions have an unusual bimodal distribution in that they affect primarily young boys (3 months to 2 years) and adult women (during the fifth to sixth decades). Typically, the lesions present as a painless abdominal mass. By definition, the lesions do not contain malignant cells but can be difficult to distinguish from a well-differentiated Wilms tumor on imaging. On ultrasound, CT, and MRI, the lesions appear as well-circumscribed, multiseptated masses (Fig. 6-32A-D). Because the lesions cannot be differentiated from malignancy at imaging, surgical resection is performed.

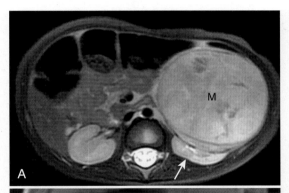

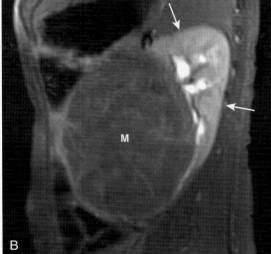

FIGURE 6-30. Wilms tumor on MRI. **A,** Axial T2-weighted image shows mass *(M)* arising from left kidney *(arrow)*. The lesion is heterogeneous in signal and is round. **B,** Sagittal post-contrast image shows low signal mass *(M)* and enhancing surrounding renal parenchyma *(arrows)*.

Mesoblastic Nephroma

Mesoblastic nephroma, or fetal renal hamartoma, is the most common renal mass in neonates. Typically, it is encountered prenatally or during the first few months of life; the mean age of

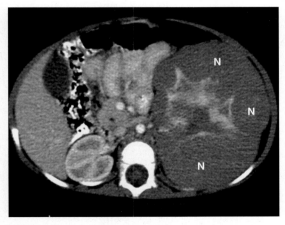

FIGURE 6-31. **Nephroblastomatosis.** CT shows peripheral plaquelike lesions *(N)* of low attenuation. The lesions circumferentially involve the left kidney and distort the central renal parenchyma. In this case, the right kidney is normal.

diagnosis is approximately 3 months. Neonates most commonly present with a nontender, palpable abdominal mass. The lesion consists of benign spindle-type cells. Ultrasound demonstrates a mixed echogenic mass that is intrarenal in location and indistinguishable from a Wilms tumor. CT demonstrates a solid intrarenal mass with variable enhancement (Fig. 6-33A, B).

Other Renal Tumors

Other, less common causes of malignant renal lesions include renal cell carcinoma, renal lymphoma, clear cell carcinoma, and rhabdoid tumor. Renal cell carcinoma is the most common cause of renal malignancy in older children, although it is still much less common than in adults. Ultrasound and CT typically show a nonspecific solid renal mass. Calcification is more common with renal cell carcinoma (25%) than with Wilms tumor.

TABLE 6-2. **Differentiating Features Between Neuroblastoma and Wilms Tumor**

Feature	Neuroblastoma	Wilms Tumor
Age	Most common before age 2 years	Peak incidence at 3 years
Calcification	Calcifications common (85% on CT) and stippled	Calcifications uncommon (15% on CT) and often curvilinear or amorphous
Growth pattern	Surrounds and engulfs vessels	Grows like ball, displacing vessels
Relation to kidney	Inferiorly displaces and rotates kidney	Arises from kidney, claw sign
Lung metastasis	Uncommon	More common (20%)
Vascular invasion	Does not occur	Invasion of renal vein/inferior vena cava

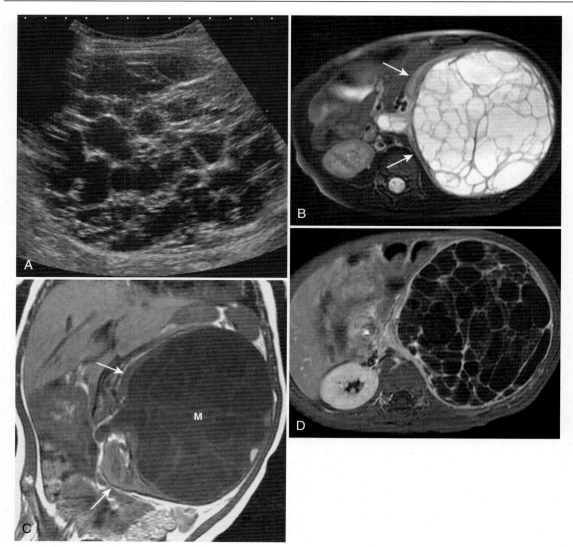

FIGURE 6-32. Multilocular cystic nephroma. **A,** Ultrasound shows a multiloculated cystic mass in the left kidney. **B,** T2-weighted, axial MR image shows multiseptated cystic mass. Note "claw sign" indicating origin of mass in left kidney *(arrows)*. **C,** T1-weighted, coronal MRI shows low signal in cystic structures within mass *(M)*. Again, note renal parenchyma *(arrows)* surrounding the medial aspect of the mass. **D,** Postcontrast, axial MR image shows only septal enhancement of cyst walls without solid components.

Angiomyolipoma

Patients with tuberous sclerosis are predisposed to developing angiomyolipomas. These lesions commonly demonstrate fatty components on imaging (Fig. 6-34A, B) and may spontaneously hemorrhage. Hemorrhage from angiomyolipomas is the leading cause of death in tuberous sclerosis patients. Angiomyolipomas bigger than 4 cm in diameter are particularly predisposed to contain dysplastic arteries and aneurysms that may hemorrhage; they are commonly treated by prophylactic embolization. The angiomyolipomas start as small echogenic foci within the kidneys during early childhood (Fig. 6-35) and grow into large infiltrative masses that enlarge the kidneys (see Fig. 6-34). Tuberous sclerosis is also associated with autosomal dominant polycystic kidney disease and renal cysts.

ADRENAL GLANDS

A number of pathologic processes can involve the adrenal glands in children. The most commonly encountered adrenal disorders are neuroblastoma and neonatal adrenal hemorrhage.

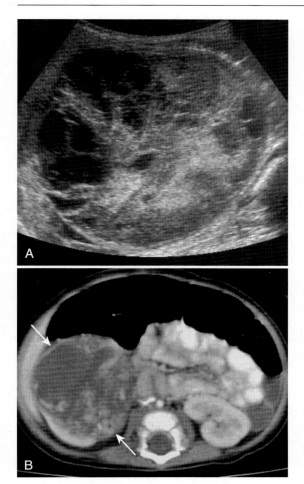

FIGURE 6-33. Mesoblastic nephroma in two neonates. **A,** Ultrasound shows a heterogeneous mass in the right kidney of a neonate. **B,** CT in another neonate shows a heterogeneously enhancing right renal mass *(arrows)*.

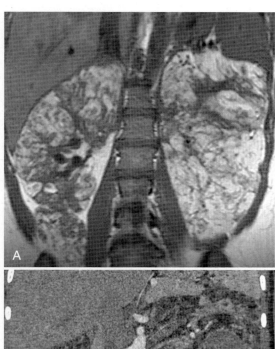

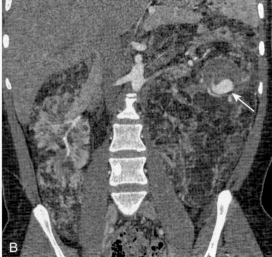

FIGURE 6-34. Advanced angiomyolipomas. **A,** T1-weighted coronal MR image shows diffuse fatty infiltration and enlargement of the bilateral kidneys. **B,** Coronal CT shows diffuse fatty infiltration and enlargement of the bilateral kidneys. There is contrast enhancement *(arrow)* within a partially thrombosed aneurysm in the left kidney.

Neuroblastoma

Neuroblastoma is a malignant tumor of primitive neural crest cells that most commonly arises in the adrenal gland but can occur anywhere along the sympathetic chain. It is differentiated from its more benign counterparts, ganglioneuroma and ganglioneuroblastoma, by the degree of cellular maturation. Neuroblastoma is an aggressive tumor with a tendency to invade adjacent tissues. The tumor metastasizes most commonly to liver and bone. It is the most common extracranial solid malignancy in children and the third most common malignancy of childhood, with only leukemia and primary brain tumors being more common. Approximately 90% to 95% of patients with neuroblastoma have elevated levels of catecholamines (vanillylmandelic acid) in their urine, a useful diagnostic tool.

Neuroblastoma is a very unusual tumor in that the prognosis and the patterns of distribution of disease depend strongly on age. In children who are less than 1 year of age, the disease tends to spread to liver and skin; they usually have a good prognosis. In those older than 1 year of age, the disease tends to spread to bone; they have a poorer prognosis. The staging (Evans) system for neuroblastoma is unique (Table 6-3). There is a special stage "IV s" that is given to children less than 1 year of age with

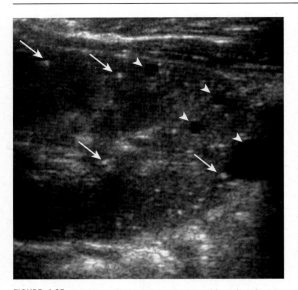

FIGURE 6-35. Angiomyolipoma in a 5 year old with tuberous sclerosis. Ultrasound shows multiple punctuate echogenic foci in the kidney. The most prominent echogenic foci are denoted by *arrows*. There are also multiple small cysts *(arrowheads)*.

metastatic disease that is confined to skin, liver, and bone marrow (Fig. 6-36A-D). Cortical bone involvement demonstrated by radiography or nuclear bone scintigraphy is not considered stage IV s. It is intriguing that patients with stage IV disease have very poor prognoses and commonly require therapy such as bone marrow transplantation, whereas patients with stage IV s disease have excellent prognoses and at many institutions are watched with imaging and

TABLE 6-3. **Evans Anatomic Staging for Neuroblastoma**

Stage	Definition	Prognosis (% survival)
I	Tumor confined to organ of origin	90
II	Tumor extension beyond organ of origin but not crossing midline	75
III	Tumor extension crossing midline	30
IV	Disseminated disease (skeleton or distant soft tissues, lymph nodes, and organs)	10
IV s	Age less than 1 year	Near 100
	Primary tumor with metastatic disease to skin, liver, or bone marrow	Often, no therapy

receive no therapy. Other factors associated with better prognoses are listed in Table 6-4.

Although neuroblastoma may be encountered initially as a mass on abdominal radiographs or ultrasound, confirmation of the diagnosis and definition of the exact extent of disease is obtained with either CT or MRI. Some investigators have advocated MRI over CT because of its superior ability to identify tumor extension into the neuroforamina. Neuroforaminal involvement is important to identify because, at many institutions, it will lead neurosurgery services to become involved in the surgical resection. In my experience, both CT and MRI are excellent in identifying neuroforaminal and spinal canal involvement.

On CT, neuroblastoma is detected with a sensitivity of nearly 100%. The tumors tend to appear lobulated and to grow in an invasive pattern, surrounding and engulfing, rather than displacing, vessels such as the celiac axis, superior mesenteric artery, and aorta (Fig. 6-37). The masses are often inhomogeneous secondary to hemorrhage, necrosis, and calcifications. Calcifications are seen by CT in as much as 85% of cases (see Fig. 6-37). On MRI, neuroblastoma, like most other malignancies, appears bright on T2-weighted images and can be heterogeneous in signal. Calcifications are less commonly seen on MRI. During the staging of neuroblastoma, most patients also undergo evaluation by metaiodobenzylguanidine (MIBG) and bone scintigraphy. The role of positron emission tomography (PET) and PET/CT is still being defined.

Other adrenal tumors that occur in childhood, but much less commonly than neuroblastoma, include pheochromocytoma and adrenal carcinoma.

Neonatal Adrenal Hemorrhage

Adrenal hemorrhage can occur in neonates secondary to birth trauma or stress. Like neuroblastoma, adrenal hemorrhage may present as an asymptomatic flank mass and may be seen on imaging as an adrenal mass. Surgical intervention is unnecessary in adrenal hemorrhage, so differentiation from neuroblastoma is important. Ultrasound is usually able to differentiate the two. Neuroblastoma typically appears as an echogenic mass with diffuse vascularity (color Doppler), whereas adrenal hemorrhage typically appears as an anechoic, avascular mass (Fig. 6-38). Performing serial ultrasounds over time (see Fig. 6-38) is an acceptable way of

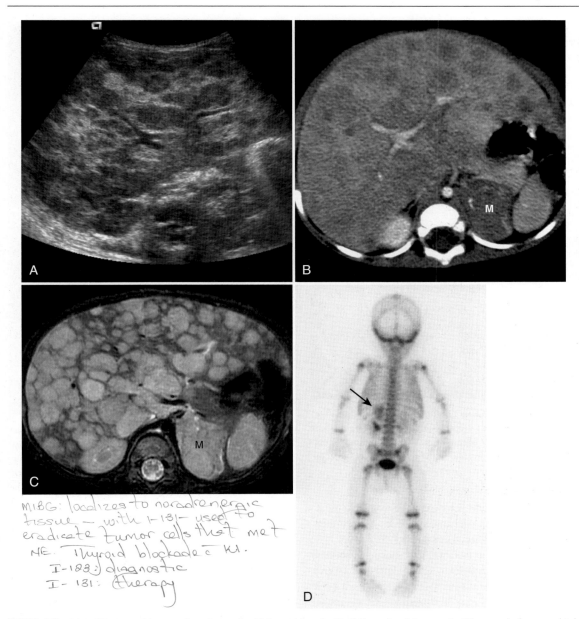

MIBG: localizes to noradrenergic
tissue — with I-131- used to
eradicate tumor cells that met
NE. Thyroid blockade c̄ KI.
 I-123: diagnostic
 I-131: therapy

FIGURE 6-36. Stage IV s neuroblastoma in a 9-month-old boy with palpable fullness in abdomen. **A,** Ultrasound shows multiple heterogeneous hypoechoic masses throughout the liver parenchyma. **B,** CT shows left suprarenal mass *(M)*. There are multiple low-attenuation metastatic lesions in the liver. **C,** T2-weighted axial MRI shows multiple liver metastatic lesions more clearly and again demonstrates left adrenal mass *(M)*. **D,** MIBG study (oriented with left side of patient on left of image) shows increased uptake in left adrenal mass *(arrow)*. There is downward displacement of the left renal collecting system.

differentiating problematic cases because the prognosis for neonates with stage I neuroblastoma is excellent. With time, adrenal hemorrhages decrease in size. MRI can also be useful in differentiating adrenal hemorrhage (low T2-weighted signal, blood product signal) from neuroblastoma (high T2-weighted signal) in very problematic cases.

PELVIC RHABDOMYOSARCOMA

Rhabdomyosarcoma is a highly malignant tumor that can occur in numerous locations throughout the body. It is the most common malignant sarcoma of childhood and typically presents during the first 3 years of life. Its most common locations include the pelvis and genitourinary tract

TABLE 6-4. Features Associated with Better Prognosis in Patients With Neuroblastoma

Age of diagnosis less than 1 year
Histologic grade
Decreased n-myc amplification
Stage IV s
Thoracic primary

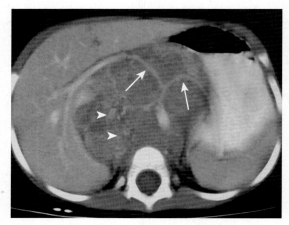

FIGURE 6-37. Neuroblastoma in a 2-year-old girl. CT shows heterogeneously enhancing retroperitoneal mass that surrounds and anteriorly displaces the abdominal aorta and engulfs and surrounds the branches *(arrows)* of the celiac artery. Note the heterogeneous calcifications *(arrowheads)*.

Bunch of Grapes

(39%) and the head and neck (39%). The most common locations within the genitourinary tract include the bladder, prostate (Fig. 6-39A, B), spermatic cord, paratesticular tissues, uterus, vagina, and perineum. It affects girls and boys equally. When the lesion involves the bladder, it typically appears as a multilobulated mass, likened to a bunch of grapes. Pelvic rhabdomyosarcoma may result in hydronephrosis.

Botryoides rhabdomyosarcoma
Walls of hollow, mucosa lined structures
urinary bladder, vagina, nasopharynx, CBD

SACROCOCCYGEAL TERATOMA

Sacrococcygeal teratomas typically present as large cystic or solid masses either on prenatal imaging or at birth. Less commonly, they present as buttock asymmetry or a presacral mass later in childhood. The majority are benign, but there is an increased risk for malignancy with delayed diagnosis. The masses can be primarily external (47%), internal within the pelvis (9%), or dumbbell-shaped, with both internal and external components (34%). On imaging, the lesions

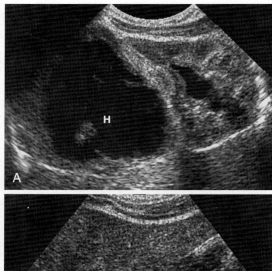

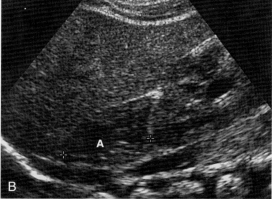

FIGURE 6-38. Adrenal hemorrhage in a 4-day-old neonate. A, Initial sonogram shows predominantly cystic-appearing, hypoechoic mass *(H)* in a suprarenal location. The kidney is displaced inferiorly. B, Follow-up ultrasound from approximately 1 month later shows marked interval decrease in the size of the adrenal gland *(A)*, a more adrenoform shape, and resolution of the cystic appearance, consistent with resolving hematoma.

f on full flw remnt of sibon

appear heterogeneous, with variable cystic, solid, and fatty components (Fig. 6-40A-E).

SCROTUM

The commonly encountered imaging issues in the pediatric scrotum include testicular neoplasm, testicular microlithiasis, and the acutely painful scrotum. Of testicular neoplasms, 90% are germ cell in origin. Less than 10% of testicular tumors are metastatic from leukemia or lymphoma. Most primary testicular tumors present with a nontender, firm scrotal mass. Ultrasound confirms an intratesticular mass (Fig. 6-41). However, there are no ultrasound findings that suggest a specific histologic diagnosis. If a scrotal mass is extratesticular in location, the most likely diagnosis is embryonal rhabdomyosarcoma arising from the spermatic cord or epididymis.

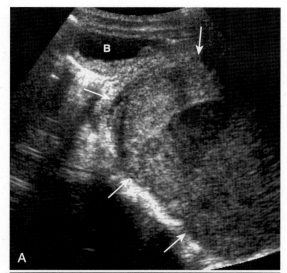

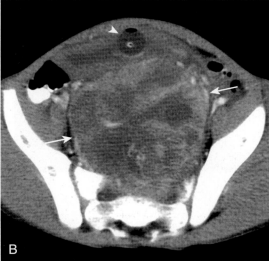

FIGURE 6-39. Rhabdomyosarcoma arising from the prostate in a boy. **A,** Longitudinal ultrasound shows large heterogeneous mass *(arrows)* arising from the pelvis and displacing the bladder *(B)*. **B,** CT shows a large heterogeneous mass *(arrows)* arising from the pelvis and displacing the bladder anteriorly (Foley catheter balloon demarcated by *arrowhead*).

Testicular Microlithiasis

Testicular microlithiasis appears on ultrasound as multiple small echogenicities within the testes (Fig. 6-42). There is often no posterior acoustic shadowing because of the small size of the calcifications. The finding is typically seen incidentally when the scrotum is being imaged for other reasons. It was initially reported that the risk for development of testicular neoplasm was

between 18% and 75% in patients with ultrasound-demonstrated testicular microlithiasis. This led to recommendations for serial screening ultrasounds in patients with testicular microlithiasis to exclude development of neoplasm. However, more recent reports have shown that testicular microlithiasis is much more common than initially suspected, occurring in about 6% of the male population between 17 and 35 years of age. These reports have also shown that the overwhelming majority of these patients will not develop malignancies. Some now advocate following such patients with physical examination rather than ultrasound.

The Acute Scrotum

Because of the possibility of testicular torsion, imaging of the acutely painful scrotum is an emergency. The major differential considerations in a child with acute scrotal pain include testicular torsion, epididymoorchitis, and torsion of the testicular appendage. Testicular hematoma is another less commonly encountered entity. The most common entities encountered in the setting of acute scrotal pain are actually epididymoorchitis and torsion of the testicular appendage. Although ultrasound examinations are performed to rule out testicular torsion, it is actually much less common than the other entities.

Testicular torsion occurs when the testis and cord twist within the serosal space and cause testicular ischemia. Prompt diagnosis and therapy are important because preservation of the testis is possible only in patients whose torsion is relieved within 6 to 10 hours. Color Doppler ultrasound has replaced testicular scintigraphy as the modality of choice in evaluating an acute scrotum. Color Doppler demonstrates absence of flow or asymmetrically decreased flow within the affected testis (Fig. 6-43A, B). Demonstration of flow within a normal testis is more difficult in children less than 2 years of age. Gray-scale ultrasound may demonstrate asymmetric enlargement and slightly decreased echogenicity of the affected testis (see Fig. 6-43). With progressive ischemia or infarction, hemorrhage and necrosis may cause increasing asymmetric heterogeneity (see Fig. 6-43). This is a late finding.

Epididymoorchitis usually occurs without an identifiable cause. In contrast to testicular torsion,

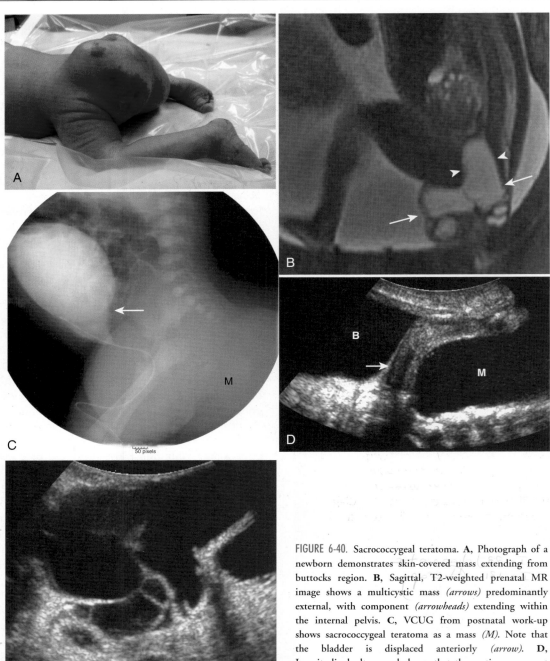

FIGURE 6-40. Sacrococcygeal teratoma. **A,** Photograph of a newborn demonstrates skin-covered mass extending from buttocks region. **B,** Sagittal, T2-weighted prenatal MR image shows a multicystic mass *(arrows)* predominantly external, with component *(arrowheads)* extending within the internal pelvis. **C,** VCUG from postnatal work-up shows sacrococcygeal teratoma as a mass *(M)*. Note that the bladder is displaced anteriorly *(arrow)*. **D,** Longitudinal ultrasound shows that the cystic component of the mass *(M)* extends superiorly to the level of the inferior bladder *(B)*. The uterus *(arrow)* is displaced posteriorly and superiorly. **E,** Ultrasound over the external portion of the mass shows its multicystic nature.

in epididymoorchitis the affected testis and epididymis demonstrate asymmetric and sometimes strikingly increased flow on Doppler ultrasound (Fig. 6-44A, B). Gray-scale ultrasound demonstrates enlargement and decreased echogenicity of the testis and epididymis. Reactive hydroceles are common.

Another cause of acute scrotum is torsion of the testicular appendage, a vestigial remnant of the mesonephric ducts. A mass of increased

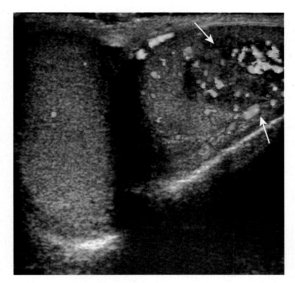

FIGURE 6-41. Testicular germ cell neoplasm. Transverse ultrasound shows focal, heterogeneous, hypoechogenic mass *(arrows)* in left testicle. Increased blood flow is shown on color Doppler.

echogenicity may be seen between the superior pole of the testis and the epididymis. Enlargement of the testicular appendage to greater than 5 mm has been touted as the best indicator of torsion. Periappendiceal hyperemia and normal testicular flow are supportive findings (Fig. 6-45A, B). Torsion of the testicular appendage is a self-limited entity and does not require surgical management. The importance of making the diagnosis is to avoid unnecessary surgical exploration.

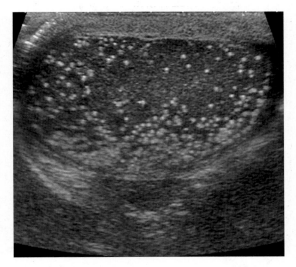

FIGURE 6-42. Testicular microlithiasis. Longitudinal ultrasound of the left testicle shows multiple punctate areas of increased echogenicity without posterior shadowing.

Trauma may result in a testicular hematoma. On ultrasound, hematomas appear as avascular masses of abnormal echogenicity. Associated hematoceles are common.

ACUTE PELVIC PAIN IN OLDER GIRLS AND ADOLESCENTS

Acute pelvic pain in older girls and adolescents is a commonly encountered problem that has many possible causes. Pain can be related to menstruation, multiple ovarian pathologies, or appendicitis. Ovarian causes of pain include ovarian cysts, hemorrhagic cysts, ectopic pregnancy, ovarian torsion, endometriosis, pelvic inflammatory disease, or other masses such as teratoma (Fig. 6-46A, B) or other neoplasms (Fig. 6-47A, B). Ovarian dermoids (mature teratoma) can show fluid/fluid levels, fat, and calcifications on imaging (see Fig. 6-46). Other ovarian neoplasms are usually large at the time of presentation (see Fig. 6-47), can have a cystic or solid appearance, and typically do not have differentiating features at imaging. In girls with right lower quadrant pain, appendicitis is also a possibility. The high incidence and variety of pathologic processes that may involve the ovaries make ultrasound the primary imaging modality for right lower quadrant pain in girls.

Hemorrhagic cysts are a common cause of pelvic pain in adolescent girls. On ultrasound, the lesions appear as echogenic masses that often have enhanced through-transmission. Sometimes the masses can be quite large. Ovarian cysts can be discovered when CT is performed to evaluate for appendicitis (Fig. 6-48).

Ovarian torsion, which is less common than hemorrhagic cysts, can appear as an enlarged and echogenic ovary secondary to edema. There can be prominent peripheral follicular cysts, which are highly suggestive of the diagnosis (Figs. 6-49A, B, 6-50). However, the most commonly encountered positive finding is asymmetric ovarian volumes, with the larger ovary located on the side of pain. Doppler ultrasound demonstration of decreased or absent blood flow has not been shown to be accurate in diagnosing or excluding ovarian torsion. Note that a hemorrhagic cyst compressing the ovarian parenchyma peripherally can have a similar appearance and at times cannot be differentiated from ovarian torsion.

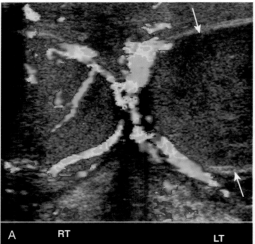

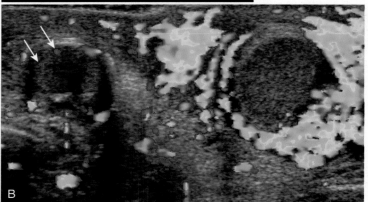

FIGURE 6-43. Testicular torsion, two examples. **A,** Transverse Doppler ultrasound showing both testes in a boy with left scrotal pain demonstrates absent flow and heterogeneous echo-texture of left testicle *(arrows)*. Note normal echo-texture and present flow on right. **B,** Later findings of torsion in different patient. Transverse Doppler ultrasound showing both testes in boy with left scrotal pain demonstrates absent flow and heterogeneous echo-texture of left testicle. Note the flow detected *(arrows)* in the right testicle. There is a large amount of flow surrounding the left testicle, related to inflammatory reaction secondary to the necrosis.

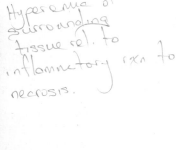

Hyperemia of surrounding tissue rel. to inflammatory rxn to necrosis.

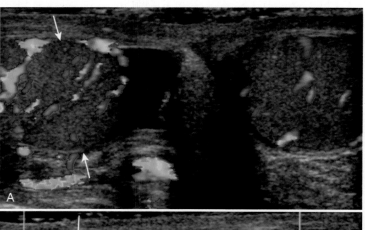

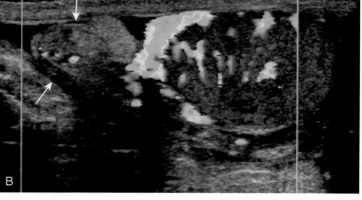

FIGURE 6-44. Epidydimoorchitis in a boy with acute onset of right scrotal pain. **A,** Transverse color Doppler ultrasound shows asymmetric increased flow to the symptomatic right testis *(arrows)*. There is a reactive hydrocele. **B,** Longitudinal color Doppler ultrasound shows enlarged epidydimis *(arrows)*. There is increased flow to both the epidydimis and the testicle.

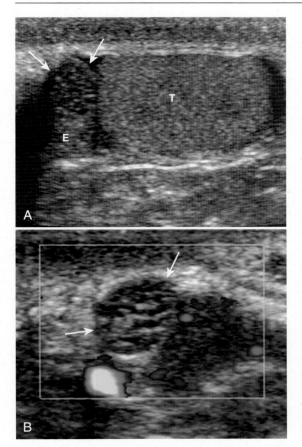

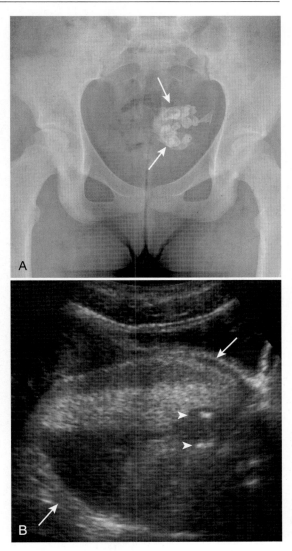

FIGURE 6-45. Torsion of the testicular appendage. **A,** Longitudinal view of the symptomatic side shows testicular appendage *(arrows)* to be enlarged (>5 mm). The appendage sits between the testicle *(T)* and the epididymis *(E)*. **B,** Color Doppler ultrasound image shows absence of flow to the testicular appendage *(arrows)*.

FIGURE 6-46. Ovarian dermoid (mature teratoma). **A,** Radiograph shows cluster of well-developed teeth in the pelvis *(arrows)*. **B,** Ultrasound demonstrates mass in left ovary *(arrows)* with fluid-fluid levels of various echogenicities. Note echogenic teeth *(arrowheads)*.

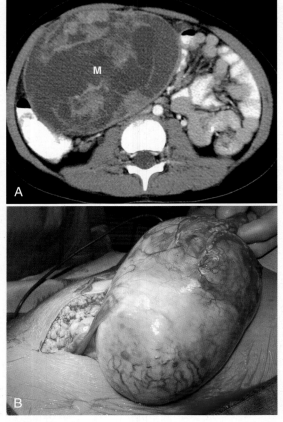

FIGURE 6-47. Sertoli cell neoplasm of the ovary. **A,** CT shows heterogeneous mass arising from right superior pelvis *(M).* **B,** Surgical photograph shows large mass arising from right ovary.

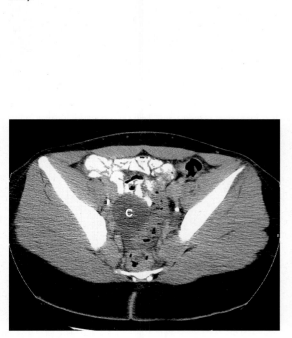

FIGURE 6-48. Hemorrhagic cyst identified on CT in a 14-year-old obese girl with right lower quadrant pain and suspected appendicitis. CT shows 5-cm cyst *(C)* in region of right adnexa.

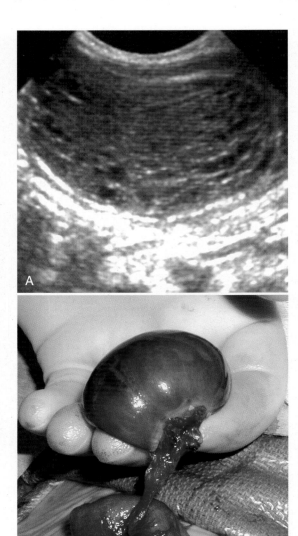

FIGURE 6-49. Ovarian torsion. **A,** Ultrasound shows asymmetrically enlarged ovary with increased echogenicity and some peripheral cysts. Doppler evaluation (not shown) showed no vascular flow. **B,** Surgical photograph showing infarcted ovary.

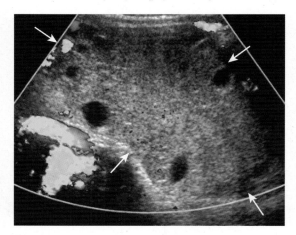

FIGURE 6-50. Ovarian torsion. Ultrasound shows asymmetrically enlarged ovary *(arrows)* with increased echogenicity and peripheral cysts. Doppler evaluation shows no vascular flow to ovary.

Suggested Readings

Daneman A, Alton DJ: Radiographic manifestations of renal anomalies, *Radiol Clin North Am* 29:351-363, 1991.

Frush DP, Sheldon CA: Diagnostic imaging of pediatric scrotal disorders, *Radiographics* 18:969-985, 1998.

Han BK, Babcock DS: Sonographic measurements and appearance of normal kidneys in children, *AJR* 145: 611-618, 1985.

Hartman DS: Renal cystic disease in multisystem conditions, *Urol Radiol* 14:13-17, 1992.

Kirks DR, Kaufman RA, Babcock DS: Renal neoplasms in infants and children, *Semin Roentgenol* 22:292-302, 1987.

Kraus SJ: Genitourinary imaging in children. *Pediatr Clin North Am* 48:1381-1424, 2001.

Lebowitz RL, Olbing H, Parkkulainen KV, et al: International system of radiographic grading of vesicoureteral reflux: International reflux study in children, *Pediatr Radiol* 15:105-109, 1985.

Ng YY, Kingston JE: The role of radiology in the staging of neuroblastoma, *Clin Radiol* 47:226-235, 1993.

Sty JR, Wells RY, Schroeder BA, Starshak RJ: Diagnostic imaging in pediatric renal inflammatory disease, *JAMA* 256:895-899, 1986.

CHAPTER SEVEN

Musculoskeletal

PEDIATRIC OBESITY

It has been well reported in the lay press that pediatric obesity has reached epidemic proportions. It is estimated that somewhere between one fifth and one third of children in the United States are obese; pediatric obesity is also becoming a worldwide trend. If you consider which pediatric diseases are common and which cause significant morbidity and mortality in adulthood, pediatric obesity may well be the number one pediatric health concern. Obesity is a multiorgan system problem, but because it is a disease of the soft tissues, it is included here in the musculoskeletal chapter.

Pediatric obesity has a well-documented association with several diseases of childhood such as slipped capital femoral epiphysis (Fig. 7-1) but is also associated with a host of other potential problems, including: psychosocial problems (poor self-esteem, depression); glucose intolerance/ type 2 diabetes (the frequency of pediatric type 2 diabetes has increased 100 times in the past 20 years in Cincinnati); hyperlipidemia; steatohepatitis; cholelithiasis; obstructive sleep apnea; hypertension; and pulmonary embolism. Many of these traditionally adult disorders are now being encountered in obese children. Perhaps most concerning, approximately 80% of obese children will go on to be obese adults and have all of the associated morbidity.

Obesity poses multiple challenges for imaging in a pediatric setting. Most children's hospitals are geared toward dealing with the small end of the human spectrum, but they have not traditionally been well equipped to deal with the large end. Issues of image quality, imaging equipment weight limits, and diameter size limits can all be problematic.

Some have suggested that pediatric radiologists can take an advocacy role in raising awareness of pediatric obesity by including mention of obesity, when obviously present, within the impression of radiology reports. Written documentation of obesity in an official report can increase caregivers' and parents' awareness of a child's obesity.

NORMAL VARIANTS AND COMMON BENIGN ENTITIES

Probably more than in any other organ system, the normal imaging appearance of the skeletal system is strikingly different in children from its appearance in adults (Fig. 7-2A-D). This is related to the changing appearance of growing and maturing bone. The most striking changes occur in the vicinity of physes and apophyses. Many of the more common mistakes made in pediatric skeletal radiology are related to the misinterpretation of normal structures as being abnormal. Textbooks are dedicated to the normal radiographic appearances and variations of bones in children. The details of the normal changes in the radiographic appearance throughout the maturing skeleton cannot be covered here. The following section describes several normal variants and commonly encountered benign entities.

Apophyseal Irregularity

In the growing child, apophyses in various parts of the body can have variable and often somewhat irregular appearances. Separate ossicles of an apophysis can mimic fragments, irregularity can mimic periosteal reaction, and mixed sclerosis and lucency can be confused with findings of an inflammatory or neoplastic process. Common apophyses that may have this appearance include tibial tuberosity, ischeal tuberosity, ischeal pubic synchondrosis, and posterior calcaneal apophysis (Fig. 7-3A-C). Irregularity and fragmentation are commonly seen in the normal tibial tuberosity. The calcaneal apophysis can often demonstrate a strikingly sclerotic appearance. The ischeal pubic synchondrosis can appear very prominent and asymmetric.

Distal Femoral Metaphyseal Irregularity

Distal femoral metaphyseal irregularity, also referred to as cortical desmoid and cortical

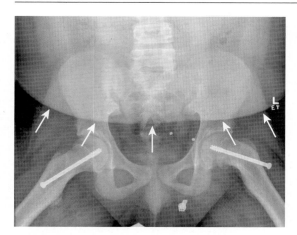

FIGURE 7-1. Obese teenager with pins previously placed for bilateral slipped capital femoral epiphyses. Note the large panniculus of abdominal fat *(arrows)*.

irregularity syndrome, refers to the presence of irregular cortical margination and associated lucency involving the posteromedial aspect of the distal femoral metaphysis. It occurs in as many as 11% of boys aged 10 to 15 years. Although debated, its presence is thought to be related to chronic avulsion at the insertion of the adductor magnus muscle. Although this lesion can be associated with pain, it is often discovered incidentally, and its significance lies in its alarming radiographic appearance. On radiography, there is cortical irregularity present along the posteromedial cortex of the distal femoral metaphysis, best seen on the lateral view (Fig. 7-4A-C). On frontal radiographs, there may be an associated lucency (see Fig. 7-4). Familiarity with the typical location, appearance, and patient age is important so that these lesions are not confused with aggressive malignancies. Because the lesions are often bilateral, confirmation of their benign nature can be made by demonstrating a similar lesion on radiographs

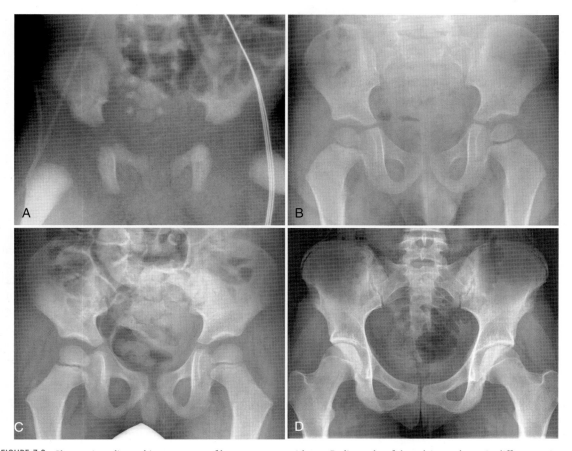

FIGURE 7-2. Changes in radiographic appearance of bony structures with age. Radiographs of the pelvis are shown in different patients. **A,** at birth; B, at 2 years of age; **C,** at 5 years of age; **D,** at 15 years of age. Note the dramatic changes in the appearance of the pelvis as structures ossify over time. At birth (in A), the femoral heads and large portions of the ischium are yet to ossify.

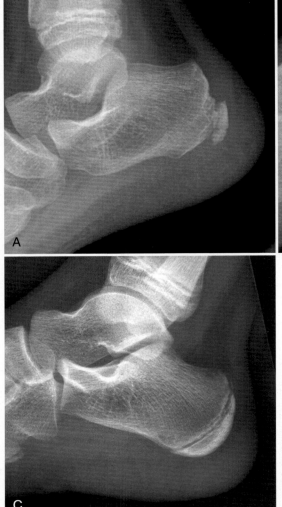

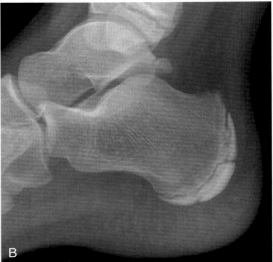

FIGURE 7-3. Apophyseal irregularity; examples of variability in the fragmented appearance of posterior apophysis of the calcaneous in three normal 10-year-old children. **A,** Ossified portion of posterior apophysis is small and appears as fragmented ossicles. **B,** Ossified portion of posterior apophysis extends along total posterior border of calcaneous and has multiple separate-appearing ossicles. **C,** Ossified portion of posterior apophysis extends along total posterior border of calcaneous and appears as one solid piece of ossified bone.

of the opposite knee. In problematic cases, computed tomography (CT) or magnetic resonance imaging (MRI) can be used to demonstrate the characteristic findings: a characteristic scooplike defect with an irregular but intact cortex; no associated soft tissue mass; and sometimes a subtle contralateral lesion (see Fig. 7-4).

Benign Cortical Defects

Benign cortical defects, or nonossifying fibromas, are commonly encountered lesions of no clinical significance. They are seen in as many as 40% of children at some time during development and are most common between 5 and 6 years of age. The term *nonossifying fibroma* is typically reserved for larger lesions. They occur most

commonly within the bones around the knee, particularly the distal femur. They appear as lucent, eccentric, well-defined lesions with thin cortical rims (Fig. 7-5) and are typically round or oval. Over time they become more sclerotic and eventually resolve. When the characteristic pattern is identified, no further imaging or follow-up is necessary.

TRAUMA

Fractures in children differ from those in adults for multiple reasons. Children's bones are more pliable and have a greater propensity to deform prior to breaking. Therefore, incomplete fractures are more common in children than adults. The incomplete fracture may be purely

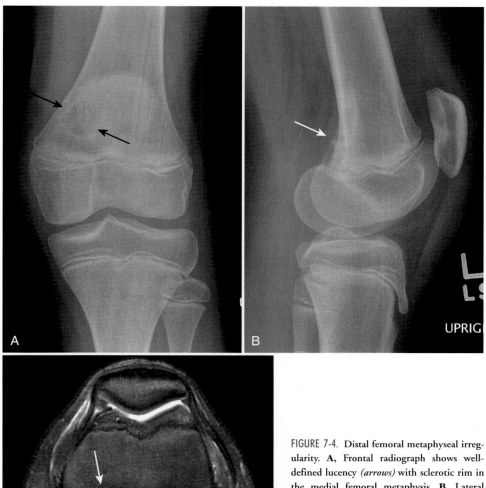

FIGURE 7-4. Distal femoral metaphyseal irregularity. **A,** Frontal radiograph shows well-defined lucency *(arrows)* with sclerotic rim in the medial femoral metaphysis. **B,** Lateral radiograph shows irregularity *(arrow)* along the posterior cortex of the distal femoral metaphysis. **C,** T2-weighted axial MRI in a different patient shows a high signal *(arrows)* internal and external to the posteromedial cortex of the distal femur in the region of the adductor magnus insertion. Note the characteristic position and lack of associated soft tissue mass.

a bowing type of fracture (Fig. 7-6), may be associated with a buckling of the cortex on the concave margin of the bowing (torus fracture), or may demonstrate an incomplete fracture along the cortex of the convex margin of the bowing (greenstick fracture; see Fig. 7-6). Buckle fractures may be subtle and may appear only as an increase in acute angulation of a normally gentler curve (Fig. 7-7).

The potential for healing and the healing rate of fractures also differ in children and adults. Younger children heal very quickly. Periosteal reaction can be expected to be radiographically present 7 to 10 days after injuries in children. Children also tend to heal completely. Nonunited fractures are very uncommon in children. Fracture remodeling is also rapid and impressively complete in fractures of pediatric long bones. Normal alignment is typically restored.

Involvement of the Physis

One of the potential problematic issues with fractures in children is involvement of the physis.

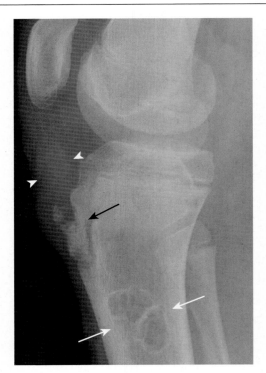

FIGURE 7-5. Nonossifying fibroma visualized incidentally in a 13-year-old child with knee pain. Radiograph shows well-defined lesion *(white arrows)* with sclerotic borders consistent with nonossifying fibroma. The cause of pain is identified as Osgood-Schlatter disease. Note fragmentation of tibial tubercle *(black arrow)* and enlargement and indistinctness of distal patellar tendon *(arrowheads)*.

The physis is involved in as many as 18% of pediatric long bone fractures. Physeal involvement may result in growth arrest of that limb and in a higher rate of necessary internal fixation. The standard classification for physeal fractures is that by Salter and Harris. It divides fractures into five types according to whether there is involvement of the physis, epiphysis, or metaphysis, as determined by radiography (Fig. 7-8). Fractures with higher numbers have a greater incidence of complications. Type 1 fractures involve only the physis. They tend to occur in children younger than 5 years of age. On radiography, the epiphysis may appear to be displaced in comparison to the metaphysis. However, type 1 fractures often reduce prior to the radiograph's being obtained, and the only imaging finding will be soft tissue swelling adjacent to the physis. Type 2 fractures involve the metaphysis and the physis but do not involve the epiphysis (Fig. 7-9A, B). They are the most common type of physeal injury (up to 75%). On radiography, there is typically a triangular

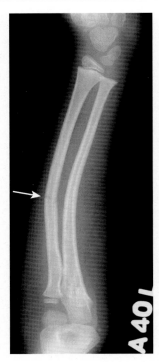

FIGURE 7-6. **Incomplete fractures of the radius and ulna.** The radius demonstrates a greenstick fracture with an incomplete fracture along the convex margin of the cortex *(arrow)*. The ulna demonstrates a bowing fracture.

fragment of bony metaphysis attached to the physis and epiphysis. Type 3 fractures involve the physis and epiphysis but not the metaphysis (see Fig. 7-9). Type 3 injuries have a greater predisposition for growth arrest. Type 4 injuries involve the epiphysis, physis, and metaphysis and, like type 3 injuries, are associated with a high rate of growth arrest. Type 5 fractures consist of a crush injury to part of or all of the physis. Posttraumatic growth arrest may be detected radiographically by demonstration of a bony bridge across the physis.

Commonly Encountered Fractures by Anatomic Location

Pediatric fractures have unique features in almost all locations. The following material reviews several of the more commonly encountered areas.

WRIST

The wrist is the most common fracture site in children. Most fractures of the distal forearm are buckle or transverse fractures of the distal

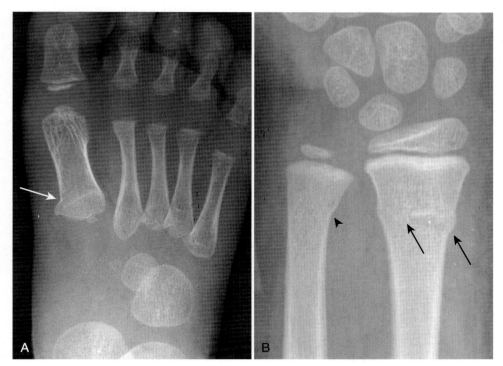

FIGURE 7-7. Buckle fractures. **A**, Radiograph shows increased angulation *(arrow)* of the medial aspect of the proximal portion of the first metatarsal bone consistent with a buckle fracture. **B**, Radiograph of the wrist shows transverse fracture through radius *(arrows)* with buckle component. Also note the buckle fracture of the ulna *(arrowhead)* shown by the increased angulation of the cortex.

metaphysis of the radius, with or without fracture of the distal metaphysis of the ulna (see Figs. 7-7, 7-9). However, the distal radius is also the most common area of physeal fracture (28% of physeal injuries occur in the distal radius). Displacement or obliteration of the pronator fat pad indicates a fracture or deep soft tissue injury. The normal pronator fat pad is visualized on a lateral view of the forearm as a thin line of fat with a mildly convex border. In most distal forearm fractures, the convexity of the pronator fat pad is increased or the fat pad becomes obliterated by soft tissue attenuation.

ELBOW

There are several unusual features that make elbow injuries in children different from those in adults. In contrast to adults, in whom fracture of the radial neck is the most common injury, children most commonly experience supracondylar fractures. They usually occur secondary to hyperextension that occurs when falling on an outstretched arm. As many as 25% of such fractures are incomplete and may be subtle on radiography. On radiographs, there can be posterior displacement of the distal fragment such that a line drawn down the anterior cortex of the humerus

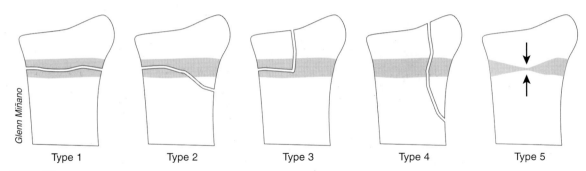

FIGURE 7-8. Diagram showing Salter-Harris classification of fractures involving the physis.

Type 1   Type 2   Type 3   Type 4   Type 5

Glenn Miñano

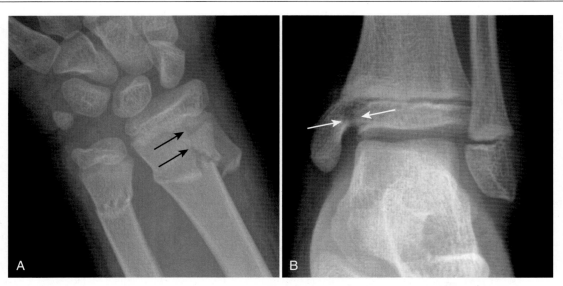

FIGURE 7-9. Examples of Salter fractures. **A,** Salter 2 fracture of the distal radius. Radiograph shows transverse fractures of the distal radius and ulna. The fracture of the radius has an associated longitudinal metaphyseal component *(arrows)* that extends into the physis, making this a Salter 2 fracture. **B,** Salter 3 type fracture of the distal tibia. Radiograph shows a vertical intraarticular fracture *(arrows)* involving the medial epiphysis of the distal tibia. The fracture extends into the physis, making this a Salter 3 fracture.

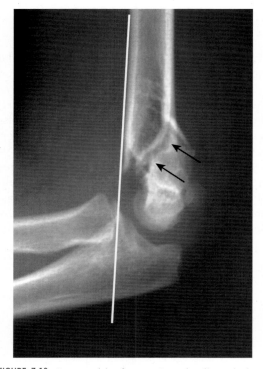

FIGURE 7-10. Supracondylar fracture. Lateral radiograph shows fracture line through the anterior cortex *(arrows)* with posterior displacement of the distal fragment. There is posterior displacement of the capitellum in relation to the anterior humeral line *(line drawn).*

(anterior humeral line) no longer bisects the middle third of the capitellum (Fig. 7-10). The fracture line is usually best seen through the anterior cortex of the distal humerus on the lateral view (see Fig. 7-10). A joint effusion is typically evident. Elbow effusions are identified when there is displacement of the posterior fat pad, resulting in its visualization on a lateral view (Fig. 7-11A, B). Normally, the posterior fat pad rests within the olecranon fossa and is not visible on a true lateral view of the elbow. The anterior fat pad, which is often visible normally, may become prominent and have a prominent apex anterior convexity.

There is much debate about the significance of a traumatic elbow effusion in the absence of a visualized fracture. It is often taught that such a joint effusion is synonymous with an occult fracture. However, studies have shown that fractures are probably present in the minority, rather than in the majority of such cases. The point is moot because traumatic injury to the elbow is treated by splinting, whether a subtle fracture is identified or not. Therefore, obtaining additional oblique views or follow-up studies to document the presence or absence of a fracture adds radiation and does not alter patient care.

Other elbow injuries include fractures of the lateral condyle (Fig. 7-12) and avulsion of the medial epicondyle (Little League elbow; Fig. 7-13). With avulsion of the medial epicondyle

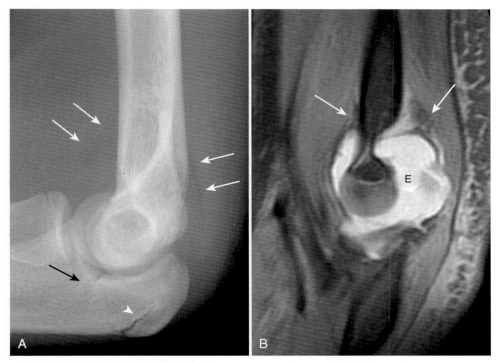

FIGURE 7-11. Traumatic elbow effusion. **A,** Lateral radiograph of the elbow shows elevation of both the anterior and posterior fat pads *(white arrows)* consistent with traumatic elbow effusion. The patient has a nondisplaced, intraarticular fracture through the olecranon *(black arrow)*. Note the normal variant line with sclerotic margins *(arrowhead)* through the more posterior olecranon. **B,** Elbow effusion demonstrated on MRI for illustrative purposes in a different patient. Sagittal T2-weighted image shows large joint effusion *(E)* that uplifts and displaces the anterior and posterior fat pads *(arrows)*. The fat pads are low in signal on this fat-saturated image. The joint effusion raises the posterior fat pad out of the olecranon fossa, making it visible on lateral radiography.

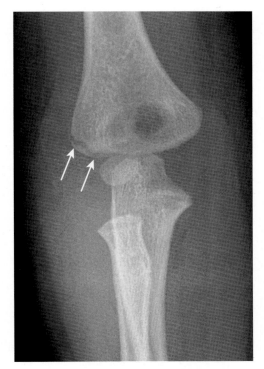

FIGURE 7-12. Fracture of the lateral condyle. Radiograph shows avulsed sliver of bone *(arrows)* arising from lateral condyle.

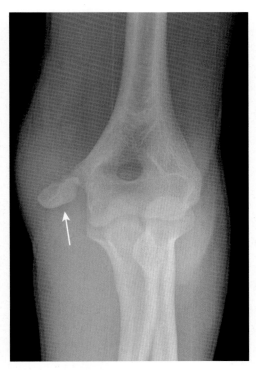

FIGURE 7-13. Avulsion of the medial epicondyle. Frontal radiograph shows displacement of medial epicondyle *(arrow)* and overlying soft tissue swelling.

(10% of elbow injuries), the medial epicondyle may become displaced. To avoid mistaking the displaced apophysis for one of the other ossicles of the elbow, it is important to know the predictable order of ossification of the elbow ossification centers. The order can be remembered by the mnemonic CRITOEcal (capitellum, radial head, internal epicondyle, trochlea, olecranon, external epicondyle). Whenever there is a fracture of the forearm, it is important to evaluate the radial-capitellar joint for potential dislocation of the radial head. The radial head should align with the capitellum. If it does not, radial head dislocation should be suspected (Fig. 7-14).

Toddler's Fracture

When a child first begins to walk, a nondisplaced oblique or spiral fracture of the midshaft of the tibia can occur (Fig. 7-15). Such an injury is common and is referred to as a toddler's fracture. Most children present with failure to continue to walk or refusal to bear weight on that extremity. Oblique views often demonstrate the fracture better than do frontal or lateral views. Toddlers can also suffer from similar types of

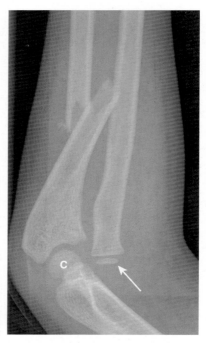

FIGURE 7-14. Monteggia fracture. Radiograph shows fracture through proximal one third of ulna. There is also dislocation of the radial head. The radial head *(arrow)* does not line up with the capitellum *(C)*.

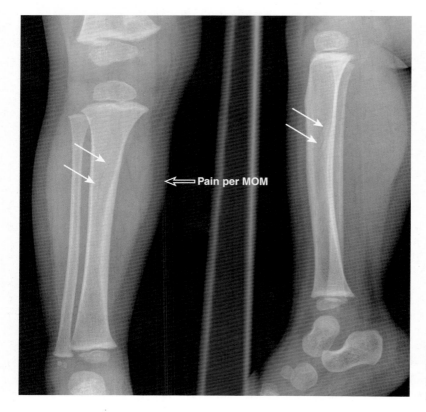

Pain per MOM

FIGURE 7-15. Toddler's fracture. Radiographs show subtle oblique, nondisplaced fracture *(arrows)* through proximal tibial shaft.

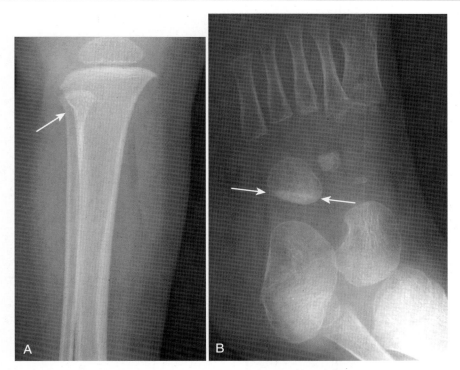

FIGURE 7-16. Toddler's fractures: other common sites. **A,** Radiograph shows buckle fracture *(arrow)* through the proximal tibia. **B,** Radiograph shows sclerotic band *(arrows)* indicating toddler's fracture of the cuboid.

fractures involving the proximal anterior tibia, calcaneus, or cuboid (Fig. 7-16A, B).

Avulsion Fractures in Adolescents

An avulsion injury is a structural failure of bone at a tendon or aponeurotic insertion and is related to a tensile force being applied by a musculoskeletal unit. Adolescents are prone to avulsive injuries because of a combination of their propensity to have great strength, their ability to sustain extreme levels of activity, and their immature, growing apophyses. The growing apophysis is often more prone to injury than the adjacent tendons. The sites of insertion of muscles capable of generating great forces are most predisposed to avulsion injuries.

Radiologists may encounter findings of chronic avulsion when patients are imaged for pain or incidentally when imaging is performed for other reasons. The irregularity and periostitis that can be associated with chronic avulsions should not be misinterpreted as suspicious for malignancy. In addition, if unwarranted biopsies of these areas are performed, the histologic changes associated with the healing callus of the avulsion injury may be misinterpreted as

malignancy. The most common sites of avulsion occur within the pelvis, where muscles capable of great force attach. Sites at which apophyseal avulsions most commonly occur, along with the associated muscular attachments, are the iliac crest (transversalis, internal oblique abdominalis, external oblique abdominalis); the anterior superior iliac spine (sartorius); the anteroinferior iliac spine (rectus femoris; Fig. 7-17A-C); the ischial apophysis (hamstring muscles: biceps femoris, gracilis, semimembranosus, semitendinosus; Fig. 7-18A, B); and the lesser trochanter (iliopsoas). The radiographic findings of avulsion injuries include displacement of the ossified apophysis from normal position and variable, and often exuberant, amounts of associated periosteal new bone formation.

The extensor mechanism of the knee consists of the quadriceps femoris muscles, the quadriceps tendon, the patella, the patellar tendon, and the patellar tendon insertion on the tibial tuberosity; this mechanism can also be involved by avulsion injuries. Chronic avulsion of the patellar tendon at its attachment to the patella is called Sinding-Larsen-Johansson syndrome. It occurs most commonly in children between the ages of 10 and 14 years of age. Symptoms include localized pain and swelling

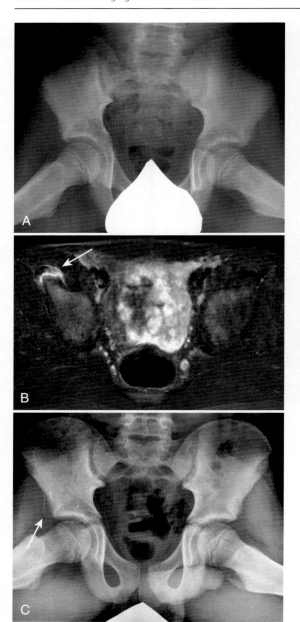

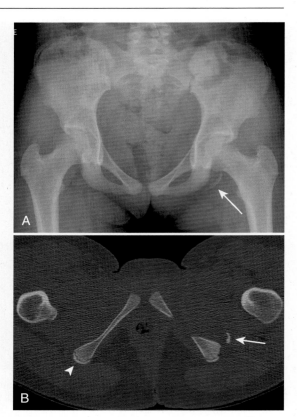

FIGURE 7-18. Avulsion injury of the ischeal apophysis associated with acute pain in a teenage high-performance athlete. **A,** Radiograph shows a crescentic fragment of bone *(arrow)* displaced from the left ischeal apophysis. **B,** CT obtained for potential pinning in this athlete shows that the anterior portion of the apophysis *(arrow)* is displaced anteriorly. Note normal-appearing right ischeal apophysis *(arrowhead).*

FIGURE 7-17. Avulsion of the right anterior inferior iliac spine associated with acute pain in a teenage athlete. **A,** Initial radiograph is normal. **B,** Axial, T2-weighted MR image obtained to evaluate acute pain shows high-signal edema and displacement of the apophysis of the right anteroinferior iliac spine *(arrow).* **C,** Follow-up radiograph 3 weeks later shows ossified callus formation *(arrow)* around the site of the injury.

over the inferior aspect of the patella associated with restricted knee motion. Radiography demonstrates irregular bony fragments at the inferior margin of the patella associated with adjacent soft tissue swelling and thickening and indistinctness of the patellar tendon (Fig. 7-19A, B). Chronic avulsive injury of the

patellar tendon at its inferior attachment is referred to as Osgood-Schlatter lesion (tibial tuberosity avulsion). It is a common disorder that most often affects active adolescent boys. Symptoms include pain and swelling over the tibial tuberosity. Radiography demonstrates bony fragmentation of the tibial tuberosity, associated adjacent soft tissue swelling, and thickening and indistinctness of the patellar tendon (Fig. 7-20A, B; and see Fig. 7-5).

Child Abuse

Child abuse, also referred to as the more politically correct and less graphic nonaccidental trauma, is unfortunately common. It is estimated that more than 1 million children are seriously injured and 5000 killed secondary to abuse each year in the United States alone. Most of the

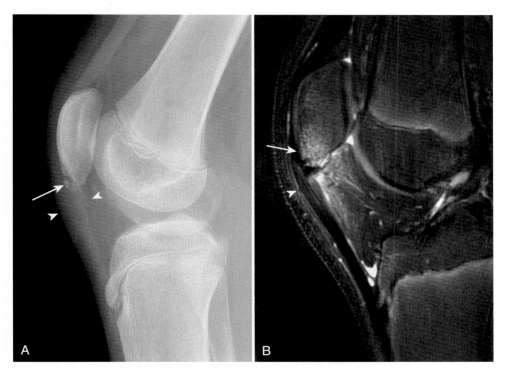

FIGURE 7-19. Sinding-Larsen-Johansson syndrome: chronic avulsion of the patellar tendon at its attachment to the patella. **A,** Radiograph shows thickening of the proximal patellar tendon *(arrowheads)* and irregularity and fragmentation at the attachment to the distal patella *(arrow).* **B,** T2-weighted, sagittal MR image shows high-signal edema within the distal end of the patella *(arrow),* the proximal patellar tendon *(arrowhead),* and in the adjacent portions of the Hoffa fat pad.

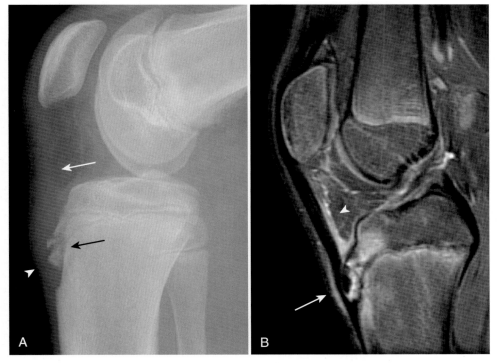

FIGURE 7-20. Osgood-Schlatter lesion: chronic avulsion of the patellar tendon at its attachment to the tibial tuberosity. **A,** Radiograph shows irregularity and fragmentation of the tibial tuberosity *(black arrow)* with overlying soft tissue swelling *(arrowhead).* Note thickening of the distal patellar tendon *(white arrow).* **B,** T2-weighted, sagittal MR image shows high-signal edema within the tibial tuberosity *(arrow)* and extending along the distal patellar tendon *(arrowhead).*

children are less than 1 year of age and almost all are less than 6 years of age. When clinical or imaging findings are suspicious for potential abuse, a radiographic skeletal survey is typically obtained. The purpose of the skeletal survey is to document the presence of findings of abuse for legal reasons so that the child can be removed from exposure to the abuser. Other tests sometimes used include a repeat skeletal survey after approximately 2 weeks to look for healing injuries not seen on the initial skeletal survey, skeletal scintigraphy, abdominal CT, and MRI of the brain. The identification and reporting of findings of child abuse by the radiologist is an important task. False-positive cases can cause a nonabused child to be removed from his or her family, whereas false-negative cases can result in a child's returning to a potentially life-threatening environment.

The radiographic findings of abuse vary in their specificity. One of the highly specific findings is the presence of posterior rib fractures occurring near the costovertebral joints (Fig. 7-21A-F). These are thought to occur when an adult squeezes an infant's thorax. Such rib fractures may be subtle prior to development of callus formation. The evaluation for rib fractures should be a routine part of the evaluation of the chest radiograph of any infant. Another finding that is highly specific for abuse is the metaphyseal corner fracture (see Fig. 7-21). This fracture extends through the primary spongiosa of the metaphysis, the weakest portion, and usually occurs secondary to forceful pulling of an extremity. The broken metaphyseal rim appears as a corner fracture (a triangular piece of bone) when seen tangentially or as a crescentic rim of bone (referred to as a bucket-handle fracture) when seen obliquely. Other fractures associated with abuse include those of the scapula, spinous process, and sternum. Spiral long bone fractures in nonambulatory children are also highly suspicious. Multiple fractures in children of various ages (some with callus and some acute) as well as multiple fractures of various body parts are highly suspicious for abuse (see Fig. 7-21). In fact, any fracture in an infant should be viewed with suspicion, because as many as 30% of fractures in infants are secondary to abuse. Extraskeletal findings seen in abuse include acute or chronic subdural hematoma, cerebral edema (asphyxia), intraparenchymal brain hematoma, lung contusion, duodenal hematoma, solid abdominal organ laceration, and pancreatitis.

The clinical and imaging findings of abuse do not usually require differential diagnosis. However, other entities that may cause multiple fractures or that may cause radiographic findings that could be confused with injury, such as periosteal reaction, should always be considered. The other disorders that may present with multiple fractures in an infant are osteogenesis imperfecta and Menkes syndrome. Both of these entities are also associated with excessive Wormian bones and osteopenia.

PERIOSTEAL REACTION IN THE NEWBORN

When periosteal reaction is encountered in a newborn, there are a number of entities that must be considered (Table 7-1). They include physiologic new bone formation; TORCH infections (osteomyelitis), prostaglandin therapy; Caffey disease; metastatic neuroblastoma; and abuse. Physiologic periosteal new bone formation is commonly seen in infants during the first few months of life. It typically involves rapidly growing long bones, such as the femur, tibia, and humerus. Differential features that support physiologic growth as the cause of periosteal reaction include symmetric distribution, benign appearance of the periosteal reaction, and appropriate age of the child. When periosteal reaction involves the femur, tibia, or humerus, the other three bones are usually involved too. Radiographs may show one or several dense lines of periosteal reaction paralleling the cortex of the diaphysis of the long bones. Neonates with congenital heart disease are commonly treated with prostaglandins to maintain patency of the ductus venosus; these children commonly demonstrate prominent periosteal reaction.

TORCH Infections

The differential diagnosis for transplacentally acquired infections can be remembered by the mnemonic TORCH: toxoplasmosis, other (syphilis), rubella, cytomegalovirus, herpes.

CONGENITAL RUBELLA SYNDROME
Rubella is the most common of the transplacental viral infections. Its features include eye abnormalities, deafness, hepatosplenomegaly,

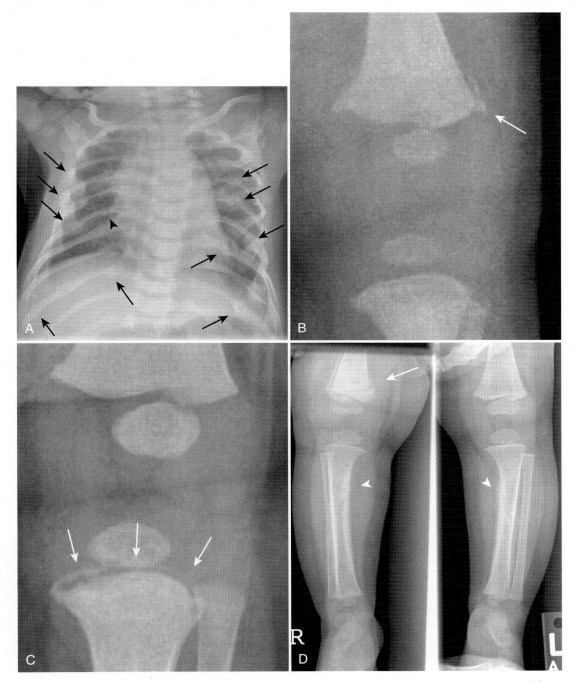

FIGURE 7-21. Musculoskeletal findings of child abuse demonstrated in multiple infants. **A,** Chest radiograph shows multiple rib fractures. Callus formation around subacute fractures is noted by *arrows.* There are also acute fractures *(arrowhead).* **B,** Metaphyseal fracture with characteristic corner fracture appearance *(arrow).* **C,** Metaphyseal fracture with characteristic bucket-handle appearance *(arrows).* **D,** Multiple fractures of bilateral lower extremities. There is a metaphyseal fracture of the right distal femur *(arrow)* and shaft fractures of the bilateral tibias *(arrowheads).*

(Continued)

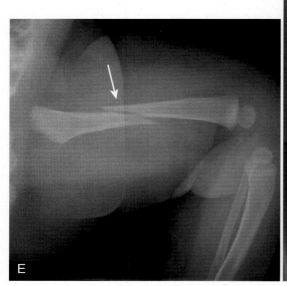
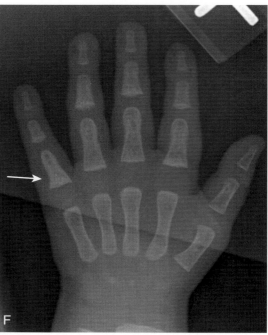

FIGURE 7-21. cont'd **E,** Midshaft fracture *(arrow)* of the femur. In a nonambulatory child, abuse must be considered. **F,** Subacute buckle fracture of the fifth proximal phalanx *(arrow).* Dedicated frontal radiographs of the hands and feet should be included in skeletal surveys for abuse.

aortic and pulmonic stenosis, and intrauterine growth retardation. Bony changes are present in as many as 50% of cases. They include irregular fraying of the metaphyses of long bones and generalized lucency of the metaphyses. The findings have been likened to a celery-stalk appearance (Fig. 7-22). These radiographic findings are most apparent during the first few weeks of life. The bony manifestations of rubella are currently extremely rare.

SYPHILIS

Congenital syphilis occurs secondary to transplacental infection, usually occurring during the second or third trimester. Clinical findings include hepatosplenomegaly, rash, rhinorrhea, anemia,

and ascites. Bony changes are present in as many as 95% of patients but often do not appear until 6 to 8 weeks after the time of infection. The radiographic findings may be present before the blood serology turns positive. Findings include nonspecific metaphyseal lucent bands and

Table 7-1. **Differential Diagnosis for Periosteal Reaction in a Newborn**

Physiologic growth
TORCH infections
   Syphilis, rubella
Prostaglandin therapy
Caffey disease (infantile cortical hyperostosis)
Neuroblastoma metastasis
Abuse

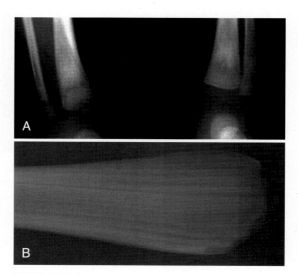

FIGURE 7-22. Congenital rubella in a 6-week-old infant. **A,** Radiograph shows irregular fraying of the metaphyses and alternating longitudinal dark and light bands of density, or "celery stalking." **B,** Radiograph of a celery stalk, for comparison.

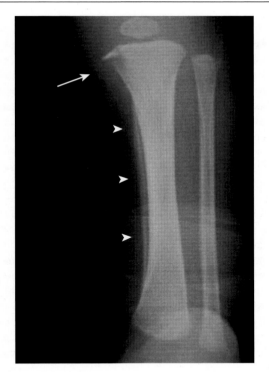

FIGURE 7-23. Congenital syphilis in a 6-week-old girl. Radiograph shows periosteal reaction along the shaft of the left tibia *(arrowheads)*. There is also characteristic lucency of the medial proximal tibial metaphysis *(arrow)*, called the Wimberger corner sign.

periosteal reaction involving multiple long bones (Fig. 7-23). The Wimberger corner sign is the most specific finding of syphilis and consists of destruction of the medial portion of the proximal metaphysis of the tibia, resulting in an area of irregular lucency (see Fig. 7-23). Bony manifestations

of syphilis are much more commonly encountered than those of rubella or other TORCH infections.

Caffey Disease (Infantile Cortical Hyperostosis)

Caffey disease is an idiopathic syndrome that consists of periosteal reaction shown on radiographs, irritability, fever, and soft tissue swelling over the areas of periosteal reaction. It occurs during the first few months of life. The bones most commonly involved include the mandible, clavicle, ribs, humerus, ulna, femur, scapula, and radius. Imaging shows periosteal new bone formation, sclerosis, and adjacent soft tissue swelling (Fig. 7-24). The disease is self-limited and currently occurs much less commonly than in the past.

LUCENT PERMEATIVE LESIONS IN CHILDREN

A bone lesion is considered permeative when it has ill-defined borders, has a wide zone of transition, and has multiple small, irregular holes centrally. As in an adult, a permeative bone lesion in a child is consistent with an aggressive inflammatory or neoplastic lesion. The finding is nonspecific. The more common causes of a permeative lesion in a child include osteomyelitis, Langerhans cell histiocytosis, neuroblastoma metastasis, Ewing sarcoma, and lymphoma/leukemia. The differential diagnosis can be further limited by considering

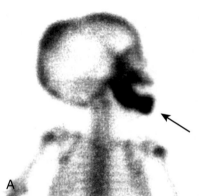

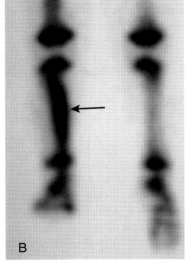

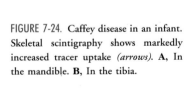

FIGURE 7-24. Caffey disease in an infant. Skeletal scintigraphy shows markedly increased tracer uptake *(arrows)*. **A,** In the mandible. **B,** In the tibia.

Table 7-2. Differential Diagnosis of a Permeative Bone Lesion in a Child on the Basis of Age

Less Than 5 years	Greater Than 5 years
Osteomyelitis	Ewing sarcoma
Langerhans cell histiocytosis	Lymphoma/leukemia
	Osteomyelitis
Neuroblastoma metastasis	Langerhans cell histiocytosis

the patient's age (Table 7-2). If the patient is younger than 5 years of age, the most likely diagnoses include osteomyelitis, Langerhans cell histiocytosis, and metastatic neuroblastoma. Ewing sarcoma and lymphoma are exceedingly rare in children younger than 5. In older children, Ewing sarcoma and lymphoma/leukemia become candidates, and metastatic neuroblastoma becomes much less likely.

Osteomyelitis

Acute osteomyelitis is a relatively common cause of clinically significant bone pathology in children. It is primarily a disease of infants and young children; one third of cases occur in children younger than 2 years of age, and one half of cases occur before 5 years of age. Because of the young age of most of the children, the presentation is often nonspecific, and diagnosis is delayed. Erythrocyte sedimentation rate is elevated in a vast majority of cases. Most cases of osteomyelitis are hematogenous in origin; many patients have a recent history of respiratory tract infection or otitis media. *Staphylococcus aureus* is the most common cause.

Osteomyelitis tends to occur in the metaphyses or metaphyseal equivalents of children. This is thought to be related to the rich and slow moving blood supply to these regions. Approximately 75% of cases involve the metaphyses of long bones; the most common sites are the femur, tibia, and humerus. The other 25% of cases occur within metaphyseal equivalents of flat bones, most typically involving the bony pelvis.

The earliest radiographic finding of osteomyelitis is deep soft tissue swelling evidenced by displacement or obliteration of the fat planes adjacent to a metaphysis. Bony changes may not be present until 10 days after the onset of symptoms. Initial bony changes consist of poorly defined lucency involving a metaphyseal area. Commonly, progressive bony destruction is present (Figs. 7-25A, B; 7-26A-C). Periosteal new bone formation begins at approximately 10 days. Osteomyelitis can appear as sclerotic, rather than lucent, when it is a chronic process (see Fig. 7-26). Other imaging modalities that are used in the evaluation of suspected osteomyelitis include skeletal scintigraphy, MRI, and occasionally CT. On skeletal scintigraphy, osteomyelitis appears as a focal area of increased activity on the angiographic, soft tissue, and skeletal phase images. Skeletal scintigraphy becomes positive early after the onset of osteomyelitis and is often positive prior to development of changes seen on radiography. Another advantage of scintigraphy is the ability to evaluate for multiple sites of involvement. MRI also demonstrates abnormal findings early after the onset of osteomyelitis. Osteomyelitis appears as an area of increased T2-weighted signal within a metaphysis. There are usually large areas of surrounding edema that are seen as an increased T2-weighted signal within the adjacent bone marrow and soft tissues. Gadolinium administration may show areas of nonenhancement suspicious for necrosis or abscess formation (see Fig. 7-26). Identification of drainable fluid for surgical planning is one of the advantages of MRI over scintigraphy.

Langerhans Cell Histiocytosis

Langerhans cell histiocytosis (LCH), also known as eosinophilic granuloma and histiocytosis X, is an idiopathic disorder that can manifest as focal, localized, or systemic disease. It remains unclear whether the disease process is inflammatory or neoplastic. It is characterized by abnormal proliferation of Langerhans cells. The disease is twice as common in boys as in girls and occurs most commonly in whites. Although there is a spectrum of disease severity ranging from focal to systemic, there are several specific disease categories.

Letterer-Siwe disease is an acute disseminated form of LCH that occurs in children less than 1 year of age. There is acute onset of hepatosplenomegaly, rash, lymphadenopathy, marrow failure, and pulmonary involvement. Skeletal involvement may not be present. The prognosis is poor; most children die within 1 to 2 years.

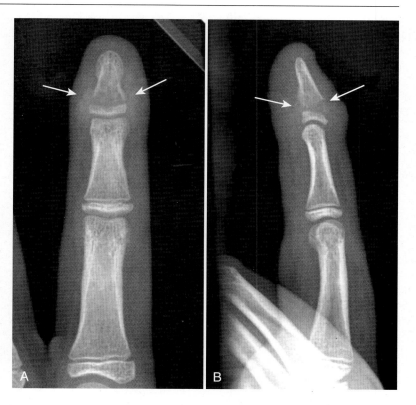

FIGURE 7-25. Osteomyelitis following nail-bed injury and distal phalanx fracture. (Fractures involving the nail bed should be considered open fractures and are at risk for development of osteomyelitis.) **A,** Frontal radiograph shows metaphyseal destruction *(arrows)* of bone contiguous with physis. **B,** Lateral view shows dorsal soft tissue swelling and metaphyseal destruction *(arrows)*. The metaphysis is slightly displaced relative to the epiphysis, a finding that is most likely related to the initial fracture.

Hand-Schüller-Christian disease is the chronic form of systemic LCH. Most of the patients with this form have skeletal involvement. Other manifestations include hepatosplenomegaly, diabetes insipidus, exophthalmos, dermatitis, and growth retardation. These patients typically present between 3 and 6 years of age. The morbidity rate is high.

In eosinophilic granuloma, the process is isolated to bone or lung. Such diagnoses make up 70% of cases of LCH, and the prognosis is excellent. Most cases have a single site of bony involvement.

The radiographic appearance of skeletal manifestations of LCH is extremely variable. Lesions may be lucent or sclerotic, may be permeative or geographic, and may have a sclerotic or poorly defined border. The most common sites of LCH, in decreasing order of frequency, are the skull (Fig. 7-27A, B), ribs, femur, pelvis, spine, and mandible. Skull lesions may have a "beveled edge," which is related to uneven destruction of the inner and outer tables of the skull. Rib lesions may be multiple and commonly have an expanded appearance. When the spine is involved, a classic finding is vertebral plana (vertebral destruction with severe collapse; Fig. 7-28A, B).

A child who presents with a lesion suspicious for LCH should be evaluated by a skeletal survey to identify other bony lesions; a chest radiograph to exclude pulmonary involvement, and often an MRI or CT to characterize and evaluate the anatomic extent of disease.

Ewing Sarcoma

Ewing sarcoma is the second most common primary malignancy of bone in children after osteosarcoma. It is an aggressive, small, round, blue cell tumor similar to primitive neuroectodermal tumor. Ewing sarcoma most commonly occurs in the second decade of life, and its occurrence in children younger than 5 years of age is exceedingly rare. The most common sites of involvement, in decreasing order of frequency, are the femur, pelvis, tibia, humerus, and ribs. Two thirds of cases involve the pelvis or femur.

The radiographic appearance of Ewing sarcoma is variable. Most lesions involve the metaphysis, but diaphyseal involvement is more common than it is in other bone malignancies. Most lesions have an aggressive appearance: a lucent lesion with poorly defined borders and a permeative appearance in the cortex (Fig. 7-29A-C). Aggressive-appearing periosteal new bone formation (spiculated, onion skin, Codman triangle) is

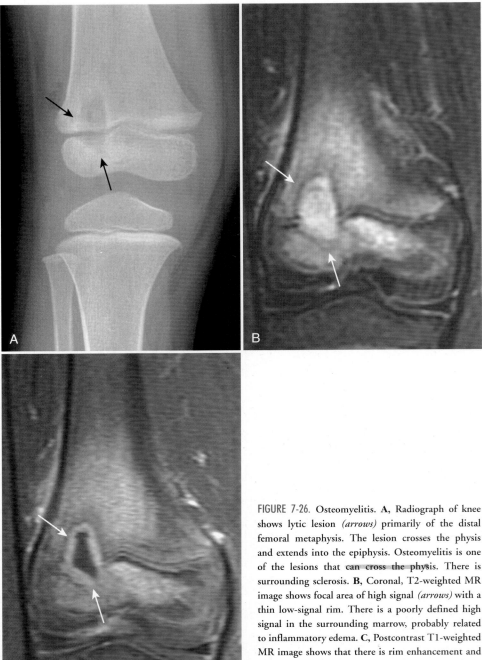

FIGURE 7-26. Osteomyelitis. **A,** Radiograph of knee shows lytic lesion *(arrows)* primarily of the distal femoral metaphysis. The lesion crosses the physis and extends into the epiphysis. Osteomyelitis is one of the lesions that can cross the physis. There is surrounding sclerosis. **B,** Coronal, T2-weighted MR image shows focal area of high signal *(arrows)* with a thin low-signal rim. There is a poorly defined high signal in the surrounding marrow, probably related to inflammatory edema. **C,** Postcontrast T1-weighted MR image shows that there is rim enhancement and lack of central enhancement of the lesion *(arrows)*. This is suggestive of an area of necrotic bone or drainable fluid (abscess).

commonly present. However, Ewing sarcoma can appear predominantly sclerotic in as many as 15% of cases. MRI demonstrates a destructive bony mass, often with an associated soft tissue component (see Fig. 7-29). The 5-year survival rate for those with Ewing sarcoma is 70% in those with localized disease and 30% in those in whom metastatic disease is present.

Metastatic Disease

In children, most cases of metastatic disease result from small, round, blue cell tumors. The most common primary neoplasms to metastasize to bone are neuroblastoma and leukemia/lymphoma. In any child younger than 3 years of age with a neoplastic bony lesion, metastatic neuroblastoma

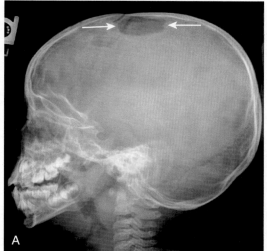

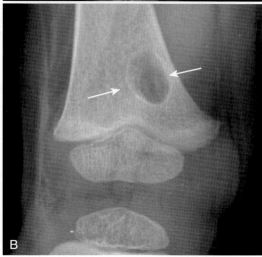

FIGURE 7-27. Langerhans cell histiocytosis. **A,** Radiograph shows a well-defined lytic lesion *(arrows)* of the skull. The lesion has a typical beveled-edge appearance. **B,** Radiograph shows lytic destructive lesion *(arrows)* of right femur. The lesion has a sclerotic border.

(Fig. 7-30A-C) should be considered and is much more likely than a primary bone neoplasm. Leukemia and lymphoma may deposit in the regions of the metaphyses and cause bony destruction. The appearance is often that of lucent metaphyseal bands (Fig. 7-31). These nonspecific bands are often referred to as leukemic lines. Primary bone lymphoma is rare in children.

FOCAL SCLEROTIC LESIONS IN CHILDREN

There are multiple causes of focal sclerotic bone lesions in children. The more common causes are listed in Table 7-3.

Osteoid Osteoma

Osteoid osteoma is a relatively common bone lesion. Most cases occur within the second decade of life and usually present with pain. Classically, the pain is worse at night and is relieved by nonsteroidal antiinflammatory medication. The lesions are more common in boys. The cause is unknown, and it is currently unclear whether the lesion is a benign neoplasm or an inflammatory lesion. Most commonly, osteoid osteomas occur within the cortex of the metadiaphyses or diaphyses of the long bones of the lower extremities.

On radiography, an osteoid osteoma appears as a lucent cortical nidus surrounded by an area of reactive sclerosis (Fig. 7-32). The nidus is typically less than 1.5 cm in diameter. Classically, a punctate radiodensity is identified within the central lucency (a dense dot within a lucent area, surrounded by sclerotic density). CT is commonly used to further characterize the lesion because the punctate central radiodensity and lucency are often better demonstrated on CT than on radiography (see Fig. 7-32), and it defines the anatomic position of the nidus. CT can be used as guidance for percutaneous drill removal of the osteoid osteoma. Skeletal scintigraphy demonstrates a "double-density sign" of intense increased uptake by the nidus, surrounded by less intense but abnormally increased uptake by the surrounding sclerotic bone.

Stress Fracture

A stress fracture is defined as an injury resulting from repetitive trauma. It usually occurs when a new or intense activity has recently been initiated. The most common sites of stress fractures in children, in decreasing order of frequency, are the tibia, fibula, metatarsals, and calcaneus. A stress fracture appears on radiographs as a transverse or oblique band of sclerosis or as a lucent line surrounded by sclerosis or periosteal new bone formation (Fig. 7-33A, B).

Table 7-3. **Common Causes of Focal Sclerotic Lesions in Children**

Osteoid osteoma
Chronic osteomyelitis
Stress fracture
Osteosarcoma

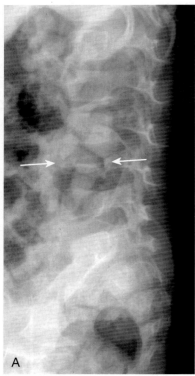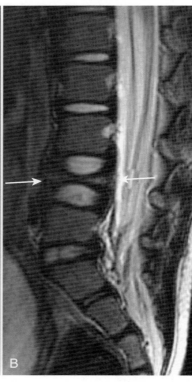

A

B

FIGURE 7-28. Langerhans cell histiocytosis in a 2-year-old boy with back pain. **A,** Radiograph of the lumbar spine shows collapse of the L4 vertebral body (vertebral plana; *arrows*). It is difficult to visualize because of bowel gas. **B,** T2-weighted, sagittal MR image confirms collapse of the L4 vertebral body *(arrows).*

Periosteal new bone formation may be the only finding. In the tibia, the most common location is the proximal posterior cortex, although the anterior cortex can also be involved. In the calcaneus, there is typically a vertical sclerotic band paralleling the posterior cortex. Calcaneal stress fractures most commonly occur when a child has had a cast removed after a preceding injury and returns to activity after a period of prolonged disuse (Fig. 7-34). Skeletal scintigraphy demonstrates a stress fracture as an area of focal increased uptake days to weeks prior to the development of radiographic findings. CT may be helpful in demonstrating the linear nature of the lesion when trying to evaluate whether a sclerotic lesion is a stress fracture, osteoid osteoma, or osteomyelitis. Stress fractures may be identified on MRI when it is performed to evaluate for pain. They appear as low-signal linear structures with surrounding high T2-weighted signal edema (see Fig. 7-33).

Osteosarcoma

Osteosarcoma, or osteogenic sarcoma, is the most common primary bone malignancy of childhood. It occurs most commonly in patients between 10 and 15 years of age and is more common in boys than in girls. Although most cases of osteosarcoma arise in otherwise healthy children, there are certain predisposing conditions, such as hereditary retinoblastoma and previous radiation therapy. Osteosarcoma is a very malignant lesion that uniquely gives rise to neoplastic osteoid and bone. The majority of osteosarcomas arise from the medullary cavity, although the lesion may arise from the surface of bone. The latter scenario gives rise to the periosteal and parosteal forms. The most common sites for development of osteosarcoma are the metaphyses of long bones. More than 60% of cases of osteosarcoma arise in the region of the knee (distal femur or proximal tibia).

The radiographic appearance of osteosarcoma is dependent on the amount of bony destruction and new bone formation. The lesions are typically large at the time of presentation. The destructive component of the tumor is demonstrated by lucent destruction of a metaphysis with aggressive features (aggressive periosteal reaction, poorly defined borders) (Figs. 7-35A-D, 7-36A, B). Tumor bone is seen in more than 90% of cases of osteosarcoma and helps to differentiate this tumor from other types of bone malignancies (see Fig. 7-35). It appears as a cloudlike density.

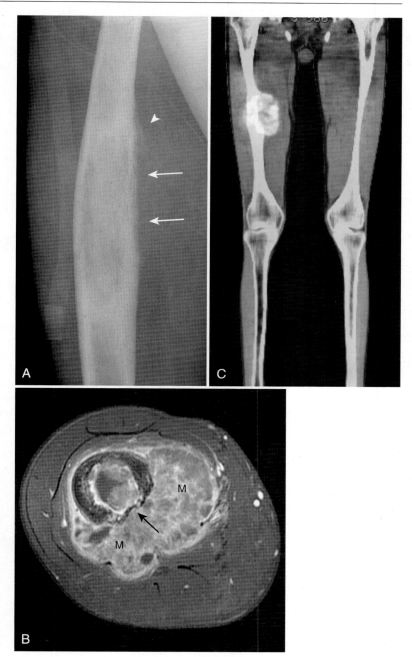

FIGURE 7-29. Ewing sarcoma of diaphysis of femur. **A,** Radiograph shows lytic lesion with poorly defined margins. There is cortical destruction *(arrows)* and a Codman triangle *(arrowhead).* **B,** Postcontrast, axial MR image shows lesion of femur with large associated soft tissue mass *(M).* There is heterogeneous enhancement. There is cortical destruction *(arrow).* **C,** Positron emission tomography and CT coronal image shows high metabolic activity within the tumor (orange color).

One feature that helps to differentiate tumor bone from sclerotic reactive bone is that tumor bone often extends beyond the expected confines of the bony shaft. In most cases of osteosarcoma, there is a large soft tissue mass present at the time of diagnosis. In poorly differentiated, very aggressive lesions, tumor bone may not be present and the lesion may appear as a nonspecific, aggressive lucent lesion.

MRI is used to evaluate the extent of bone and soft tissue involvement for presurgical planning.

The extent of marrow abnormality, soft tissue mass, and cortical destruction is well demonstrated as abnormal increased T2-weighted signal on MRI. However, MRI is not accurate in differentiating peritumoral marrow edema from tumor-involved marrow. Therefore, all abnormal signals in the marrow are generally considered to be involved by tumor for the sake of surgical planning. MRI is accurate in depicting the relationship between the soft tissue mass and adjacent nerves and vascular structures. It is important to image the

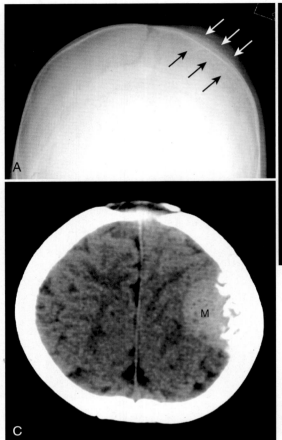

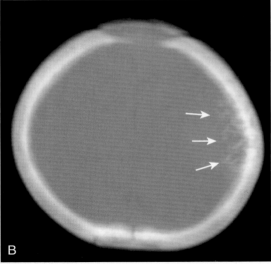

FIGURE 7-30. Metastatic neuroblastoma in a 1-year-old child presenting with a lump on the head. **A,** Radiograph shows soft tissue lump with aggressive hair-on-end-appearing periosteal reaction *(arrows)* by underlying bone. **B,** CT at bone windows shows permeative appearance of bone and associated aggressive periosteal reaction *(arrows)*. **C,** CT at brain windows shows associated soft tissue mass *(M)* arising from bone and associated periosteal reaction.

entire length of the long bone involved by the tumor because osteosarcoma can occasionally have discontinuous bone involvement (skip lesions), and identification of such skip lesions affects surgical planning. Surgery in conjunction with chemotherapy is standard therapy; limb-salvage procedures are currently being performed in as much as 80% of patients. The 5-year survival has increased to 77% in recent years. Often, a course of chemotherapy is administered and the patient is reimaged prior to surgery. MRI has been shown to be useful in documenting chemotherapeutic response by demonstrating decrease in the size of the soft tissue mass and the amount of peritumoral edema. The most common type of metastatic disease is pulmonary (lung nodules), which is evaluated by CT. Skeletal metastatic disease is reported to be present in as many as 15% of patients and is evaluated by skeletal scintigraphy.

MULTIFOCAL BONE LESIONS IN CHILDREN

The presence of multifocal involvement narrows the differential diagnosis for bone lesions in

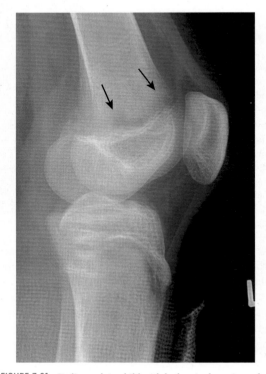

FIGURE 7-31. Radiograph in child with leukemia shows irregular, lucent metaphyseal band (leukemic line; *arrows*) involving the distal tibia.

children (Table 7-4). Osteomyelitis, Langerhans cell histiocytosis, and metastatic disease have already been discussed. In addition, there are several hereditary syndromes that cause multifocal bone lesions in children.

In multiple hereditary exostoses (osteochondromatosis), there is a propensity to develop multiple bilateral osteochondromas. Osteochondromas appear as bony growths that arise from the metaphysis and are continuous with the adjacent bony cortex (Fig. 7-37A-C). They have a tendency to point away from joints. The most common location is the bones surrounding the knee. With osteochondromatosis, the lesions can lead to a number of problems, including limb shortening, leg length discrepancy, bowing and deformity, compression of adjacent nerves and vessels, and malignant degeneration into chondrosarcoma (5%).

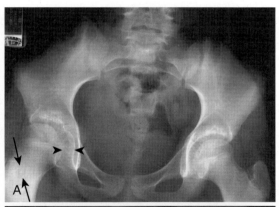
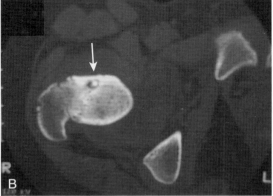

FIGURE 7-32. Osteoid osteoma in an 11-year-old girl. **A,** Radiograph shows increased sclerosis of intertrochanteric region of the right femur. Within this area of sclerosis is a round central lucency *(arrows)* containing a central punctate density. There is associated joint effusion identified by asymmetric widening of the right joint space *(arrowheads).* **B,** CT scan shows dense nidus *(arrow)* within central lucency and surrounding sclerosis.

The more proximal lesions have a greater propensity for malignant degeneration.

With enchondromatosis (Ollier disease), there is a propensity to develop multiple enchondromas. Although they most commonly occur bilaterally, it is possible for all the lesions to be located on one side of the body. Solitary enchondromas tend to occur in the hands and feet (Fig. 7-38), whereas lesions of enchondromatosis tend to be located within the metaphyses of long bones. With growth, the lesions may take on an oblong or flame-shaped, linear configuration perpendicular to the physis (Fig. 7-39). Malignant degeneration occurs more commonly than in osteochondromatosis, occurring in approximately 30% of lesions. When soft tissue venous malformations are seen in conjunction with multiple enchondromas, the syndrome is called Maffucci syndrome. In those patients, phleboliths may be seen within the soft tissue masses on radiographs. Patients with Maffucci syndrome have higher incidences of malignant degeneration than do those with Ollier syndrome and are also at increased risk for malignant neoplasms of the abdomen and central nervous system.

McCune-Albright syndrome is the presence of polyostotic fibrous dysplasia, skin pigmentation abnormalities, and endocrine abnormalities. The most common endocrine abnormality is precocious puberty in girls. Polyostotic fibrous dysplasia most commonly involves the facial bones, pelvis, spine, and proximal humeri. The lesions tend to be unilateral. Many patients present with pathologic fracture by 10 years of age (Fig. 7-40A-C). There is no predisposition to malignancy. Fibrous dysplasia has a variable appearance radiographically. It can be purely lytic or sclerotic and can be expansile or nonexpansile. The classic description is that of "ground-glass opacity" (see Fig. 7-40), which is a smudged and somewhat dense appearance of the central portion of the lesion. Periosteal reaction should be present only if there is a pathologic fracture.

CONSTITUTIONAL DISORDERS OF BONE

The term *constitutional disorders of bone* refers to any developmental abnormality of bone resulting in diffuse skeletal abnormality. The skeletal dysplasias, mucopolysaccharidoses, and osteogenesis imperfecta fall into this category.

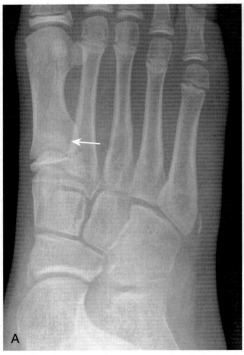

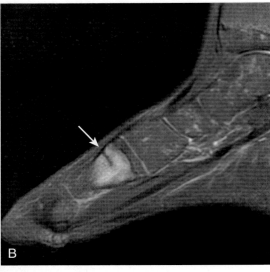

FIGURE 7-33. Stress fracture of the base of the first metatarsal bone. **A,** Radiograph shows sclerotic, transversely oriented band *(arrow)* through base of first metatarsal bone. **B,** Sagittal T2-weighted MR image shows stress fracture as linear low-signal band *(arrow)* with surrounding high-signal edema.

Skeletal Dysplasias

For some reason, many people think that those trained in pediatric radiology have a textbook knowledge of skeletal dysplasias. This unfortunate rumor could not be farther from the truth. Most pediatric radiologists deal with skeletal

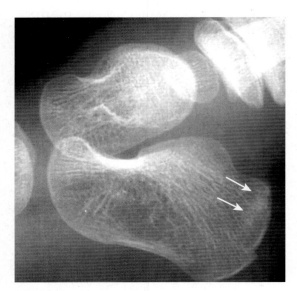

FIGURE 7-34. Stress fracture of the calcaneus in a 10-year-old boy with pain following return to activity after his lower extremity was casted for a different fracture. Radiograph shows vertical sclerotic band *(arrows)* in the posterior calcaneus.

dysplasia fairly infrequently and typically know only enough to be able to recognize that a dysplasia is present and that they need help. Most pediatric institutions have one person who is enthralled with and knowledgeable about skeletal dysplasias, and that person is consulted whenever a dysplasia arises. Anyone who is in a situation in which such a person is not available should consult the excellent textbooks available. I recommend the text by Taybi and Lachman. It is practical to have an understanding of the approach to the dysplasias and to know something about the more common ones. The radiographic identification of a particular dysplasia can be helpful for prognostication and genetic counseling for the parents (is the identified dysplasia a dominant or recessive trait?).

Radiographic evaluation of dysplasia requires images of the skull, spine, thorax, pelvis, and extremities. An important feature for categorization is identifying whether the extremities are shortened and, if so, which portion is short. Extremity shortening can be classified as rhizomelic, mesomelic, or acromelic (Fig. 7-41). *Rhizomelic* refers to proximal shortening (humerus, femur) and is seen in achondroplasia and thanatophoric dwarfism. *Mesomelic* refers to middle narrowing (radius-ulna, tibia-fibula). Most of the mesomelic dysplasias are quite rare. *Acromelic* refers to distal shortening

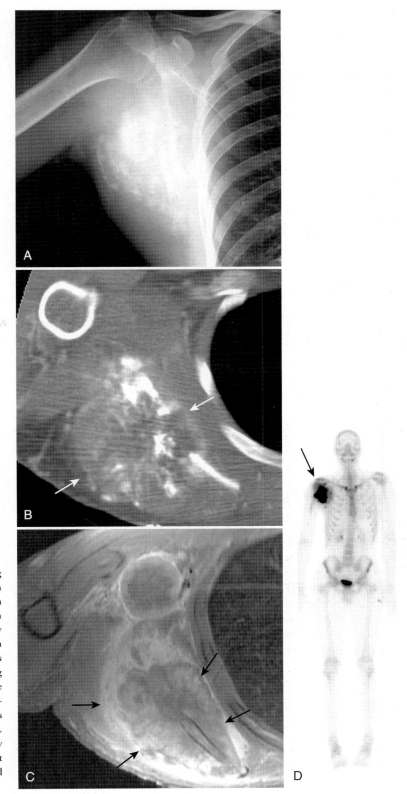

FIGURE 7-35. Osteosarcoma arising from right scapula. **A,** Radiograph shows tumor bone formation as a cloud of high density emanating from the right scapula. There is poorly defined lucency and cortical destruction in the scapula. **B,** CT shows mass *(arrows)* arising from and destroying the cortex of the right scapula. Note tumor bone formation. **C,** Axial post-contrast T1-weighted MR image shows mass *(arrows)* arising from the scapula. **D,** Bone scan shows dramatically increased uptake in region of right scapula *(arrow)* but no other abnormal sites of increased uptake.

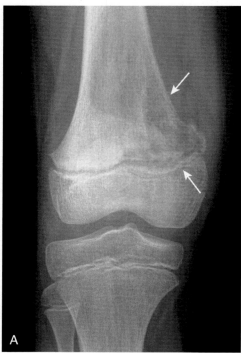

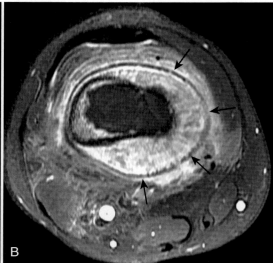

FIGURE 7-36. Osteosarcoma arising from right femur. **A,** Radiograph shows metaphyseal lucent lesion *(arrows)* with associated cortical destruction. **B,** Axial, contrast-enhanced T1-weighted MR image shows mass arising from the marrow of the right femur. Note enhancing mass displacing and extending external to the periosteum *(arrows)*, which appears as a low-signal curvilinear structure.

and is seen with asphyxiating thoracic dystrophy (Jeune syndrome) and chondroectodermal dysplasia (Ellis-van Creveld syndrome). Other features helpful in categorizing dysplasias include determining whether there are skull enlargement, short ribs (Fig. 7-42), a short spine, abnormal vertebral bodies (see Fig. 7-42), and an abnormal pelvic configuration (Fig. 7-43). The pelvis may demonstrate abnormalities in the configuration of the iliac wings or in the appearance of the acetabulum. The iliac wings may be abnormally tall or short or may have a squared appearance. The acetabular roof may appear horizontal (a decreased acetabular angle). *Trident acetabulum* refers to a case in which the acetabulum is seen to have three inferior pointing spikes resembling an upside-down trident. This is a buzz word for Jeune syndrome but also can be seen in Ellis-van Creveld syndrome and thanatophoric dysplasia. Some of the more common dysplasias and their radiographic manifestations are described in Table 7-5.

Table 7-4. Multifocal Bone Lesions in Children

Multifocal osteomyelitis
Langerhans cell histiocytosis
Metastatic disease
Multiple hereditary exostoses (osteochondromatosis)
Enchondromatosis (Ollier disease, Maffucci syndrome)
Polyostotic fibrous dysplasia (McCune-Albright syndrome)
Neurofibromatosis

ACHONDROPLASIA

Achondroplasia is discussed in greater detail because it is the most common short-limbed dwarfism. It is an autosomal dominant disease in which the heterozygous form demonstrates the clinical manifestations, and the homozygous form is lethal. Patients with achondroplasia have rhizomelic limb shortening (see Fig. 7-41). They also have craniofacial disproportion, an enlarged skull, a small skull base, and a small foramen magnum and jugular foramina. The last may result in brain stem compression. In the spine, the vertebral bodies are short and decreased in anterior-to-posterior diameter. The disk spaces are too tall. There is a decrease in the interpediculate distance (left to right), with this distance being narrower in the more inferior lumbar spine than in the more superior lumbar spine (the opposite of normal; see Fig. 7-42). The pedicles are also short in the anterior to posterior diameter. Because of these findings, achondroplasts are prone to spinal stenosis. The shortened long bones show metaphyseal flaring (see Fig. 7-41). In infancy, there is commonly space between the middle fingers, resulting in a trident appearance of the hand. The iliac

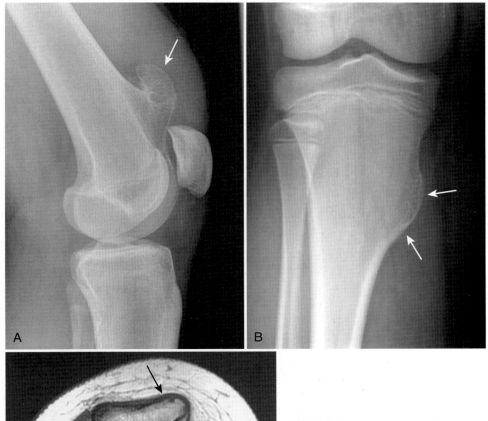

FIGURE 7-37. Osteochondroma of the knee in two children. **A,** Radiograph shows osteochondroma as bony growth *(arrow)* extending from the anterior cortex of the femur. Note that the lesion points away from the joint. **B,** Radiograph in another patient shows osteochondroma as a bony outgrowth *(arrows)* from the medial, proximal tibia. The lesion is more sessile than the lesion shown in A. **C,** Axial, T1-weighted MR image on same patient as in B shows that the lesion *(arrows)* is contiguous with the bony cortex and the marrow cavity. There is no associated soft tissue mass.

bones are short in height and the acetabular roof is horizontal (a decreased acetabular angle), making the iliac bones resemble old-fashioned tombstones (see Fig. 7-43).

Mucopolysaccharidoses

Mucopolysaccharidoses are a group of hereditary disorders manifested by defects in lysosomal enzymes. They include such disorders as Hunter, Hurler, and Morquio syndromes. The skeletal findings in this group of diseases are similar and have been referred to as dysostosis multiplex. The vertebral bodies are oval in shape and often have an anterior beak in the anterior cortex (Fig. 7-44). This is located in the midportion of the vertebral bodies in Morquio syndrome and in the inferior portion in Hurler syndrome. Beaking is most prominent in the lumbar vertebral bodies. There can be focal kyphosis (gibbous deformity; see Fig. 7-44). The clavicles and ribs are commonly thickened. The ribs are narrower posteromedially, giving them a "canoe-paddle" appearance. The appearance of the pelvis is essentially the

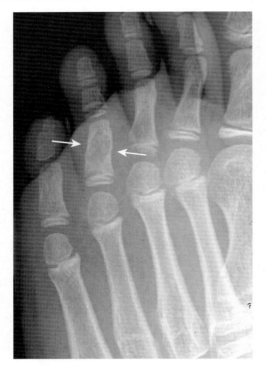

FIGURE 7-38. Enchondroma. Radiograph shows well-defined lytic lesion *(arrows)* of the fourth proximal phalynx. There appears to be some internal calcified matrix.

opposite of that in achondroplasia. The iliac wings are tall and flared and the acetabuli are shallow (increased acetabular angles; see Fig. 7-44). The femoral heads are dysplastic, and femoral necks are gracile and demonstrate coxa valga (loss of angle between the neck and

the shaft of the femur). The hands have a characteristic appearance that includes proximal tapering of the metatarsal bones (see Fig. 7-44).

Osteogenesis Imperfecta

The term *osteogenesis imperfecta* (OI) represents a heterogeneous group of genetic disorders that result in the formation of abnormal type 1 collagen. In all types, there is osteopenia and a propensity for fracture. There is commonly evidence of multiple fractures of various ages. In such cases, other findings such as osteopenia should be clues to a diagnosis of OI rather than child abuse. There is a spectrum of clinical presentations and radiographic appearances that have historically been divided into the often fatal recessive congenital form and the dominant tarda form. In classic congenital cases, there are thick tubular bones (Fig. 7-45) that result from the healing of multiple fractures, resulting in short-limb dwarfism. In the tarda form, there are thin gracile bones with undertubulation (Fig. 7-46A, B). OI tarda cases are commonly treated with bisphosphonate therapy to increase bone calcium deposition. Such therapy can result in a striking pattern of alternating sclerotic and lucent bands within the metaphyses of fast-growing bones (see Fig. 7-46). Multiple wormian bones (small ossicles along the cranial sutures), blue sclera, and thin skin are also commonly noted in association with OI. In OI and some other disorders,

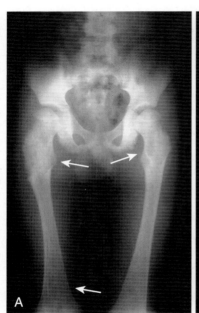

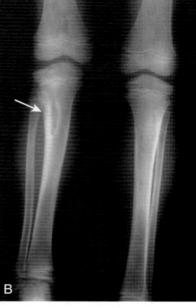

FIGURE 7-39. Enchondromatosis shown as multiple lucent lesions *(arrows)* predominantly on the right side. **A,** Involvement of the femurs. **B,** Involvement of the tibia. The lesions have a flamed-shaped appearance perpendicular to the physis.

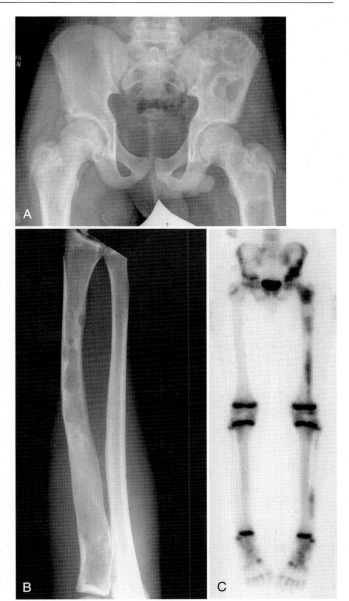

FIGURE 7-40. Polyostotic fibrous dysplasia. **A,** Radiograph of the pelvis. **B,** Radiograph of the forearm. Both show multiple unilateral left lesions within the pelvis, left femur, and radius, consistent with fibrous dysplasia. Note the ground-glass appearance, especially in the lesion in the radius. The lesions are expansile. **C,** Bone scan shows increased uptake in multiple lesions in left pelvis, femur, and fibula.

the number of wormian bones along the sutures is increased beyond normal (up to 12) and may number in the dozens.

Osteopetrosis

Osteopetrosis is a rare bone disorder in which the osteoclasts are defective in resorbing and remodeling bone. As a result, bone is laid down and not resorbed. This results in dense bony sclerosis. There is often a bone-within-bone appearance on radiographs (Fig. 7-47A, B). The skull base is thickened and encroachment upon the cranial nerves is a common complication. Although the total body calcium stores are increased, serum calcium levels are often paradoxically low, and radiographic findings of superimposed rickets are not uncommon. Lack of normal marrow space results in pancytopenia which often leads to complications and death.

HIP DISORDERS

There are a number of unique abnormalities that can involve the pediatric hip.

(Text continues on page 188.)

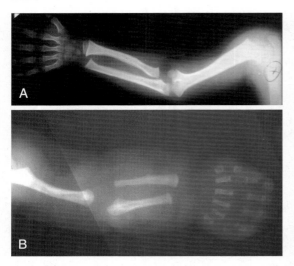

FIGURE 7-41. Abnormal configurations of the extremities associated with skeletal dysplasias. **A,** Rhizomelic (proximal) limb shortening demonstrated in achondroplasia, with the most severe limb shortening involving the humerus. Note the associated metaphyseal flaring. **B,** Acromelic (distal) limb shortening in chondroectodermal dysplasia, with the most severe shortening involving the bones of the hands, radius, and ulna. Note the polydactyly, which is also associated with chondroectodermal dysplasia.

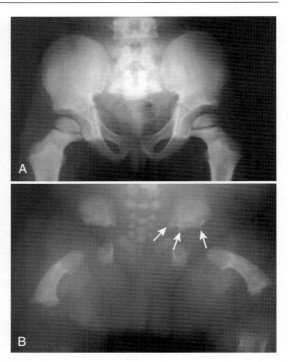

FIGURE 7-43. Abnormal configurations of the pelvis seen in skeletal dysplasias. **A,** Achondroplasia. The radiograph shows the acetabuli to be more horizontal than normal (decreased acetabular angles). The iliac angles are steep. The iliac bones are short and have rounded tops. The combination of these findings gives the iliac bone a "tombstone" appearance. **B,** Trident acetabulum. The radiograph shows three downward spikes *(arrows)* forming an upside-down trident. Trident acetabulum is a buzz word associated with Jeune syndrome, but the acetabulum often has a similar appearance in thanatophoric dysplasia and chondroectodermal dysplasia. In this patient with thanatophoric dysplasia, also note telephone-receiver-shaped femurs.

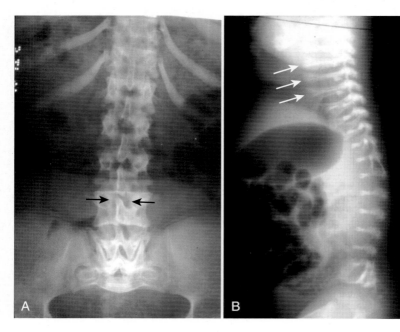

FIGURE 7-42. Abnormal configurations of the spine seen in skeletal dysplasias. **A,** Achondroplasia. Frontal radiograph shows that the interpediculate distance *(arrows)* becomes narrower inferiorly. **B,** Thanatophoric dysplasia. The vertebral bodies demonstrate platyspondyly. Also note the short ribs *(arrows),* resulting in a narrow anterior-to-posterior diameter of the chest and a protuberant abdomen.

Table 7-5. **Radiographic Manifestations of Several Skeletal Dysplasias**

Dysplasia	Type of Extremity Shortening	Pelvis	Short Ribs	Spine	Enlarged Skull	Other
Achondroplasia	Proximal	Squared iliac wings Small sacroiliac notch Decreased acetabular angle (looks like tombstones)	Yes	Short vertebral bodies Narrow interpediculate distance	Yes	Metaphyseal flaring
Thanatophoric dysplasia	Proximal	Squared iliac wings Decreased acetabular angle Trident acetabulum	Yes	Platyspondyly	Yes	Early death Metaphyseal flaring "Telephone-receiver" femurs
Chondrodysplasia punctata	Proximal	Normal	No	Stippled epiphysis	No	Stippled epiphyses
Diastrophic dysplasia	Proximal	Normal	No	Normal	No	Metaphyseal enlargement Hitchhiker thumb Enlarged ears
Mesomelic dysplasia	Middle	Normal	No	Normal	No	Mandibular hypoplasia
Asphyxiating thoracic dystrophy (Jeune)	Distal	Decreased acetabular angle Trident acetabulum	Yes	Normal	No	Very short ribs Respiratory distress Metaphyseal irregularity and beaking
Chondroectodermal dysplasia (Ellis-van Creveld)	Distal	Decreased acetabular angle Trident acetabulum	Yes	Normal	No	Polydactyly, abnormal nails Congenital heart disease Amish community
Cleidocranial dysplasia	All	Squared iliac wings Decreased acetabular angle Widened pubic symphysis	No	Abnormal ossification	Yes	Absent/small clavicles Widened pubic symphysis Wormian bones
Camptomelic dysplasia	All	Tall, narrow iliac wings Increased acetabular angle	No	Ossification defects	Yes	Bowing of long bones (campto, bent limb) Airway obstruction

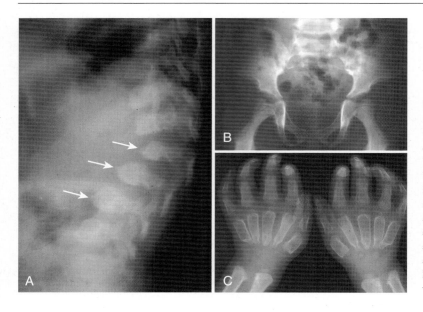

FIGURE 7-44. Radiographic findings in mucopolysaccharidosis (dysostosis multiplex). **A,** Radiograph of the spine demonstrates the vertebral bodies to be oval and to have anterior inferior beaks *(arrows).* There is an associated focal lumbar kyphosis (gibbous deformity). **B,** Radiograph of the pelvis shows increased acetabular and iliac angles, giving the pelvis a flared appearance. The femoral necks are gracile and show coxa valgus. **C,** Radiograph of the hands shows squared metacarpal bones with tapered proximal ends.

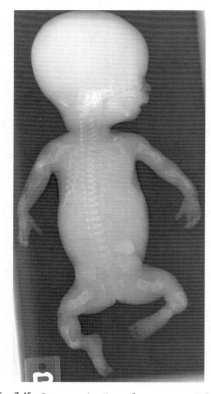

FIGURE 7-45. Osteogenesis imperfecta, congenital form. Babygram shows multiple fractures of the long bones and ribs, resulting in thick, tubular long bones. Note the near complete lack of ossification of the skull. The lungs are not aerated. The radiograph was obtained post mortem.

Developmental Dysplasia of the Hip

Development dysplasia of the hip (DDH), also previously referred to as congenital hip dislocation, refers to a condition related to abnormal development and configuration of the acetabulum and to increased ligamentous laxity around the hip. The cause is debated. DDH is much more common in females (in a ratio of as much as 9:1), in whites, and in children born in breech deliveries. One third of children with DDH are affected bilaterally. Clinical evaluation for DDH is part of routine neonatal screening. Neonates may demonstrate asymmetric gluteal folds, limited abduction, or a positive click felt on Ortolani (relocation) or Barlow (dislocation) maneuvers. If not detected and treated in infancy, DDH can lead to chronic abnormalities of the hip.

Ultrasound is used to evaluate the hips of children who have clinical findings suggestive of DDH. Both the morphology of the acetabulum and any abnormal mobility of the hip are evaluated. Because there is physiologic ligamentous laxity during the first days of life, it is better to wait 2 weeks before performing hip ultrasound. The static morphologic evaluation is performed with the ultrasound probe coronal to the hip. Stress (Barlow) maneuvers are performed while evaluating the hip in the axial plane. On the static coronal view, the anatomy simulates that seen on a frontal radiograph of the pelvis (Fig. 7-48A-C). On such a view, the iliac bone appears as an echogenic line. This line should

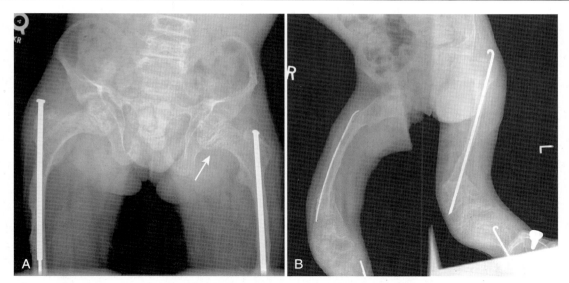

FIGURE 7-46. Osteogenesis imperfecta, tarda form. **A**, Radiograph of the pelvis. **B**, Radiograph of the femurs. Both show gracile, thin bones. There is deformity and internal hardware due to multiple previous fractures. There is extreme osteopenia. Note the alternating sclerotic and lucent bands in the metaphyses, most prominent in the proximal femurs *(arrow)*, resulting from bisphosphonate therapy.

Iliac line should bisect the femoral head

bisect a nondislocated femoral head. A dislocated femoral head will be positioned posterior and lateral to the iliac line (see Fig. 7-48). The angle created between lines drawn along the straight part of the iliac bone and the acetabular

Posterolateral displacement

roof form what Graf calls the alpha angle (see Fig. 7-48). Normally, the alpha angle is greater than 60 degrees (55 degrees in newborns). In DDH the acetabulum is shallow, resulting in a decreased alpha angle on ultrasound, which

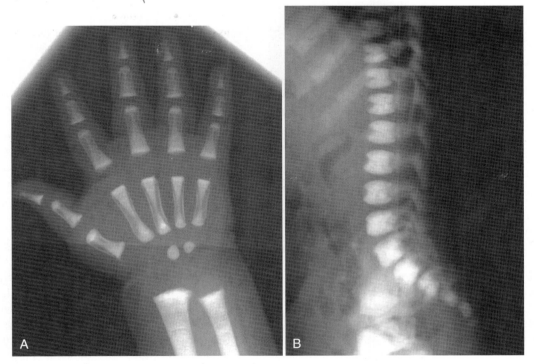

FIGURE 7-47. Osteopetrosis. **A**, Radiograph of hand shows severe bony sclerosis with bone-in-bone appearance. **B**, Radiograph of spine shows severe sclerosis of vertebral bodies.

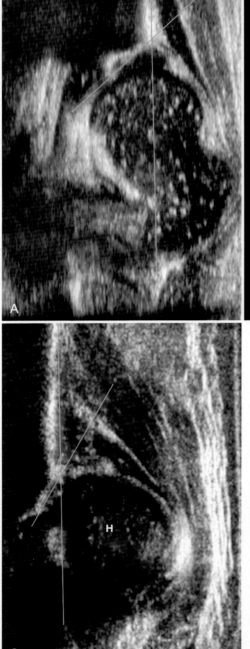

FIGURE 7-48. Coronal ultrasound of the hip in three babies. The ultrasounds are oriented in the plane correlating with a hip radiograph. The iliac bone forms a straight echogenic line that bisects the femoral head. The *alpha* angle is shown between a line drawn parallel to the roof of the acetabulum and a line drawn parallel to the iliac bone. With a shallow acetabulum, this angle is decreased. **A,** Normal. The alpha angle is 66 degrees, denoting a normally developed acetabular roof. The femoral head is bisected by the vertical line drawn along the iliac crest, denoting a nondislocated femoral head. **B,** Immature acetabulum without dislocated femoral head. The acetabulum is shallow and has an alpha angle of 48 degrees. The femoral head is not dislocated. **C,** Poorly developed acetabulum and dislocated femoral head. The acetabulum is very shallow and has a small alpha angle. The femoral head *(H)* is lateral to the iliac line, indicating that it is completely dislocated from the acetabulum.

correlates with an increased acetabular angle on radiographs (see subsequent material). A decreased alpha angle may be followed on repeat static ultrasound during therapy to evaluate for morphologic improvement.

DDH can also be evaluated by radiography. Radiographs are particularly useful after the femoral heads begin to ossify, rendering ultrasound of limited value. Also, it is important to know the radiographic findings of DDH so that such abnormalities may be identified when seen incidentally on other neonatal imaging studies that include the hips such as abdominal radiographs. Because the femoral epiphysis and portions of the acetabulum are cartilaginous and not directly visualized on radiographs of the

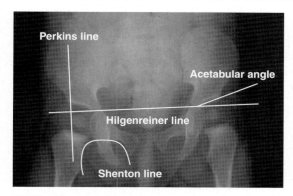

FIGURE 7-49. Radiograph of the normal pelvis demonstrating anatomic landmarks including Hilgenreiner, Perkins, and Shenton lines.

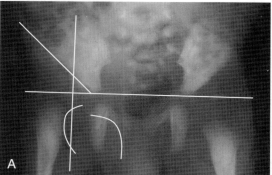

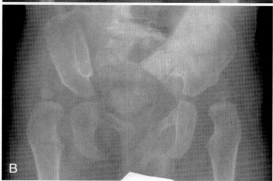

FIGURE 7-50. Developmental dysplasia of the hip in two patients. **A,** Developmental dysplasia of the hip on the right. The femoral heads are not yet ossified. The right metaphysis is displaced laterally compared to the Perkins line, and the Shenton arc is not continuous. The acetabular angle is greater than 30 degrees. **B,** Bilateral developmental dysplasia in a 1-year-old child. The femoral heads are ossified. Both femoral heads are displaced laterally. The acetabula are shallow and the acetabular angles are increased.

pelvis in the newborn period, landmarks are used to determine whether the hip is dislocated. With increasing age and ossification of the femoral head, direct visualization of a dislocated femoral head can be seen. Lines used to evaluate for DDH include the Hilgenreiner (Y-Y) line, the Perkins line, the Shenton arc, and the acetabular angle (Fig. 7-49). The Hilgenreiner line is a line drawn through the bilateral triradiate cartilages, touching the inferior medial aspect of each acetabulum. A second line is then drawn connecting the inferior medial and superolateral aspects of the acetabulum, outlining the acetabular roof. The angle made between these two lines is the acetabular angle. Normally, the acetabular angle is just less than 30 degrees at birth and decreases to 22 degrees at 1 year of age. With DDH, acetabular angles are abnormally increased. Another cause of increased acetabular angles is neuromuscular disorders. Abnormally decreased acetabular angles can be seen during the first year of life in Down syndrome and in multiple dysplasias, including achondroplasia (see Fig. 7-43). The vertical line of Perkins is drawn such that it is perpendicular to Hilgenreiner line and traverses the superolateral corner of the acetabulum. When the femoral head is ossified and visible, it should lie medial to the Perkins line. When the head is not ossified, the Perkins line should bisect the middle third of the metaphysis. If the metaphysis is lateral to this position, the hip is subluxed or dislocated (Fig. 7-50A, B). The Shenton arc is a continuous smooth arch connecting the medial cortex of the proximal metaphysis of the femur and the inferior edge of the superior pubic ramus. In DDH and dislocation, the arc is discontinuous (see Fig. 7-50).

Chronic Hip Subluxation

In patients with neuromuscular disorders such as cerebral palsy, development of progressive hip subluxation/dislocation may occur. Radiographs (Fig. 7-51) are used to evaluate how much the bony acetabulum covers the femoral head (% coverage), the degree of coxa valga (loss of angle between the neck and shaft of the femur), and the presence of complete dislocation.

Proximal Focal Femoral Deficiency

Proximal focal femoral deficiency (PFFD) is a congenital disorder consisting of a range of hypoplasias to the absence of the proximal portions of the femur (Fig. 7-52). In its most severe form, the acetabulum, femoral head, and proximal femur may be absent. A varus deformity is

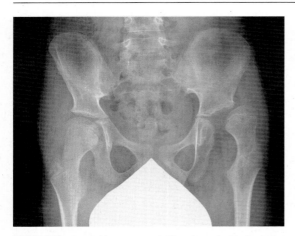

FIGURE 7-51. Hip subluxation in child with cerebral palsy. Note loss of normal angle (straight appearance) between the femoral neck and the shaft bilaterally (coxa valga). There is subluxation of the left hip, with only approximately 30% acetabular coverage. On the right, there is near complete acetabular coverage of the femoral head.

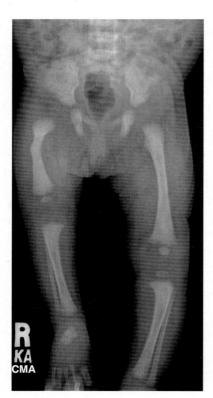

FIGURE 7-52. Proximal focal femoral deficiency shown on radiograph as hypoplastic right femur. Note elevated position of right knee compared to left.

commonly associated with the deficiency. It is important not to confuse the milder forms of PFFD with developmental dysplasia of the hip. In the latter, the femur is of normal length. PFFD can be associated with ipsilateral fibular hemimelia and deformity of the foot.

Septic Arthritis

There are many potential causes of painful hips in children (Table 7-6). Many of these diagnoses present at specific ages, so the differential diagnosis can often be limited on the basis of age (see Table 7-6).

Septic arthritis is the most urgent diagnosis to exclude in a patient with a painful joint, because delay in diagnosis can lead to destruction of the joint. In children, septic arthritis is thought to occur most commonly as a result of extension of infection from the adjacent metaphysis. In younger children, it usually occurs secondary to bacterial sepsis, and the most common organisms are *Staphylococcus aureus* (more than 50% of cases) and group A streptococci. Most cases of septic arthritis are monoarticular and involve large joints. The hip is the most common joint involved, followed by the knee.

In septic arthritis of the hip, children usually present with pain, limp, or failure to bear weight. Radiographs of the pelvis and hips are usually obtained to exclude other diagnoses.

Table 7-6. **Potential Causes of Hip Pain in Children**

Diagnosis	Typical Age at Presentation
Septic arthritis	Any age; most common in infants and teenagers
Toxic synovitis	<10 years
Osteomyelitis	<5 years
Langerhans cell histiocytosis	Any age, but pelvic bone involvement typically seen in those <5 years
Slipped capital femoral epiphysis	12-15 years
Legg-Calvé-Perthes disease	5-8 years
Juvenile rheumatoid arthritis	1-3 years
Ewing sarcoma	Second decade
Osteoid osteoma	Second decade

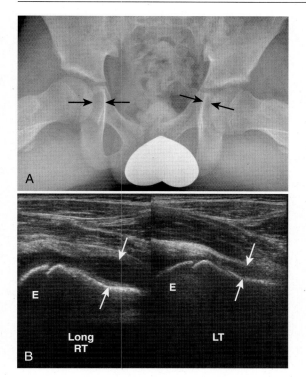

shaft of the proximal femur and the joint capsule is diagnostic of a joint effusion (see Fig. 7-53). The absence of fluid does exclude a diagnosis of septic arthritis. When fluid is present, ultrasound guidance can be used to tap the effusion. There are causes of joint effusion other than septic arthritis. They include toxic synovitis, noninfectious arthritis, and Legg-Calvé-Perthes disease.

Toxic Synovitis

Toxic synovitis is the name given to cases in which children present with pain or limping, have a joint effusion, have no findings of organisms in joint aspiration, and have symptoms that subside with rest. It occurs in children less than 10 years of age. It is a diagnosis of exclusion and is always in the differential diagnosis of septic arthritis. It is thought to be secondary to viral infection.

Legg-Calvé-Perthes Disease

Legg-Calvé-Perthes disease (LCP) is idiopathic avascular necrosis of the proximal femoral epiphysis. It occurs more commonly in boys than in girls (4:1), most commonly in whites, and typically between 5 and 8 years of age. Affected children present with pain in the groin, hip, or ipsilateral knee. The disease can be bilateral in as many as 13% of cases. It is often associated with skeletal immaturity (decreased bone age). Radiographs are usually positive, even early in the disease. Early findings include an asymmetric, small, ossified femoral epiphysis, widening of the joint space as a result of either joint effusion or synovial hypertrophy, and a subchondral linear lucency. The subchondral linear lucency (crescent sign) is best seen on frog-leg views and represents a fracture through the necrotic bone (Fig. 7-54A-D). When the diagnosis is suspected and radiographs are nondiagnostic, the diagnosis of LCP can be made on MRI (high T2-weighted signal marrow edema, loss of fatty marrow signal on T1-weighted images, asymmetric decreased enhancement with gadolinium) or bone scintigraphy (asymmetric lack of uptake; see Fig. 7-54). Later changes in LCP include changes in the femoral epiphysis, such as fragmentation, areas of increased sclerosis and lucency, and loss of height (collapse; see Fig. 7-54). Lucencies may

FIGURE 7-53. Septic arthritis of the right hip. **A,** Radiograph shows marked asymmetry of the hip joint spaces (arrows), with the right greater than the left. **B,** Longitudinal ultrasound of right and left hips, performed with an anterior approach, shows asymmetric widening (arrows) of right joint space as compared to left, consistent with right effusion. E, epiphysis.

The primary radiographic finding of septic arthritis is asymmetric widening of the hip joint space by more than 2 mm on a nonrotated film (Fig. 7-53A, B). The joint spaces are evaluated by measuring the distance between the teardrop of the acetabulum and the medial cortex of the metaphysis of the femur. Unfortunately, this finding, although important when positive, is not sensitive for a joint effusion. Fluid tends to accumulate in the anterior recess of the hip joint prior to displacing the femur laterally. When septic arthritis is associated with osteomyelitis or another cause of soft tissue swelling, displacement or obliteration of the fat pads surrounding the hip may be noted. These include the obturator internus, gluteus muscle, and iliopsoas fat pads. Abnormalities of the fat pads are also insensitive. Therefore, a normal pelvic radiograph in no way excludes a diagnosis of septic arthritis.

The presence of hip joint effusion is evaluated by ultrasound. The probe is placed longitudinally anterior to the hip joint. Asymmetric widening of a hypoechoic space between the

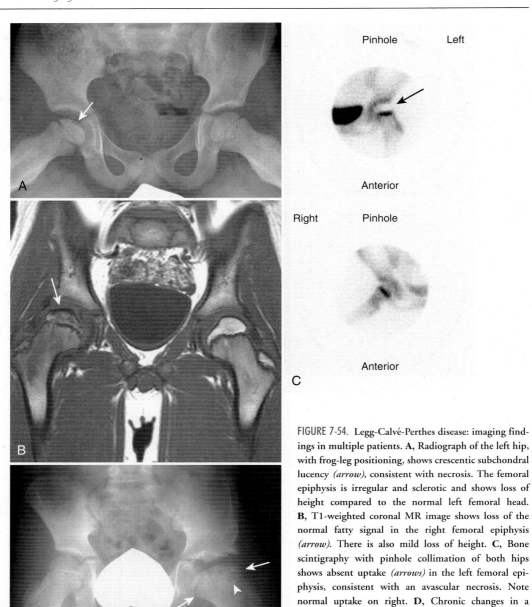

FIGURE 7-54. Legg-Calvé-Perthes disease: imaging findings in multiple patients. **A,** Radiograph of the left hip, with frog-leg positioning, shows crescentic subchondral lucency *(arrow)*, consistent with necrosis. The femoral epiphysis is irregular and sclerotic and shows loss of height compared to the normal left femoral head. **B,** T1-weighted coronal MR image shows loss of the normal fatty signal in the right femoral epiphysis *(arrow)*. There is also mild loss of height. **C,** Bone scintigraphy with pinhole collimation of both hips shows absent uptake *(arrows)* in the left femoral epiphysis, consistent with an avascular necrosis. Note normal uptake on right. **D,** Chronic changes in a node-fragmented, shortened capital femoral epiphysis with metaphyseal "cyst" *(arrowhead)*. Note widening of femoral head and neck (coxa magna; *arrows*). There has been left surgical acetabular reconstruction to create acetabular coverage of the enlarged left femoral head.

be seen in the adjacent metaphysis in as many as one third of patients. Chronic LCP may result in a broad, overgrown femoral head (coxa magna; see Fig. 7-54); a short femoral neck; and physeal arrest. Problems arise when the overgrown femoral head is not covered by the acetabulum, and this scenario may require surgical reconstruction of the acetabulum.

Slipped Capital Femoral Epiphysis

Slipped capital femoral epiphysis (SCFE) is an idiopathic Salter type 1 fracture through the proximal physis of the femur that results in displacement (slippage of the femoral epiphysis). It is more common in boys than in girls (2.5:1), in African Americans, and in obese children. Certain groups

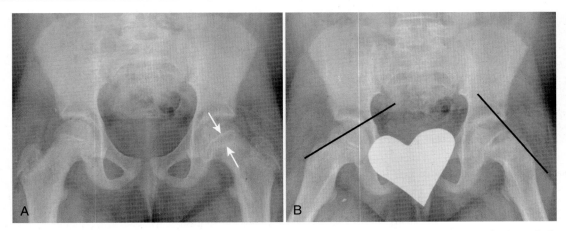

FIGURE 7-55. Slipped capital femoral epiphysis in a 12-year-old child with hip pain. **A,** Frontal, neutrally positioned radiograph shows asymmetric widening and indistinctness of the physis *(arrows)* of the left proximal femur. **B,** Radiograph with frog-leg lateral positioning shows posterior displacement of the epiphysis in relation to the physis. A line drawn along the lateral cortex of the metaphysis does not bisect the left epiphysis, whereas a similar line on the normal right side does.

such as those with renal osteodystrophy are predisposed. The hips can be involved bilaterally in up to one third of patients. However, both hips do not usually present at the same time. The typical age of diagnosis is 12 to 15 years.

The slippage of the femoral head in SCFE is posterior and to a lesser extent medial. Because of this, findings are more prominent on the frog-leg lateral view than on the frontal anteroposterior radiograph. On the frog-leg lateral view, the epiphysis is seen to be posteriorly displaced in comparison to the metaphysis. The image has been likened to an ice cream cone with the dip of ice cream falling off the cone. A line drawn tangential to the lateral cortex of the metaphysis on the frog-leg lateral view should bisect a portion of the ossified epiphysis

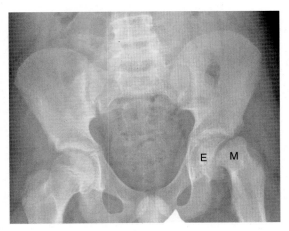

FIGURE. 7-56. Slipped capital femoral epiphysis. Radiograph shows complete slip of left epiphysis *(E)* in relation to left metaphysis *(M)*.

(Figs. 7-55A, B, 7-56). If the physis is medial to this line, it has slipped. Findings of SCFE can be very subtle on the frontal view. They include asymmetric widening of the physis and indistinctness of the metaphyseal border of the physis (see Fig. 7-55). SCFE is typically treated with pin fixation to prevent further slippage, but the epiphysis is not moved back to its normal position. Potential complications of SCFE include avascular necrosis of the femoral head and chondrolysis.

METABOLIC DISORDERS

Rickets

Rickets is the bony manifestations of a heterogeneous group of problems resulting from a relative or absolute insufficiency of vitamin D or its derivatives. It may result from dietary deficiency, malabsorption, renal disease, or lack of end-organ response. The lack of vitamin D results in insufficient conversion of growing cartilage into mineralized osteoid and buildup of nonossified osteoid. The radiographic manifestations are most prominent in rapidly growing bones, and skeletal surveys to evaluate for rickets can be confined to frontal views of the knees and wrists. Radiographic findings include metaphyseal fraying, cupping, and irregularity along the physeal margin (Fig. 7-57). There is osteomalacia with unsharp, smudged-appearing trabecular markings. Patients may be predisposed to insufficiency fractures (Looser zones) and slipped capital femoral epiphyses.

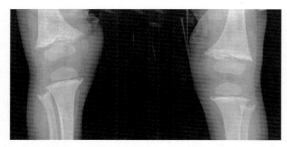

FIGURE 7-57. Rickets. Radiograph of bilateral knees shows metaphyseal cupping, fraying, and irregularity.

Lead Poisoning

Lead poisoning most commonly occurs in children younger than 2 years of age secondary to consumption of lead-containing substances such as old paint chips. Broad sclerotic metaphyseal bands (lead lines) may be seen in areas of rapid growth such as the knee. Unfortunately, dense metaphyseal bands can be seen as a normal variant. One discriminating factor is that lead lines tend to affect all of the metaphyses surrounding the knee, whereas the normal variant type of dense bands tends to spare the proximal fibula.

MISCELLANEOUS DISORDERS

Scoliosis

Scoliosis is defined as lateral curvature of the spine. Radiographic evaluation for spinal curvature after suspicion is raised on routine physical examination is a common occurrence in children. Most often, scoliosis is idiopathic in origin; the following discussion pertains to idiopathic scoliosis unless otherwise indicated. Idiopathic scoliosis is typically S-shaped, with the upper (thoracic) curvature convex to the right. Congenital scoliosis occurs secondary to abnormal vertebral segmentation and is often associated with more abrupt short-segment curves than those found in idiopathic cases. Neuromuscular scoliosis results from neurologic impairment or muscular dystrophy and is typically C-shaped. Idiopathic scoliosis is usually identified in late childhood or adolescence and is much more common in girls (M:F = 1:7). In 80% of cases, diagnosis is made between the ages of 10 years and maturity. The degree of curvature may change quickly during times of rapid growth such as puberty. Severe scoliosis can be associated with respiratory compromise, neurologic symptoms, and pain.

Radiographic evaluation is typically performed by means of a frontal view of the thoracolumbar spine, obtained on a single cassette. Studies are obtained with the patient standing (when possible) and in the posteroanterior projection to decrease the radiation dose to the breast. Depending on the situation, the frontal view may be complemented by a lateral view, bilateral bending views, or distraction views. When dictating scoliosis studies, it is important to mention the following in the technical factors of the dictation: the views obtained; whether the patient was lying down, sitting, or standing for the images; and whether the patient had an external brace on when the images were obtained. Braces typically have radiopaque snaps that are visible on radiographs.

The curvature of the spine is measured by calculating the Cobb angle. Lines are drawn parallel to the endplates of two vertebral bodies (Fig. 7-58). The angle between those two lines represents the angle of curvature. It is important to select the two

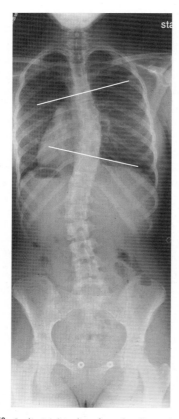

FIGURE 7-58. Scoliosis. Standing frontal radiograph of the thoracolumbar spine shows 28 degrees of apex rightward curvature from the superior aspect of T5 to the superior aspect of T10. White lines have been drawn parallel to endplates to calculate the angle. There are no vertebral anomalies. The entire iliac apophysis is ossified but not yet fused (Risser 4).

vertebral body endplates that create the greatest angle. Curves less than 7 degrees are considered normal. Curves less than 25 degrees are often treated by applying an external brace. Rapidly progressive curves or curves greater than 40 degrees are typically treated surgically.

When reporting findings, it is important to note whether any vertebral anomalies are present (Fig. 7-59A, B), the degree of spinal curvature, any change in curvature compared to previous studies, and the Risser index. The Risser index is used to define skeletal maturity by the degree of ossification of the iliac apophysis: grade 1, lateral 25%; grade 2, lateral 50%; grade 3, lateral 75%; grade 4, entire apophysis; grade 5, fusion of ossified apophysis to iliac wing. The more skeletally mature, the less chance there is of further progression of the spinal curvature. In follow-up of postoperative cases, it is also important to evaluate for fracture or change in position of hardware and change in curvature (see Fig. 7-59).

Abnormalities of Skeletal Maturity: Bone Age

Clinical indications for evaluating whether a child's skeletal maturity matches the child's true age include short stature, growth hormone deficiency, premature puberty, postmature puberty, and preoperative evaluation for orthopedic surgery (scoliosis, leg length discrepancy).

In such cases, a single frontal view of the left hand is typically obtained and compared with a set of image standards (Greulich and Pyle). The degree of epiphyseal ossification is compared with the standards. The pattern of ossification of the more distal physes of the fingers is considered more accurate than the more proximal finger physes or carpal bones. When reporting such studies, the patient's chronologic age, gender, bone age based on the standards of Greulich and Pyle, calculated standard of deviation of bone age for chronologic age, and whether the bone age falls outside of two standard deviations (i.e., whether it is abnormal) should be included.

Juvenile Rheumatoid Arthritis

Juvenile rheumatoid arthritis (JRA) is an idiopathic systemic disease that affects primarily the musculoskeletal system. It differs from adult rheumatoid arthritis in many ways. In JRA, most cases are seronegative and the

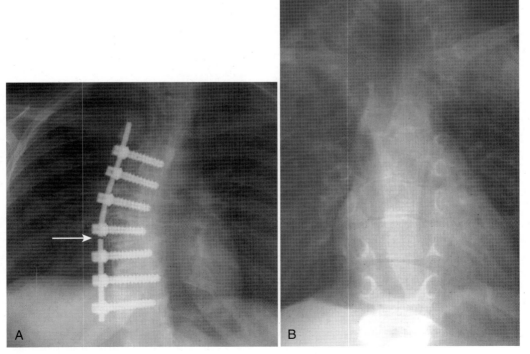

FIGURE 7-59. Imaging findings related to scoliosis. **A,** Radiograph shows fracture of hardware *(arrow)* on follow-up postoperative radiograph for spinal fusion. **B,** Radiograph shows multiple segmental vertebral and associated rib anomalies.

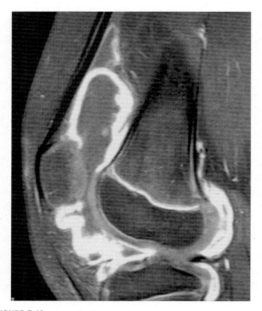

FIGURE 7-60. Juvenile rheumatoid arthritis of knee. Sagittal, contrast-enhanced, T1-weighted MR image shows markedly enhanced and thickened synovium. There is an associated joint effusion.

diagnosis is made clinically. In contrast to adult disease, in which small joint involvement predominates, large joint involvement is more common in children. The joints most commonly involved, in descending order, are the knee, ankle, wrist, hand, elbow, and hip. In most cases, the disease is pauciarticular, with between two and four joints involved. Prior to development of radiologic findings, MRI with gadolinium enhancement may show abnormally enhancing thickened synovium in involved joints (Fig. 7-60). This may be used to aid in diagnosis and in monitoring therapy. Initial radiographs may be normal or may show only soft tissue swelling or joint effusion. With more advanced disease in the knee, there may be joint effusion, epiphyseal overgrowth, widening of the intracondylar notch, and accelerated bony maturation (Fig. 7-61A, B). There can be associated periosteal reaction. In the cervical spine, there is often ankylosis of the apophyseal joints. When the hands and wrists are involved, the disease is typically most severe in the carpal bones (see Fig. 7-61). Findings include small, square-appearing carpal bones and narrowing of the intercarpal joint spaces. Later changes include erosions and ankylosis. Children may also have splenomegaly or pleural effusions. Still disease is an acute form of JRA in which children present with fever, rash,

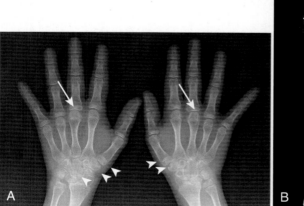

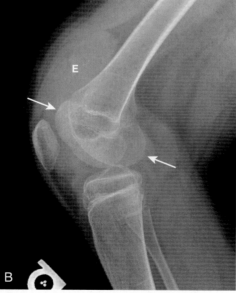

FIGURE 7-61. Juvenile rheumatoid arthritis: radiographic findings in several patients. **A,** Radiograph of the hands shows marked narrowing of intercarpal joints, erosions of several carpal bones *(arrowheads)*, and narrowing of the third metacarpophalangeal joints *(arrows)*. The findings are bilateral and symmetric. **B,** Radiograph of the knee shows large joint effusion *(E)* and bony overgrowth of the distal femoral epiphysis *(arrows)*.

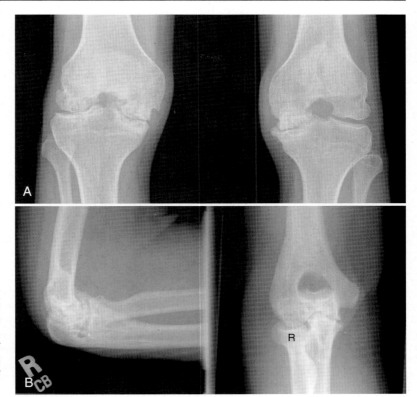

FIGURE 7-62. Hemophilia. **A,** Radiograph of the bilateral knees shows severe joint irregularity, joint-space narrowing, and widening of the intracondylar notch. **B,** Radiographs of elbow show irregularity and narrowing of the joint space and overgrowth of radial head (R).

hepatosplenomegaly, and lymphadenopathy. Skeletal involvement is rare in these children.

Hemophilia

With hemophilia, recurrent bleeding into a joint can result in a debilitating arthropathy. The joints most commonly involved include (in decreasing order of frequency of occurrence) the knee, elbow, and ankle. The recurrent hemorrhage deposits hemosiderin within the synovium, and there is associated hypertrophy of the synovium and destruction of the underlying articular cartilage. On radiography, epiphyseal overgrowth may be seen, and in the knee there is often squaring of the margin of the patella and widening of the intracondylar notch (Fig. 7-62A, B). These findings can appear similar to those in JRA. On MRI, there is destruction of articular cartilage and hypertrophy of the synovium. The hypertrophied synovium may be dark on T2-weighted images secondary to the hemosiderin deposition (Fig. 7-63), giving rise to an appearance similar to pigmented villonodular synovitis. Recurrent hematoma formation can also lead to the formation of pseudotumors, which usually occur in the

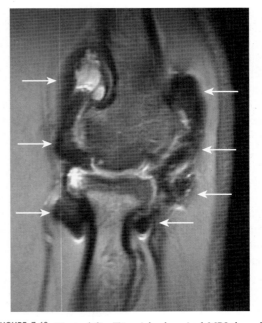

FUGURE 7-63. Hemophilia. T2-weighted, sagittal MRI through the radial-capitellar joint shows markedly thickened and low-signal synovium (arrows), consistent with hemosiderin deposition. There is associated irregularity of the capitellar joint surface.

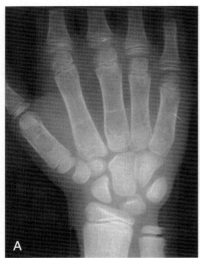
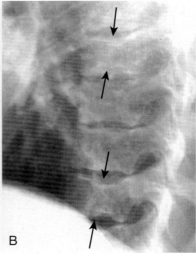

FIGURE 7-64. Bone changes in childhood anemias. **A,** Radiograph demonstrates expansion of the marrow cavities with associated expansion and thinning of the cortex, particularly in the metacarpal bones, of a child with thalassemia. **B,** Lateral radiograph shows Lincoln Log appearance of the spine in a child with sickle cell anemia. The superior and inferior endplates of multiple vertebral bodies show concavities *(arrows).*

soft tissues but can cause pressure necrosis and lucency of adjacent bone.

Sickle Cell Anemia and Thalassemia

With severe causes of anemia, such as sickle cell anemia or thalassemia, skeletal changes related to marrow expansion may be seen on radiography. Findings include thinning of the cortex, coarsening of the trabeculae, and bony remodeling (Fig. 7-64). The ribs appear widened. In the skull, the diploic space can become widened and have a hair-on-end appearance, particularly with thalassemia. In sickle cell anemia, there are often areas of bone infarction that may appear as either sclerotic or lucent areas. The vertebral bodies in sickle cell anemia often demonstrate indented and flat portions of the superior and inferior end plates, giving the vertebral bodies a "Lincoln log" appearance (see Fig. 7-64).

With severe anemia, other imaging findings may include cardiomegaly, gallstones, and splenomegaly (or conversely, in sickle cell anemia there may be autoinfarction of the spleen and a small, calcified spleen). Extramedullary hematopoiesis and a predisposition to osteomyelitis may also be noted.

Radial Dysplasia

Radial dysplasia, often referred to as radial ray syndrome, refers to a variable degree of hypoplasia or aplasia of the radius (Fig. 7-65). Often the first metatarsal or thumb may be hypoplastic or absent as well. Radial ray syndrome may be seen in conjunction with a number of syndromes, including association with VATER complex, Holt-Oram syndrome, Fanconi pancytopenia, and thrombocytopenia-absent radius syndrome.

Blount Disease

Blount disease is excessive medial bowing of the tibias (tibia vara), most commonly occurring during infancy. It is an idiopathic disease but is thought to be related to excessive pressure on the medial metaphysis of the tibia, resulting in delayed endochondral ossification. It can be differentiated from physiologic bowing of the tibias both by the degree of angulation and the appearance of the medial metaphysis of the tibia. With Blount disease, there is irregularity, fragmentation, and beaking of the medial tibial metaphysis (Fig. 7-66). Severe cases may require tibial osteotomy.

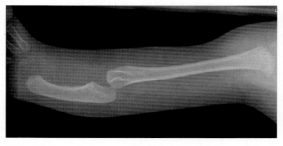

FIGURE 7-65. Radial dysplasia. Radiograph of upper extremity shows absent radius and short dysplastic ulna in a patient with Fanconi anemia. The thumb is also absent.

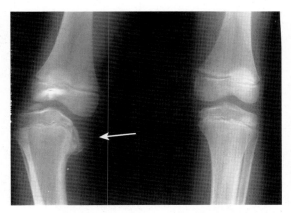

FIGURE 7-66. **Blount disease.** Radiograph demonstrates bowing of the tibia in association with irregularity and fragmentation of the medial tibial metaphysis *(arrow)*.

Neurofibromatosis

The nonmusculoskeletal aspects of neurofibromatosis type 1 are discussed in Chapter 8. Many changes can occur in the bones of patients with this disorder, and most of them are thought to be related to mesodermal dysplasia. The bones may demonstrate overgrowth, bowing (Fig. 7-67),

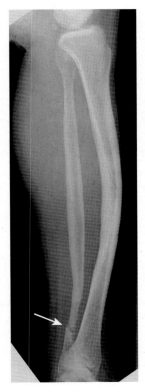

FIGURE 7-67. **Neurofibromatosis.** Lateral radiograph of tibia and fibula shows marked anterior bowing and patchy sclerosis of the tibia. There is a pseudoarthrosis of the fibula *(arrow)*.

areas of sclerosis, and numerous cortical defects. Characteristic findings include pseudoarthrosis formation (see Fig. 7-67), commonly within the tibia, and twisted-appearing (ribbonlike) ribs. The vertebral bodies may demonstrate posterior scalloping due to either dural ectasia or multiple neurofibromas. There is often kyphoscoliosis.

Clubfoot (Talipes Equinovarus)

Talipes equinovarus, or clubfoot, refers to a common congenital abnormality of the foot. In order to understand both clubfoot and other congenital abnormalities of the foot, it is important to understand the descriptive terminology. The terms *valgus* and *varus* refer to the bowing of the shaft of a bone and bowing at a joint. The name given to the bowing is determined by whether the distal part is more lateral or more medial than normal. *Valgus* refers to lateral (think: the L in valgus stands for lateral) and *varus* refers to medial. In hind-foot varus, the distal bone of the hind-foot (calcaneus) is angled too far medially in relationship to the more proximal bone of the hind-foot (talus) as seen on the anteroposterior view of the foot (Fig. 7-68A-D). Normally, this angle is approximately 30 degrees. With clubfoot, this angle is decreased. Also, on the lateral view of the foot, the lateral talocalcaneal angle is normally about 30 degrees. With clubfoot, there is a decrease in the lateral talocalcaneal angle, with the talus and calcaneus being closer to parallel to each other.

This same terminology is used to describe other parts of the body as well. Therefore, genu varum is the bowing of the knee, with the distal part (tibia) being more medial than normal, and coxa valgus is bowing at the hip, with the distal part (femur) being more lateral than normal. The terms *equinus* and *calcaneus* refer to the relationship between the ankle (tibia) and the hind-foot (calcaneus) as viewed on a lateral radiograph. Equinus is fixed plantarflexion of the calcaneus (distal end pointing down, as a deer walks), and calcaneus is fixed dorsiflexion (distal end of the calcaneus pointing up). With clubfoot, or talipes equinovarus, there is hind-foot varus, hind-foot equinus, and forefoot varus (see Fig. 7-68). Normally, a line drawn through the long axis of the talus on an anteroposterior view of the foot passes through the mid to the medial section of the metatarsal bones. With forefoot varus, the distal bones (the metatarsals) are located more medial to this drawn line.

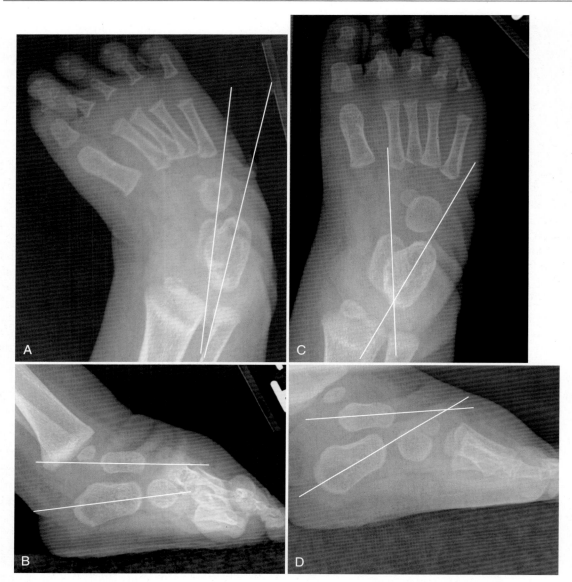

FIGURE 7-68. Foot angles in clubfoot and normal comparison (left and right foot in same child). **A,** Clubfoot. On frontal view, there is hindfoot varus. The frontal talocalcaneal angle is decreased (9 degrees). There is forefoot varus. A line drawn along the axis of the talus lies lateral to all of the metatarsal bones. **B,** Clubfoot. On the lateral view, the lateral talocalcaneal angle is decreased (9 degrees). The two bones are almost parallel. There is also equinus (plantar flexion of the hind-foot in relationship to the tibia). **C,** Normal. On the frontal view, the talocalcaneal angle is approximately 30 degrees. A line drawn along the axis of the talus traverses the midportion of the metatarsals. **D,** Normal. The lateral talocalcaneal relationships are normal; the lateral talocalcaneal angle is 30 degrees.

Tarsal Coalition

Tarsal coalition is an abnormal fibrous or bony connection between two of the tarsal bones of the feet. Patients with tarsal coalition can present with chronic foot pain or a propensity for ankle injury. It is a common abnormality affecting approximately 1% of the population and usually presents during adolescence. Although there is debate concerning which of the tarsal coalitions is the most common, talocalcaneal and calcaneonavicular coalitions are by far more common than other types. More than half of cases are bilateral. Calcaneonavicular coalition is easily demonstrated on radiographs of the foot. It is best visualized on the oblique view, in which the direct connection (bony coalition) or close proximity and irregularity of the joint margins (fibrous coalition) of the calcaneus and navicular bones (Fig. 7-69A, B) is best depicted. On the lateral

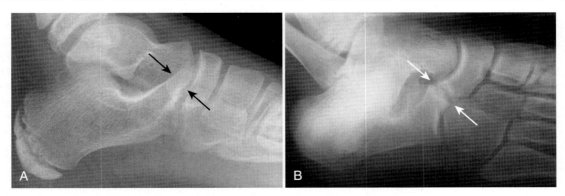

FIGURE 7-69. Calcaneonavicular coalition. **A,** Lateral radiograph demonstrates the superior calcaneus to be elongated *(arrows),* appearing to look like an anteater's nose. **B,** Oblique radiograph demonstrates close proximity and irregularity of the margins of the calcaneonavicular joint *(arrows),* consistent with fibrous coalition.

view, the anterior superior calcaneus appears longer than normal as it extends toward the navicular bone. The appearance has been likened to an anteater's nose (see Fig. 7-69). Rarely, cross-sectional imaging may be needed to confirm the diagnosis. In contrast, findings of talocalcaneal coalition can be subtle on radiography, and CT is performed to make the diagnosis. Radiographic findings include secondary signs such as talar beaking, poor visualization of the space within the talocalcaneal joint, and a prominent C-shaped band of overlapping bone overlying the calcaneus. On the lateral view, if space can be seen within the talocalcaneal joint, talocalcaneal coalition is not present. However, this space may not be seen within a normal joint on an oblique film. On coronal (short-axis) CT images, talocalcaneal coalition is visualized as

bony fusion or irregularity and close proximity (fibrous coalition) between the middle facet of the talus and the sustentaculum tali of the calcaneus (Fig. 7-70). Treatment options include surgical excision of the coalition.

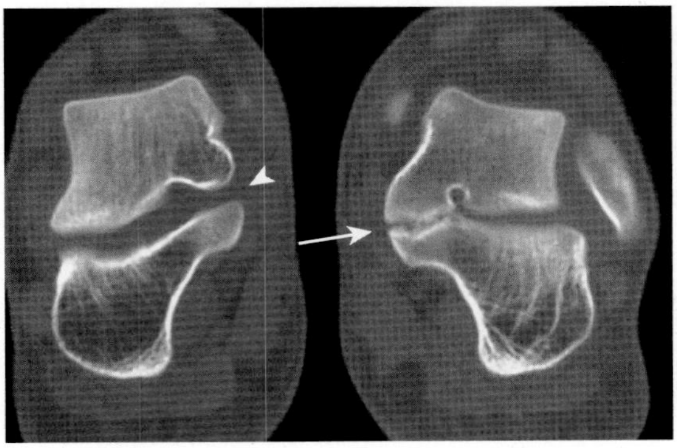

DISORDERS AFFECTING PRIMARILY SOFT TISSUES
Vascular Malformations

Vascular malformations and hemangiomas can cause significant morbidity and even mortality in both children and adults. For a number of reasons, there is often confusion regarding these lesions. The classification of and nomenclature used to describe endothelial malformations have been a source of confusion. Historically, lesions were named according to the sizes of channels within the lesions and the type of fluid the lesion contained. Blood-containing lesions were called hemangiomas and lymph-containing lesions were referred to as lymphangiomas or cystic hygromas. This classification system has been replaced by one described in 1982 by Mulliken and Glowacki. The system separates endothelial malformations into two large groups, hemangiomas and vascular malformations, on the basis of their natural history, cellular turnover, and histology (Table 7-7).

INFANTILE HEMANGIOMAS
Hemangiomas are the most common tumors of childhood, occurring in 12% of infants. Hemangiomas undergo a characteristic two-stage process of growth and regression. At birth, the lesions are commonly small and

FIGURE 7-70. Talocalcaneal coalition in the left foot. Coronal CT shows irregularity, sclerosis, close proximity, and abnormal oblique orientation of the middle facet of the left talocalcaneal joint *(arrow),* consistent with fibrous coalition. The normal right middle facet *(arrowhead)* shows smooth cortex between the talus and sustentaculum tali of the calcaneus.

Table 7-7. Differentiating Features of Hemangiomas and Vascular Malformations

Hemangiomas	Vascular Malformations
Exhibit cellular proliferation	Are composed of dysplastic vessels
Are small or absent at birth	Are present at birth
Exhibit rapid growth during infancy	Grow proportional to child
Show involution during childhood	Show no regression

inconspicuous; 60% are not visualized at birth. Shortly after birth, the phase of rapid proliferation occurs, and it can last for several months. The typical hemangioma begins to involute at approximately 10 months of age, with 50% of lesions being completely resolved by 5 years of age. Most hemangiomas require no therapy. However, potential complications include

Kasabach-Merritt syndrome (consumptive coagulopathy), compression of vital structures (e.g., airway, orbital structures), fissure formation, ulceration, and bleeding. In most cases, the diagnosis of hemangioma can be made on the basis of the temporal growth history and the appearance on physical inspection. Therefore, imaging is usually not required. Imaging may be obtained to characterize the lesion and evaluate the anatomic extent of disease and the potential compromise of adjacent vital structures. Ultrasound, MRI, or CT can be used to evaluate lesions (Fig. 7-71A-D). Imaging of a proliferating hemangioma typically shows a discrete lobulated mass. On MRI, the lesions are hyperintense on T2-weighted images (see Fig. 7-71) and isointense to muscle on T1-weighted images. Typically, prominent draining veins are identified as both central and peripheral high-flow vessels. Hemangiomas typically enhance diffusely with contrast and show increased flow on Doppler ultrasound. During the proliferative phase, hemangiomas show increased

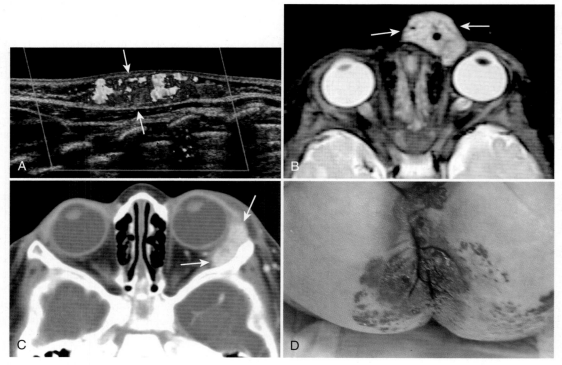

FIGURE 7-71. Infantile hemangioma: imaging characteristics in multiple patients. **A,** Ultrasound of hemangioma of back shows well-defined echogenic mass *(arrows)* confined to subcutaneous tissues. Color Doppler shows increased flow within the lesion. **B,** Axial, T2-weighted MR image of face shows a lobulated, well-defined mass *(arrows)* in the region of the nose and left orbit. There are flow voids within the lesion, consistent with prominent draining veins. **C,** Axial contrast-enhanced CT shows an enhancing, well-defined mass in the lateral aspect of the left orbit *(arrows)*. **D,** Photograph of an infant with extensive hemangioma of the gluteal region. Note the red areas of hemangioma.

arterial flow on T2* gradient echo imaging. Involuting hemangiomas can demonstrate areas of fibrofatty tissue with an associated high signal on T1-weighted images and demonstrate less contrast enhancement than proliferating hemangiomas. Unfortunately, many of the soft tissue malignancies of infancy, such as fibrosarcoma and rhabdomyosarcoma, can show an imaging appearance similar to that of proliferating hemangiomas. Therefore, cases that do not exhibit the typical appearance and growth patterns of hemangioma are often biopsied to exclude malignancy.

Low-Flow Vascular Malformations

Vascular malformations are always present at birth and enlarge in proportion to the growth of the child. They do not involute; they remain present throughout the patient's life. Vascular malformations can be subcategorized into lymphatic, capillary, venous, arteriovenous, or mixed malformations on the basis of the histologic makeup of the lesion. MRI can be used to classify vascular malformations into one of the previously mentioned categories; however, a more pertinent issue is classifying vascular malformations as either low-flow or high-flow lesions because their treatment options differ. Malformations with arterial components are considered high-flow lesions and those without arterial components are considered low-flow lesions. Low-flow vascular malformations include primarily venous, lymphatic, and mixed malformations.

Venous malformations are dysplasias of small and large venous channels. Many venous malformations cause pain; they may also cause decreased range of motion and deformity. Symptoms tend to increase in late childhood or early adulthood. Treatment options for venous malformations include elastic compression garments, percutaneous sclerosis, and surgical excision.

Lymphatic malformations consist of chyle-filled cysts lined with endothelium. The most common locations of lymphatic malformations are the neck (75%) and axillae (25%). When lymphatic malformations occur in the neck and axillae, they are often called cystic hygromas. Most lymphatic malformations present early in life; 65% are present at birth and 90% are found by the age of 2. Therapy for lymphatic malformations includes percutaneous sclerotherapy or surgical excision.

The appearance of a low-flow vascular malformation on MRI is determined by the composition of the lymphatic and venous components. The venous portions of a malformation appear as a collection of serpentine structures separated by septations. These serpentine structures represent slow-flowing blood within the venous channels and appear as high signals on T2-weighted images and intermediate signals on T1-weighted images (Fig. 7-72A-C). Phleboliths may be present; they appear as round, low-signal-intensity lesions on MRI. Gadolinium-enhanced T1-weighted images show enhancement of the slow-flowing venous channels. Lymphatic components of the malformation may contain cystic structures of various sizes, ranging from macrocystic to microcystic (Fig. 7-73A, B). These cystic structures typically appear as high in signal intensity on T2-weighted MRI and do not exhibit central enhancement with gadolinium. Fluid-fluid levels are often present. Another characteristic imaging finding in vascular malformations is that they tend to be infiltrative, without respecting fascial planes, and they often involve multiple tissue types, such as muscle and subcutaneous fat.

High-Flow Vascular Malformations

Any vascular malformation that has arterial components is considered a high-flow malformation. They include arteriovenous malformations and arteriovenous fistulae. During the proliferating stage, infantile hemangiomas may also be considered high-flow lesions. Arteriovenous malformations are direct connections between the arterial and venous systems. The lesions may present in childhood or adulthood and are often exacerbated during puberty or pregnancy. Presenting symptoms include congestive heart failure, embolism, pain, bleeding, and ulceration. High-flow vascular malformations are much less common than low-flow vascular malformations. On MRI, the lesions appear as a tangle of multiple-flow voids (Fig. 7-74A-C) that demonstrate high flow on gradient echo images. Although the lesions can be associated with surrounding edema or fibrofatty stroma, there is usually no focal, discrete, soft tissue mass. Color Doppler ultrasound demonstrates arterial waveforms in the adjacent venous structures. The most effective treatment for arteriovenous malformations is transarterial embolization.

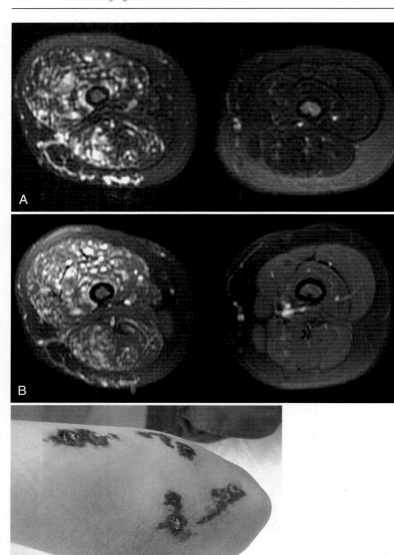

FIGURE 7-72. Venous malformation of the thigh. **A,** Axial T2-weighted MR image shows serpentine areas of high signal within the musculature throughout the right thigh. **B,** Axial contrast-enhanced T1-weighted MR image shows the serpentine areas to enhance diffusely with contrast, consistent with slow-moving venous blood. **C,** Photograph of cutaneous manifestations of venous malformation in the forearm in another patient. Note purplish, raised skin lesions.

Dermatomyositis

Dermatomyositis is an autoimmune disease that involves the skeletal muscle and skin. Children typically present with weakness and rash. MRI has been used to aid in making the diagnosis, directing biopsies to high-yield areas and monitoring the response to therapy. On T2-weighted fat-saturated images, there is increased signal intensity in the involved muscles, myofascial planes, and subcutaneous tissues (Fig. 7-75A-C). The most commonly involved muscles are those within the anterior compartment of the thigh and those surrounding the hip. There is typically rapid resolution of the abnormal high signal

after therapy has been instituted. In patients with chronic dermatomyositis, calcifications may be seen in the soft tissues on radiography (see Fig. 7-75).

Soft Tissue Malignancies

Primary malignancies of the soft tissues are uncommon in children. MRI is the imaging modality of choice for evaluating soft tissue masses. The likely diagnosis is related to the patient's age. In infants, fibrosarcoma is the most common soft tissue malignancy, whereas rhabdomyosarcoma is the most common in

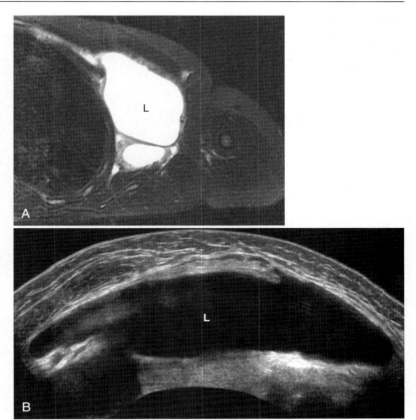

FIGURE 7-73. Lymphatic malformation in the left axilla. **A,** Axial, T2-weighted image shows multiloculated, cystic-appearing mass *(L)* in region of left axilla. **B,** Ultrasound shows dominant cystic area *(L)* that is anechoic. Ultrasound was performed as imaging guidance for percutaneous sclerosis.

older children (Fig. 7-76). Other potential malignancies include primitive neuroectodermal tumors and synovial sarcomas. Synovial sarcomas tend to occur around joints and are notoriously and deceptively benign-appearing on imaging studies, with smooth, well-defined borders.

Aggressive fibromatosis is a fibroproliferative disorder that is locally aggressive but does not metastasize. The lesions usually involve older children and occur in the deep soft tissues. On MRI, the lesions tend to be high-signal on T2-weighted images (Fig. 7-77) despite their fibrous nature. After resection, there is a tendency to recurrence along the proximal margin of the resection.

Mimickers of Soft Tissue Malignancies

There are a number of benign entities that can present as palpable masses on physical examination and may lead to a request for imaging to rule out a malignant soft tissue mass. Knowledge of these entities will lead to accurate diagnosis and avoid potentially unnecessary or wrong procedures.

Such entities include myositis ossificans, chronic foreign body, posttraumatic fat necrosis, and fibromatosis colli.

Myositis Ossificans

Myositis ossificans typically presents as a tender soft tissue mass. It is thought to be related to an organizing hematoma, but a history of trauma may be difficult to elicit. Eventually (2 to 6 weeks after the event), calcifications within the soft tissues become evident and progress into a sharply circumscribed egg-shell appearance. Initial radiographs may fail to show calcifications (Fig. 7-78A-C), and MRI performed at that time may show a nonspecific soft tissue mass (see Fig. 7-78). A low-signal ring may be seen on MRI on gradient echo sequences. CT may show calcifications before they are seen on radiography.

Chronic Foreign Body

A child may experience a penetrating trauma that introduces a small foreign body, but the trauma may not be remembered. Such a child may present months later with a palpable soft tissue mass related to formation of granulation tissue around the foreign body and be imaged

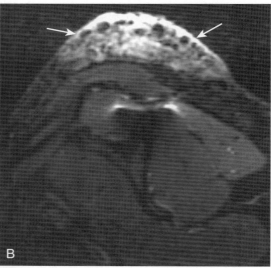

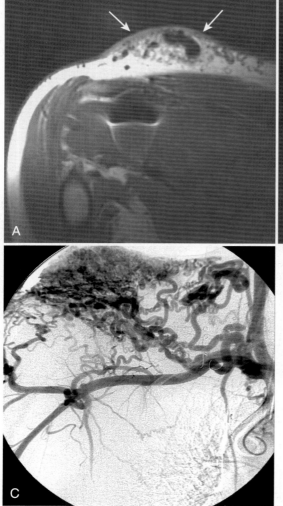

FIGURE 7-74. High-flow vascular malformation of the right shoulder. **A,** Coronal T1-weighted image shows tubular flow voids *(arrows)* in subcutaneous tissues of shoulder. There is no associated solid, soft-tissue mass. **B,** Sagittal T2-weighted image shows flow voids with surrounding high-signal edema *(arrows)*. **C,** Frontal arteriogram after injection of the arch shows a tangle of arterial structures over the right shoulder, documenting arteriovenous malformation.

for workup of a soft tissue mass. Typical locations for chronic foreign bodies are those predisposed to trauma, including the plantar aspect of the foot, the anterior portion of the knee, and the buttocks. When MRI is performed to evaluate such a soft tissue mass, the foreign body may appear as a low-signal structure surrounded by soft tissue mass (Fig. 7-79).

POSTTRAUMATIC FAT NECROSIS

As a result of minor trauma, children may develop fat necrosis in the area of the injured subcutaneous tissue. Months after the event, there may be scar formation in the area of fat necrosis, and it may present as a firm mass on physical examination. At the time of presentation, the traumatic event is usually not remembered.

The most common locations for posttraumatic fat necrosis are in the thin layer of subcutaneous tissue anterior to the tibia (take a look at any 8-year-old's shins; most have bruising) and the buttocks. On MRI, posttraumatic fat necrosis appears as a linear area of high T2-weighted signal and enhancement (Fig. 7-80). It is confined to the subcutaneous tissues, is associated with volume loss in the involved subcutaneous tissues, and is not associated with a discrete soft tissue mass. There is a similar condition known as subcutaneous granuloma annulare that also involves the subcutaneous tissues anterior to the tibia and is thought to be related to trauma, but does have soft tissue mass related to granulation tissue. My guess is that these two entities are points along a spectrum.

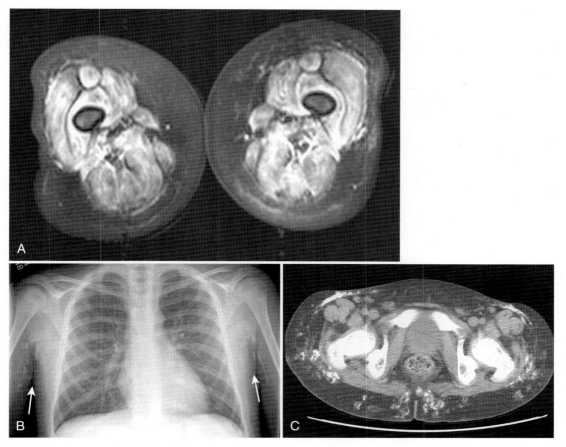

FIGURE 7-75. Dermatomyositis: imaging findings in multiple children. **A,** Axial T2-weighted image through the thigh shows marked abnormally increased signal throughout the anterior and posterior musculature of the thigh. Normally, the muscles are low in signal on this sequence. **B,** Chest radiograph shows calcifications *(arrows)* diffusely within the subcutaneous tissues. **C,** Axial CT image shows heterogeneous calcifications in the subcutaneous tissues of the lower pelvis and upper thigh.

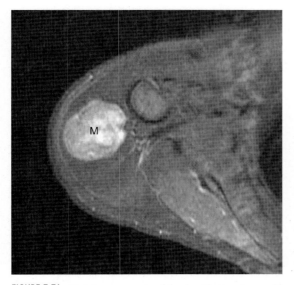

FIGURE 7-76. Rhabdomyosarcoma of the shoulder in a 5-year-old boy. Axial, postcontrast MR image shows well-defined, heterogeneously enhancing mass *(M)* in right deltoid muscle. The lesion has some deceivingly benign-appearing imaging characteristics: well-defined borders and round shape.

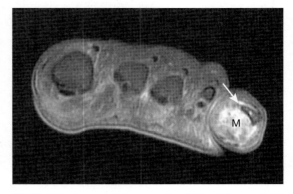

FIGURE 7-77. Aggressive fibromatosis of the fifth toe. Axial T2-weighted image shows nonspecific, heterogeneous high-signal, intramuscular soft tissue mass *(M)*. Note the deformity of the adjacent fifth phalanx *(arrow)*.

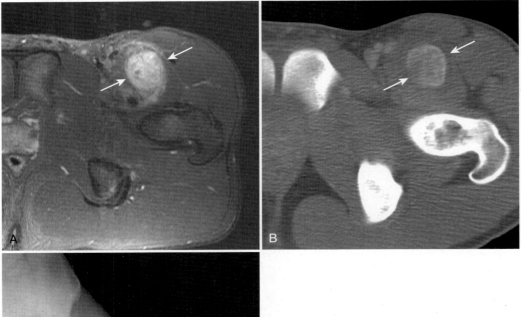

FIGURE 7-78. Myositis ossificans. **A,** Initial MRI was performed for palpable soft tissue mass. Radiographs at that time were normal. Axial postcontrast MR image shows heterogeneous, enhancing, intramuscular mass *(arrows)*. The lesion is a nonspecific soft tissue mass. **B,** CT performed to further evaluate for potential calcifications because of the possibility of myositis ossificans demonstrates calcifications throughout the mass *(arrows)*. **C,** Radiograph several weeks later shows development of calcifications *(arrow)* within well-defined peripheral borders, characteristic of myositis ossificans.

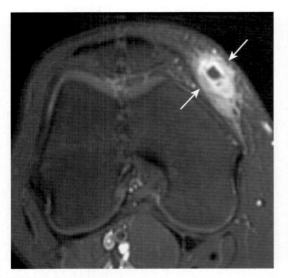

FIGURE 7-79. Chronic foreign body. Axial, postcontrast T1-weighted MR image, obtained because of palpable soft tissue mass on physical examination, shows heterogeneous enhancing mass *(arrows)* in the subcutaneous tissues of the knee. There is a central low-signal, square structure. The lesion proved to be a chronic foreign body with surrounding granulomatous formation.

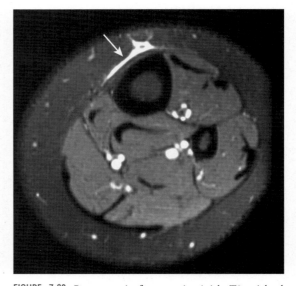

FIGURE 7-80. Posttraumatic fat necrosis. Axial, T2-weighted MRI of the knee, obtained because of palpable soft tissue mass on physical examination, shows linear area of increased signal *(arrow)* immediately anterior to the anterior surface of the tibia. There is no associated soft tissue mass. Position and appearance are characteristic of posttraumatic fat necrosis.

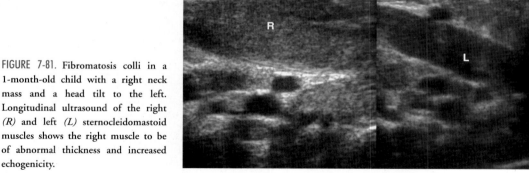

FIGURE 7-81. Fibromatosis colli in a 1-month-old child with a right neck mass and a head tilt to the left. Longitudinal ultrasound of the right *(R)* and left *(L)* sternocleidomastoid muscles shows the right muscle to be of abnormal thickness and increased echogenicity.

FIBROMATOSIS COLLI

Fibromatosis colli is a term that should not be confused with the more aggressive fibrotic processes of childhood. It is a benign mass in the sternocleidomastoid muscle in neonates who present with torticollis. The cause is poorly understood. Typically, ultrasound is performed to confirm the diagnosis. Ultrasound shows asymmetric fusiform thickening of the sternocleidomastoid muscle (Fig. 7-81), the echogenicity of which is typically heterogeneous and asymmetric but may be increased or decreased compared to the contralateral normal muscle. Most symptoms resolve over time with stretching exercises, and surgical intervention is rarely required.

Suggested Readings

Donnelly LF, Bisset GS III, Helms CA, Squire DL : Chronic avulsive injuries of childhood, *Skel Radiol* 78:138-144, 1999.

Donnelly LF, Adams DM, Bisset GS III: Centennial dissertation: vascular malformations and hemangiomas: a practical approach in a multidisciplinary clinic, *AJR* 174: 597-608, 2000.

Harcke HT, Grissom LE: Performing dynamic sonography of the infant hip, *AJR* 155:837-844, 1990.

Helms CA: *Fundamentals of skeletal radiology,* ed 2, Philadelphia, WB Saunders, 1995.

Keats TE, Joyce JM: Metaphyseal cortical irregularities in children: a new perspective on a multi-focal growth variant, *Skel Radiol* 12:112-118, 1984.

Kleinman PK: Diagnostic imaging in infant abuse, *AJR* 155:703-712, 1990.

Kozlowski K: The radiographic clues in the diagnosis of bone dysplasias, *Pediatr Radiol* 15:1-3, 1985.

Mulliken JB, Glowacki J: Hemangiomas and vascular malformations in infants and children: a classification based on endothelial characteristics, *Plast Reconstr Surg* 69: 412-422, 1982.

Oestreich AE, Crawford AH: *Atlas of pediatric orthopedic radiology,* Stuttgart, Thieme, 1985.

Ozonoff MB: *Pediatric orthopedic radiology,* ed 2, Philadelphia, WB Saunders, 1992.

Rogers LF, Poznanski AK: Imaging of epiphyseal injuries, *Radiology* 191:297-308, 1994.

Taybi H, Lachman RS: *Radiology of syndromes, metabolic disorders, and skeletal dysplasias,* ed 4, St. Louis, Mosby, 1996.

CHAPTER EIGHT

Neuro

Pediatric neuroimaging is a distinct subspecialty. Anatomic areas included in neuroimaging include the skull, brain, meninges, orbits, sinuses, neck, and spine. At many children's hospitals, dedicated neuroradiologists perform and interpret all of the neuroimaging. The large amount of information included in neuroradiology is beyond the scope of this textbook. However, this chapter is a review of some of the more commonly encountered entities.

PEDIATRIC NEUROIMAGING MODALITIES: MAGNETIC RESONANCE, COMPUTED TOMOGRAPHY, AND ULTRASOUND

In pediatric neuroimaging, magnetic resonance imaging (MRI), computed tomography (CT), and ultrasound are all used, with some overlap, in the imaging indications. In general, MRI has become the definitive test in evaluating intracranial abnormalities. It is the test of choice for evaluating brain involvement in neoplasms, vascular lesions, inflammatory disorders, and developmental abnormalities, as well as for the evaluation of neurodegenerative disorders, focal seizures, unexplained hydrocephalus, and neuroendocrine disorders. CT is typically reserved for the evaluation of trauma and acute neurologic symptoms, such as those associated with ventriculoperitoneal shunt malfunction. Sinus disease, orbital cellulitis, temporal bones, and head and neck abnormalities are also often evaluated by CT. Head ultrasound is reserved for evaluating premature infants and newborns.

BASIC REVIEW OF ADVANCED MRI TECHNIQUES IN PEDIATRIC NEUROIMAGING

A number of advanced MRI techniques are playing an increasing role in the neuroimaging of children. Such techniques are summarized here, basic vocabulary is reviewed (which is

half the battle), and applications in pediatric patients are discussed.

Functional MRI

Functional MRI (fMRI) is a noninvasive method of evaluating regional neuronal activity within the brain. Neuronal activity increases metabolic activity, which results in increased blood flow to that region and a relative increase in the ratio of oxygenated hemoglobin to deoxygenated hemoglobin. Deoxyhemoglobin is paramagnetic; therefore, a change in the ratio affects the magnetic state of the tissue and as a result, changes the local MRI signal. This phenomenon is called the BOLD (blood oxygenation level-dependent) effect. fMRI techniques show these changes superimposed on anatomic information. fMRI is used to document regional neuronal activity during a specific activity: language (Fig. 8-1), memory, or motor function. It has been a very useful research tool in increasing our understanding of brain function during various tasks. Clinically, fMRI has been used in areas such as the evaluation of patients with seizures and the planning of surgical approaches to brain tumors.

MR Spectroscopy

Proton (hydrogen) MR spectroscopy is a tool that is now routinely used to help characterize a number of pediatric neurologic conditions. Most often, single-voxel spectroscopy is created using a 1 cubic centimeter sample area. The results of spectroscopy are typically depicted as a spectrum, with each metabolic peak characterized by resonance frequency, height, width, and area (Fig. 8-2). Metabolic profiles depicted on MR spectroscopy have been much less specific than originally hoped. However, the information obtained does provide useful information that complements the information derived from MRI in many pediatric disorders, including neoplasms, ischemia, and white matter diseases.

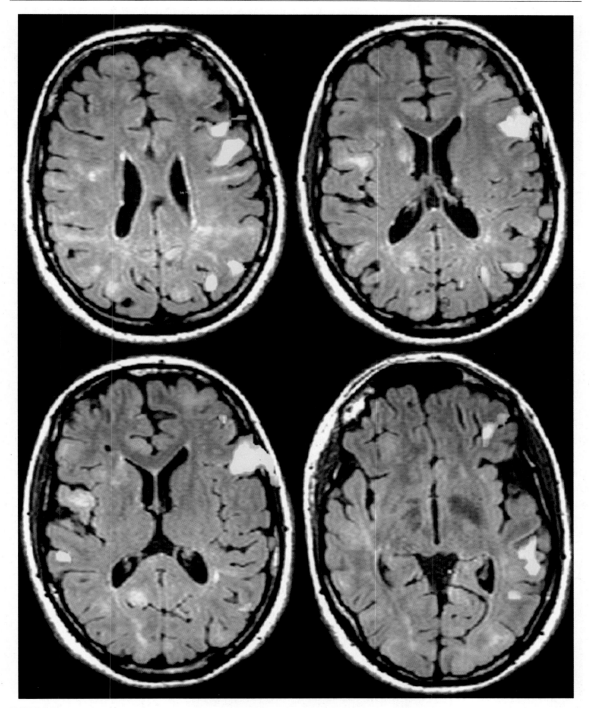

FIGURE 8-1. Functional MRI. Right-handed 18-year-old with tuberous sclerosis and chronic seizures imaged for preoperative evaluation of hemispheric language dominance. Auditorily presented noun-covert verb generation. Areas of significant BOLD-related signal change (orange-yellow areas) during silent verb production with auditorily presented noun are noted to be predominately left-sided in the left inferior frontal lobe and left temporal parietal regions, consistent with left hemispheric language dominance. Multiple areas of signal increase are noted on the (FLAIR) sequence used as an anatomic overlay, consistent with cortical and subcortical tuber formation. (Images courtesy of James L. Leach, MD.)

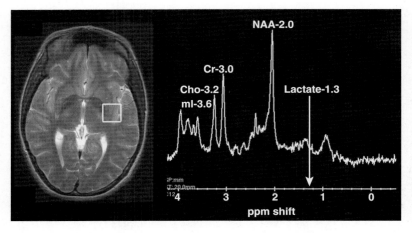

FIGURE 8-2. Normal single voxel ^{1}H-MR spectroscopy. Left image shows single voxel placement. Right image shows spectra. Note the normal stair-step relationship of choline (Cho; 3.2 ppm); creatine (Cr; 3.0 ppm); and *NAA* (NAA; 2.0 ppm) peaks. A peak related to myoinositol is also noted (Ml; 3.6 ppm). Location of pathologic lactate peak (not present in this normal example of deep gray matter) is denoted by the *arrow* (1.3 ppm). (Images courtesy of James L. Leach, MD)

The commonly evaluated brain metabolites include *N*-acetyl aspartate (NAA), creatine, choline, and lactate (see Fig. 8-2). NAA is a neuronal marker and is decreased in most disorders that destroy brain tissues, such as neoplasms (Fig. 8-3), infarcts, radiation injuries, and seizures. NAA is markedly elevated in Canavan disease. Choline compounds reflect the synthesis and degradation of cell membranes; therefore, increased choline is seen when there is high cellular turnover, as occurs with most tumors (see Fig. 8-3). Lactate is typically elevated in the setting of acute ischemia, infarction, and many high-grade tumors and severe infections (Fig. 8-4; and see Fig. 8-3). Creatine remains stable in the presence of many disorders but can be increased in hypometabolic states and decreased in hypermetabolic states.

Diffusion-Weighted Imaging

Diffusion-weighted imaging (DWI) images are determined by the variability in the diffusivity of water in tissues. Molecules move randomly in fluid (Brownian motion). In tissues, there is variable restriction of the movement of water molecules relative to tissue structure (cell membranes, vascular structures, density of cells, axons). Pathologic states alter the diffusion characteristics of brain water and therefore affect the appearance of the image. DWI images are created by applying two additional magnetic field gradients. The first dephases the spins and the second rephases the spins, if no movement occurs. If there is free movement of molecules, such as in the free-moving water in the cerebrospinal fluid (CSF), the protons lose spin coherence and

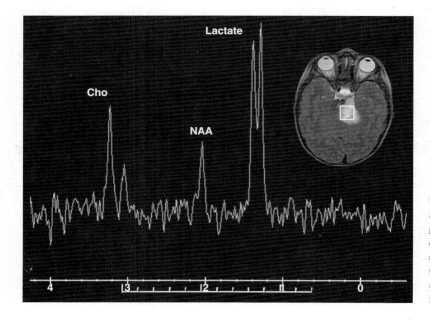

FIGURE 8-3. Abnormal spectroscopy in a 5-year-old child with left brainstem glioblastoma multiforme. Note large choline (Cho) peak, diminished *NAA*, and markedly elevated lactate peak, typical of high-grade glial neoplasm. (Images courtesy of James L. Leach, MD)

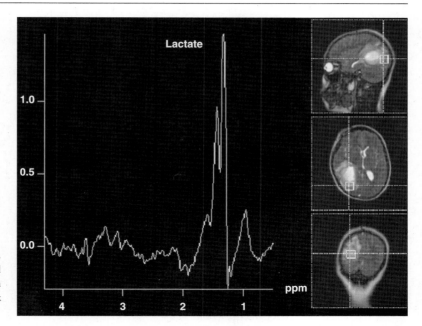

FIGURE 8-4. Abnormal spectroscopy. 12-year-old child with right parietal abscess. Note absence of normal brain metabolites and large lactate peak consistent with necrosis.

there is signal loss. If movement is restricted, the movement of molecules is less random and more signal is returned.

Images in DWI are influenced not only by diffusion but also by other tissue properties such as T2. In order to eliminate the influences on imaging appearance of factors unrelated to diffusion, the data are frequently processed, most commonly by a technique called an apparent diffusion coefficient (ADC) map. Therefore, for each DWI sequence, two sets of images are often created: the DWI images and the ADC map. What the bright and low areas mean on these two sets of images can be confusing, because they are the opposites of each other. In a pathologic process in which there is restricted diffusion, the involved area appears high in signal on the DWI images and

low in signal on the ADC map. Therefore, for clarification: restricted diffusion = bright signal on DWI = dark signal on ADC map = diminished ADC. Conversely, in pathologic processes in which there is increased diffusion, there is a dark signal on DWI images and a high signal on the ADC map. Table 8-1 shows a glossary of terms related to DWI and diffusion tensor imaging (DTI).

Pathologic processes that show restricted diffusion include acute infarction; cellular edema (such as that caused by acute ischemia or nonhemorrhagic traumatic injury); purulent fluid collections (Fig. 8-5); epidermoid cysts; and hypercellular tumors such as medulloblastoma. Processes that show increased diffusion include vasogenic edema and CSF collections such as those in an arachnoid cyst.

Table 8-1. Glossary of Terms in Diffusion-Weighted and Diffusion Tensor Imaging

Term	Definition
Isotropy	Uniformity of physical properties of a molecule in all directions; in other words, the absence of any kind of polarity
Anisotropy	The opposite of isotropy; having polarity or directionality
Eigenvalue	The mathematical property of a tensor (vector) related to magnitude and direction
Fractional anisotropy	A metric measuring the degree of anisotropy (0 for isotropy and 1 for full anisotropy)
Apparent diffusion coefficient (ADC)	A measure of the freedom of water diffusion in a particular tissue; increased ADC = increased diffusivity
Tractography	A postprocessing method of creating images representing axonal fiber tracts from diffusion tensor data
Tensor	The magnitude and direction of diffusion; is used similarly to the term *vector*. A 3 × 3 matrix is used to calculate a tensor

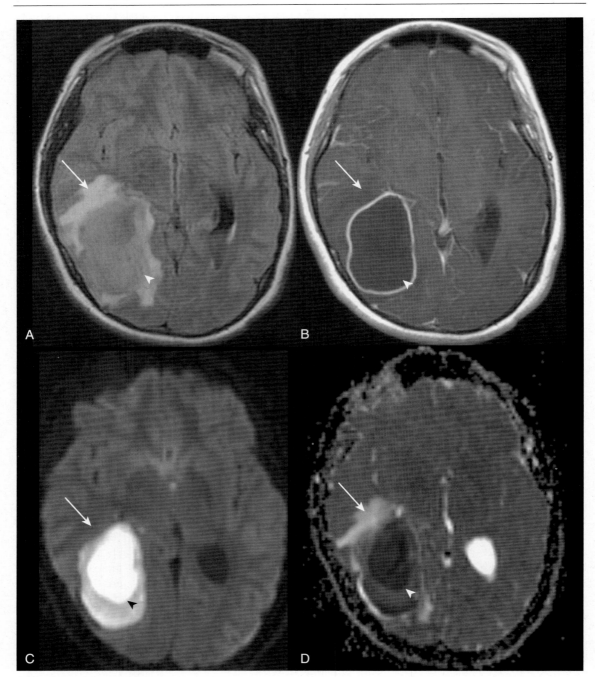

FIGURE 8-5. DWI. Brain abscess in a 12-year-old male. The *arrow* points to vasogenic edema. The *arrowhead* points to the abscess cavity. (A) Axial FLAIR sequence shows relatively low-signal area with surrounding vasogenic edema. (B), Contrast-enhanced axial T1-weighted image shows large ring enhancing the lesion identified in the right parietal lobe. (C) DWI. Abscess cavity has high signal probably related to increased T2 properties. Surrounding edema has increased diffusion and is high in signal. (D) ADC map. Abscess cavity is low in signal, consistent with restricted diffusion from purulent fluid. Surrounding vasogenic edema is high in signal, consistent with increased diffusion. (Images courtesy of James L. Leach, MD)

DWI has become a commonly used tool in neuroimaging. One of its major advantages is its high sensitivity for ischemia and infarction; it often reveals them before such findings are seen in conventional MR sequences. It is also helpful in differentiating among posterior fossa tumors. The hypercellular medulloblastoma has restricted diffusion, whereas ependymoma and astrocytoma typically do not.

Diffusion Tensor Imaging

By applying diffusion gradients in at least six directions during a diffusion MRI sequence, DTI techniques enable the identification of the location, orientation, and directionality of the white matter tracts. DTI provides several capabilities not previously possible. (1) Large individual white matter tracts can be depicted as discrete anatomic structures. The three-dimensional postprocessing technique used to create such images is called tractography. (2) Metrics describing the microarchitecture of tissue can be calculated. They include fractional anisotrophy and diffusivity.

Tractography images are typically shown in color. By convention, white matter tracts oriented left to right are shown as red, cephalocaudad as blue, and anterioposterior as green (Fig. 8-6).

DTI and tractography can be used to evaluate myelination. Increased myelination increases anisotrophy. Therefore, in normal infants, anisotrophy increases with age. Most disease states that affect white matter decrease anisotrophy. DTI has been used to evaluate stroke, brain tumor (Fig. 8-7), trauma, and demyelinating disorders. DTI and tractography have also been used to study and depict the white matter tract abnormalities associated with congenital brain anomalies and in the presurgical evaluation of brain tumors (see Fig. 8-7).

NEONATAL HEAD ULTRASOUND

Neonatal head ultrasound is performed through the open anterior fontanel of neonates and infants using a high-frequency sector transducer. Images are commonly obtained in the sagittal and coronal planes (Fig. 8-8). Head ultrasound is most commonly used to diagnose and follow up, in premature infants, intracranial complications, such as germinal matrix hemorrhage and periventricular

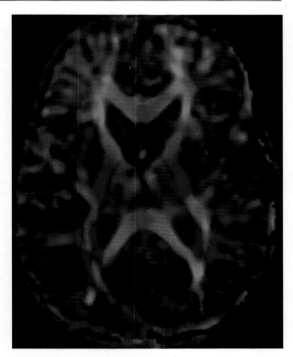

FIGURE 8-6. **Eigenvalue map showing white matter tracts. Note that red denotes tracts oriented left to right; blue denotes cephalocaudad; and green denotes anteroposterior. (Images courtesy of James L. Leach, MD)**

leukomalacia. It can also be used to screen for congenital abnormalities and hydrocephalus. Another common indication is evaluation of an infant with a large head circumference.

Germinal Matrix Hemorrhage

The germinal matrix is a fetal structure that is a stem source for neuroblasts. It typically involutes by term but is still present in premature infants. The germinal matrix is highly vascular and is subject to hemorrhaging. The germinal matrix lies within the caudothalamic groove (the space between the caudate head and the thalamus). Germinal matrix hemorrhage most commonly occurs in premature infants during the first 3 days after birth. Potential complications include destruction of the precursor cells within the germinal matrix, hydrocephalus, and hemorrhagic infarction of the surrounding periventricular tissues.

On ultrasound, germinal matrix hemorrhage is seen as an ovoid echogenic mass within the caudothalamic groove (Figs. 8-9, 8-10A, B, 8-11). For those not well acquainted with head ultrasound, there may be confusion in differentiating germinal

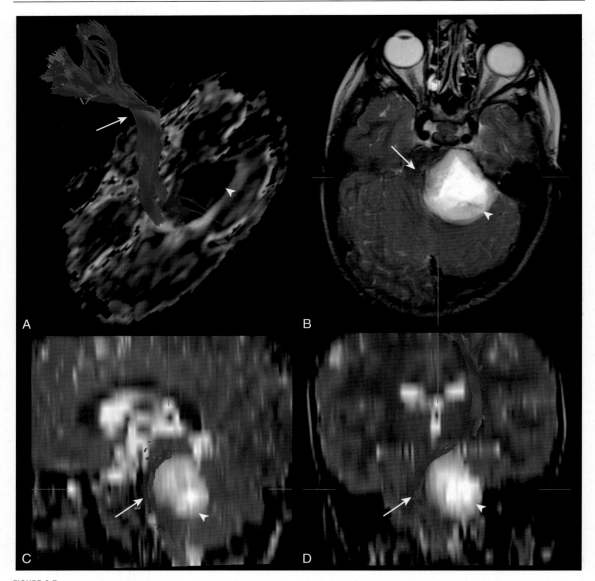

FIGURE 8-7. DTI. Left brainstem glioblastoma multiforme in 5-year-old male extending into the brachium pontis. Tractography (A) and three-dimensional fiber representation of the left corticospinal tract (B, axial; C, sagittal; D, coronal) obtained for surgical planning. Left corticospinal tract *(arrows)* overlaid on anatomic images. Note the corticospinal tract *(arrows)* displaced medially by the large brainstem mass *(arrowhead)*. (Images courtesy of James L. Leach, MD)

matrix hemorrhage from the normally echogenic choroid plexus. In contrast to germinal matrix hemorrhage, normal choroid plexus should never extend as anterior as the caudothalamic groove on a parasagittal view. Hemorrhage may extend into the ventricular system and lead to hydrocephalus. Germinal matrix hemorrhage is categorized into one of four grades (Table 8-2). Intraparenchymal hemorrhage (grade IV) is actually thought to be secondary to venous infarction rather than a direct extension of hemorrhage (see Fig. 8-11). Grades I and II hemorrhages tend

to have good prognoses. In contrast, grades III and IV hemorrhages tend to have poor prognoses, including high incidences of neurologic impairment, hydrocephalus, and death.

Periventricular Leukomalacia

Perinatal partial asphyxia can result in damage to the periventricular white matter, the watershed zone of the premature infant. This is termed periventricular leukomalacia. It most

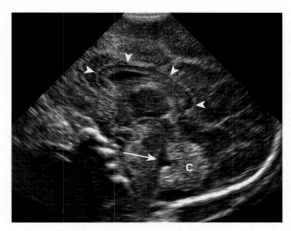

FIGURE 8-8. **Normal findings in a premature neonate on sagittal ultrasound of the head. Midline sagittal view demonstrates normal midline structures, including corpus callosum** (arrowheads), **cerebellar vermis** (C), **and fourth ventricle** (arrow).

commonly affects the white matter adjacent to the atria and the frontal horns of the lateral ventricles. It is associated with neurologic sequelae, such as movement disorders, seizures, and spasticity. On ultrasound, increased heterogeneous echogenicity is seen within the periventricular white matter. In severe cases, there may be cystic necrosis and development of periventricular cysts (Fig. 8-12A, B). With time, there is

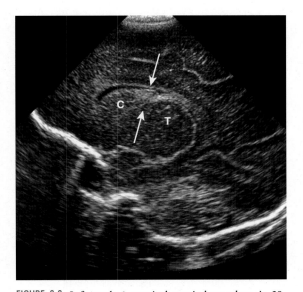

FIGURE 8-9. **Left, grade 1 germinal matrix hemorrhage in 29-week gestational age, premature infant. Off-midline sagittal ultrasound demonstrates echogenic mass** (arrows) **in left caudothalamic groove. The lateral ventricle is not dilatated. C, caudate nucleus; T, thalamus.**

often volume loss of the involved white matter (Fig. 8-13).

Benign Macrocrania

Benign macrocrania is a diagnosis of exclusion. The term refers to children with large heads (head circumference greater than 97% for age). Typically, such children present between 6 months and 2 years of age. After 2 years of age, the head size usually normalizes and the children have no long-term consequences. The parents of such children often have large heads or had large heads as infants. On imaging, there is prominent size of the lateral ventricles and extraaxial spaces (Fig. 8-14). Imaging is otherwise normal. Imaging findings alone cannot differentiate between benign macrocrania and communicating hydrocephalus.

DEVELOPMENTAL ABNORMALITIES

Developmental abnormalities can be classified on the basis of the embryologic event that fails, causing the abnormality (Table 8-3). Categories include abnormalities of dorsal induction, ventral induction, migration and cortical organization, neuronal proliferation and differentiation, and myelination. Abnormalities can also result from destruction of already formed structures. The type of developmental lesion often reflects the timing of the disturbance that occurred during development. Often, multiple distinct developmental abnormalities are present simultaneously.

Chiari Malformations

Chiari Malformation Type 1

Chiari malformation type 1 is the presence of an abnormally inferior location of the cerebellar tonsils at least 5 mm below the foramen magnum (Fig. 8-15). The medulla and fourth ventricle are in normal positions. Complications of Chiari type 1 malformation include hydrocephalus and hydrosyringomyelia (up to 25%; see Fig. 8-15). It may be suspected on CT when the foramen magnum appears "full" of soft tissue. It is best visualized on sagittal T1-weighted MR images. The cerebellar tonsils are seen positioned inferiorly and typically appear elongated rather than round. MR cine sequences are used to show movement of the tonsils into the foramen magnum.

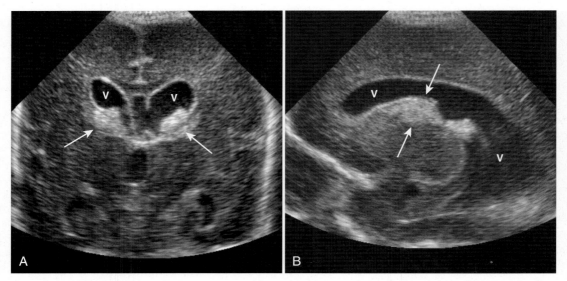

FIGURE 8-10. Bilateral grade III germinal matrix hemorrhage in 25-week gestational age, premature infant. **A,** Coronal ultrasound shows bilateral echogenic masses *(arrows)* in the region of the caudothalamic groove. There is dilatation of the lateral ventricles *(V)*, making the lesion grade 3. Note the smooth-appearing brain with sulcation consistent with the 25-week gestational age. **B,** Right sagittal off-midline ultrasound shows echogenic mass *(arrows)* in the region of the caudothalamic groove. Note ventricular dilatation *(V)*.

CHIARI MALFORMATION TYPE 2

Chiari malformations type 2 are almost always associated with myelomeningoceles. Conversely, almost all patients with myelomeningoceles have Chiari type 2 malformations. Patients with these lesions have small posterior fossae and associated inferior displacement of the cerebellum, medulla,

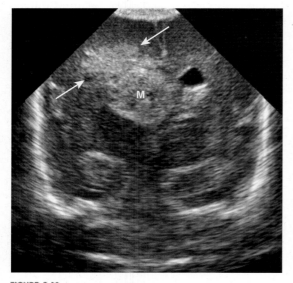

FIGURE 8-11. Right, grade IV germinal matrix hemorrhage. On coronal ultrasound, there is a large echogenic mass *(M)* in the region of the right germinal matrix and increased echogenicity extending into the adjacent white matter *(arrows)*.

and fourth ventricle into the upper cervical canal (Figs. 8-16, 8-17). Associated imaging findings include a kinked appearance of the medulla, colpocephaly (disproportionate enlargement of the posterior body of the lateral ventricles), fenestration of the falx associated with interdigitation of gyri across the midline, enlargement of the massa intermedia, inferior pointing of the lateral ventricles, and tectal beaking (a pointed appearance of the quadrigeminal plate). Chiari type 2 malformations are usually associated with hydrocephalus.

Chiari type 3 and type 4 malformations are very rare.

Holoprosencephaly

Holoprosencephaly results from lack of cleavage of the brain into two hemispheres.

Table 8-2. Grades of Germinal Matrix Hemorrhage

Grade	Morphologic Findings
I	Hemorrhage confined to germinal matrix
II	Intraventricular hemorrhage without ventricular dilatation
III	Intraventricular hemorrhage with ventricular dilatation
IV	Intraparenchymal hemorrhage

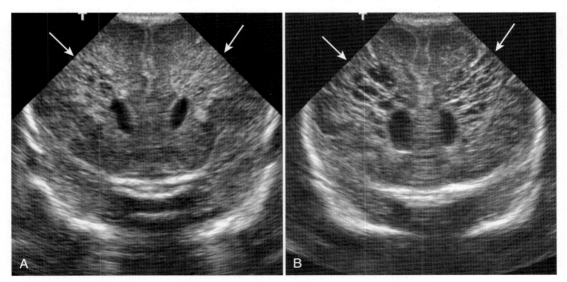

FIGURE 8-12. Periventricular leukomalacia in a 29-week premature infant. **A,** Coronal ultrasound shows heterogeneous echogenicity in the frontal periventricular white matter *(arrows).* **B,** A repeat ultrasound 20 days later shows development of cystic necrosis in the bilateral frontal white matter *(arrows),* consistent with cystic periventricular leukomalacia.

Although there is a continuous spectrum of severity, holoprosencephaly is classically classified into one of three distinct groups: alobar, semilobar, or lobar. The severity of the brain abnormality is reflected in the severity of the midline facial abnormality.

Alobar holoprosencephaly is the most severe form and is characterized by a monoventricle. The thalami are fused and there is no attempt at cleavage of the cerebral hemispheres. There is no falx cerebri or corpus callosum. There is a single anterior cerebral artery. These infants are stillborn or die soon after birth.

With the intermediate form, semilobar holoprosencephaly (Fig. 8-18A-D), the cerebral

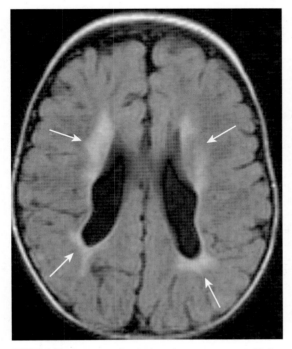

FIGURE 8-13. Periventricular leukomalacia in a 2-year-old formerly premature infant. Axial FLAIR images show volume loss and increased signal *(arrows)* in the periventricular white matter.

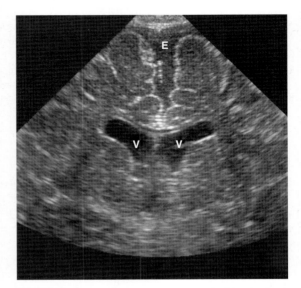

FIGURE 8-14. Benign macrocrania in a 3-month-old with a large head. The image from coronal ultrasound shows prominent extraaxial spaces *(E)* and prominence of the lateral ventricles *(V).* In most infants, the lateral ventricles are slitlike.

Table 8-3. Common Development and Congenital Abnormalities of the Brain

Abnormality	Mechanism (abnormality of)	Description	Associated Imaging Findings
Chiari malformation type 1	Dorsal induction	Inferior displacement of cerebral tonsils below level of foramen magnum	Hydrocephalus Hydrosyringomyelia
Chiari malformation type 2	Dorsal induction	Small posterior fossa with inferior displacement of cerebellum, fourth ventricle, and brainstem into cervical canal; associated with myelomeningocele	Colpocephaly Fenestrated falx Large massa intermedia Tectal beaking Cervicomedullary kink
Holoprosencephaly	Ventral induction	Failure in cleavage of brain into two cerebral hemispheres	Alobar type: Single ventricle Fused thalami Absent corpus callosum and falx
Dandy-Walker malformation	Ventral induction	Complete or partial agenesis of the cerebellar vermis in conjunction with a retrocerebellar cyst communicating with the fourth ventricle	Posterior fossa enlarged (torcula superior to lambdoid) If normal size, is a Dandy-Walker variant
Gray matter heterotopia	Migration	Arrested migration of neurons, resulting in heterotopic areas of gray matter within the white matter	Subependymal or subcortical Nodular or laminar appearance Isointense to gray matter
Schizencephaly	Migration	Gray matter lined cleft extending from lateral ventricle to cerebral surface	Entire cleft lined by gray matter Agenesis of corpus callosum
Lissencephaly (agyria)	Migration	Failure of development of gyri and sulci	Smooth cortical surface Cortical thickening Rarely isolated finding
Pachygyria	Migration	Broad, flat gyri with shallow sulci	Lumpy cortical surface Cortical thickening Rarely an isolated finding
Dysgenesis of the corpus callosum	Ventral induction	Complete or partial (anterior part present) absence of the corpus callosum	Squared lateral ventricles Bundles of Probst Colpocephaly High-riding third ventricle
Vein of Galen malformation	Unknown	Arteriovenous fistula to vein of Galen resulting in marked dilatation of the vein	Vascular mass in region of posterior third ventricle Hydrocephalus Congestive heart failure
Hydranencephaly	Injury of formed structures	Destruction of the cerebrum secondary to infarct from bilateral internal carotid artery occlusion	Cerebrum replaced by thin-walled sacks of CSF Falx present Thalami separated
Porencephaly	Injury of formed structures	Cyst formation from injury to brain parenchyma during first or second trimester	Thin-walled CSF cyst No septations

hemispheres are partially cleaved from each other posteriorly. The temporal horns may be formed but there is a single ventricle anteriorly. There is partial separation of the thalami. Midline structures such as the falx and corpus callosum may be present posteriorly but not anteriorly.

Lobar holoprosencephaly is the least severe form. The occipital and temporal horns are well formed but there is failure of cleavage of the frontal lobes. The septum pellucidum is absent and the corpus callosum may be absent or dysplastic.

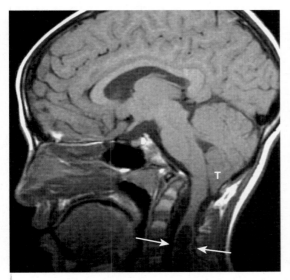

FIGURE. 8-15. Chiari 1 malformation with associated hydrosyringomyelia. Sagittal T1-weighted MRI shows the cerebellar tonsils *(T)* to be pointed and extending inferiorly into the foramen magnum. There is a large associated hydrosyringomyelia *(arrows)*.

Septooptic Dysplasia

Septooptic dysplasia is another type of ventral induction malformation, analogous to mild holoprosencephaly. It is characterized by absence of the septum pellucidum and hypoplasia of the optic nerves. It is often associated with schizencephaly, heterotopia, and hypothalamic and pituitary dysfunction. In septooptic dysplasia, the frontal horns of the lateral ventricles have a squared appearance and point inferiorly on coronal MR images.

Posterior Fossa Cystic Malformations

Posterior fossa cystic malformations include a spectrum of abnormalities. They can be divided into four groups: Dandy-Walker malformation, Dandy-Walker variant, mega cisterna magna, and arachnoid cyst.

Dandy-Walker malformation is complete or partial agenesis of the cerebellar vermis in conjunction with the presence of a posterior fossa cyst that communicates with the fourth ventricle (Fig. 8-19A, B). The posterior fossa is enlarged such that the torcular is elevated above the lambda (see Fig. 8-19). The falx cerebelli is absent. Often there are also supratentorial

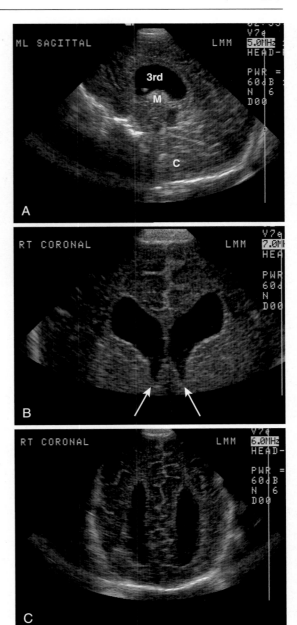

FIGURE 8-16. Chiari 2 malformation shown on ultrasound in a newborn infant with myelomeningocele. **A,** Midline sagittal ultrasound shows inferior displacement of the cerebellum *(C)*. The fourth ventricle is effaced and not visualized. There is a prominent massa intermedia *(M)*. The third ventricle *(3rd)* is dilatated secondary to hydrocephalus. **B,** Coronal image shows inferior pointing of the lateral ventricles *(arrows)*. There is obstructive hydrocephalus, with dilatation of the lateral ventricles. **C,** A more posterior coronal image shows interdigitation of the cerebral gyri, secondary to fenestration of the falx cerebri.

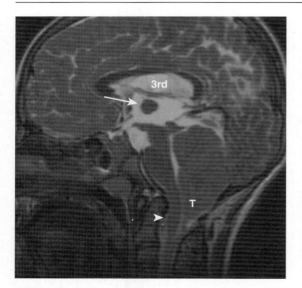

FIGURE 8-17. Chiari 2 malformation. Sagittal T2-weighted image shows downward displacement of cerebellar tonsils *(T)* and medulla *(arrowhead)*. The fourth ventricle is compressed. The third ventricle *(3rd)* is dilatated. There is a prominent massa intermedia *(arrow)*.

abnormalities, including holoprosencephaly, agenesis of the corpus callosum, polymicrogyria, and heterotopias. Hydrocephalus is common.

Dandy-Walker variant is considered present when some but not all of the criteria for the classic malformation are present. Most commonly, the cerebellar vermis is hypoplastic but present, and there is a posterior fossa cyst, but the posterior fossa is not enlarged (Fig. 8-20). When an enlarged posterior fossa CSF cyst is present in the presence of a fully developed cerebellar vermis, there are two possibilities. If the cyst exhibits no mass effect on the cerebellum, a mega cisterna magna is considered to be present. If the cyst does exhibit mass effect on the cerebellum, an arachnoid cyst is considered to be present (Fig. 8-21).

Gray Matter Heterotopias

Heterotopias are abnormalities of neuronal migration characterized by arrest in migration of the neurons from the subependymal area to the cortex. Typically, heterotopias are associated with other migrational disorders, such as schizencephaly, lissencephaly, or polymicrogyria. When a heterotopia occurs as an isolated abnormality, it typically presents with focal seizures. On CT and MRI, the lesions appear as nodular (Fig. 8-22A, B)

or linear (Fig. 8-23) areas within the white matter, most typically in the subcortical or subependymal regions. Heterotopias tend to be isointense, with gray matter on all pulse sequences.

Schizencephaly

Schizencephaly is another migrational disorder. The term refers to a cleft in the cerebral hemisphere lined with gray matter (Fig. 8-24A, B). The cleft typically extends from the lateral ventricle to the surface of the brain. Schizencephaly is often characterized as being open-lipped or close-lipped. However, this has little clinical relevance. The lesion can be unilateral or bilateral and can occur anywhere in the cerebral hemispheres. In most cases, there is associated agenesis of the corpus callosum.

The presence of gray matter lining the entire cleft is the diagnostic feature that separates schizencephaly from other causes of clefts, such as porencephaly (see later material). In cases of porencephaly, the cleft is lined by (extends through) both gray and white matter.

Lissencephaly

Lissencephaly refers to arrest of migration of neurons, resulting in either total failure of development of sulci and gyri (agyria; Fig. 8-25) or development of abnormally broad and flat gyri with abnormally shallow sulci (pachygyria) (Fig. 8-26A, B). Agyria and pachygyria are best visualized with MR imaging. There is often thickening of the associated cortex. Neither lesion typically appears in isolation; there are usually patchy areas of both agyria and pachygyria. These abnormalities are commonly associated with other migrational abnormalities and also occur as part of a number of rare syndromes.

Polymicrogyria is similar disorder that results in small, disorganized gyri. It too is usually associated with other migrational abnormalities. There is controversy as to whether polymicrogyria is a disorder of migration or is a cortical dysplasia.

Dysgenesis of Corpus Callosum

Dysgenesis of the corpus callosum includes both complete and partial absence. The corpus

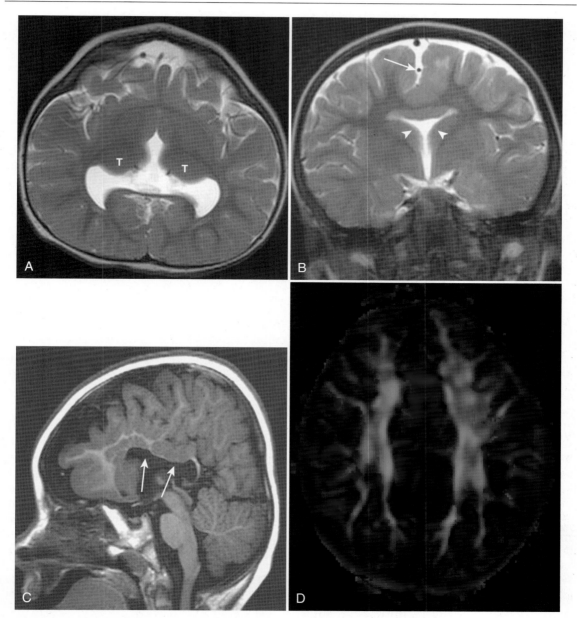

FIGURE 8-18. Semilobar holoprosencephaly. **A,** Axial T2-weighted image shows separation of the thalami *(T)* and separated occipital lobes but fusion of the frontal lobes. There is a single monoventricle and absence of the septum pellucidum. **B,** Coronal T2-weighted image shows monoventricle frontally *(arrowheads)*. Note the single anterior cerebral artery *(arrow)*. **C,** Sagittal T1-weighted image shows absence of the corpus callosum *(arrows)*. There is brachycephaly. **D,** Eigenvalue map shows decreased left-to-right tracts (absence of red tracts).

callosum normally develops from anterior to posterior. As a result, with partial absence, it is the more anterior part of the corpus callosum that is present. Absence of the corpus callosum can occur as an isolated lesion or in conjunction with many of the other developmental lesions of the brain already described in this chapter (see Fig. 8-18). On coronal MR images, the lateral ventricles are separated, and the third ventricle extends more superiorly than normal, positioned between the lateral ventricles. The white matter tracts that normally cross the midline via the corpus callosum run along the medial surface of the lateral ventricles and form the bundles of Probst, which can be seen at imaging. Colpocephaly is often present. Midline masses, such as lipoma and arachnoid cyst, can also be associated.

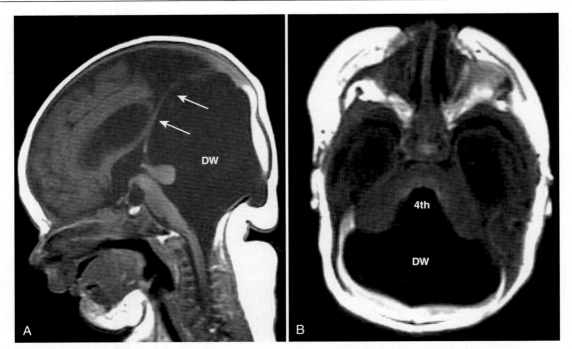

FIGURE 8-19. Dandy-Walker malformation in a newborn infant. **A,** Sagittal, T1-weighted MR image shows large posterior fossa cyst *(DW)* enlarging the posterior fossa. The cerebellar vermis is absent. The torcular *(arrows)* is elevated. **B,** Axial, proton-density-weighted MR image shows large posterior fossa cyst *(DW)* that communicates with the fourth ventricle *(4th)*.

Vein of Galen Malformations

With vein of Galen malformation, also known as vein of Galen aneurysm, there is an arteriovenous fistula connecting one or multiple cerebral arteries and the vein of Galen. Most of these malformations present during the neonatal period with congestive heart failure resulting from the associated left-to-right shunting of blood. On chest radiography, there is cardiomegaly, signs of congestive heart failure, and widening of the superior mediastinum secondary to vascular enlargement caused by the increased blood flow to and from the head.

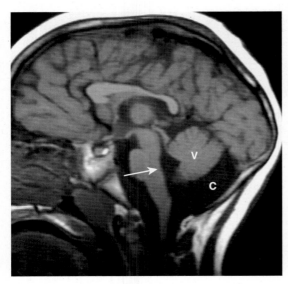

FIGURE 8-20. Dandy-Walker variant. Sagittal, T1-weighted MR image shows a posterior fossa cyst *(C)* that communicates with the fourth ventricle *(arrow)*. The vermis is hypoplastic but present. The posterior fossa is not enlarged.

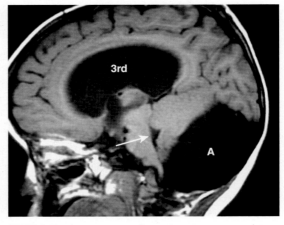

FIGURE 8-21. Posterior fossa arachnoid cyst. Sagittal T1-weighted MR image shows posterior fossa cyst *(A)* that does not communicate with the fourth ventricle *(arrow)*. There is mass effect on the cerebellum. The third ventricle *(3rd)* is markedly dilatated.

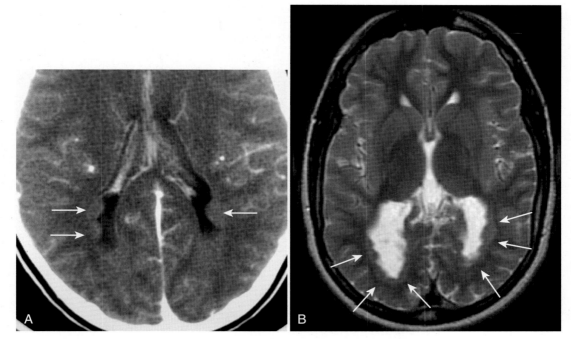

FIGURE 8-22. Heterotopic gray matter in two different patients. **A,** CT shows nodular areas *(arrows)* adjacent to the lateral ventricles. The nodules have the same attenuation as gray matter. **B,** Axial T2-weighted MRI shows nodular areas *(arrows)* lining the occipital horns of the lateral ventricles. Nodules have the same signal as gray matter, consistent with heterotopic gray matter. There is associated colpocephaly (enlargement of the occipital horns of the lateral ventricles).

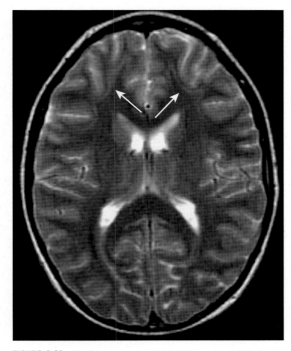

FIGURE 8-23. Band heterotopia. Axial, T2-weighted MR image shows heterotopias as linear structures *(arrows)* within the frontal white matter that are isointense to gray matter.

Imaging studies demonstrate a large mass in the region of the posterior third ventricle. Doppler imaging, MR arteriography, or contrast enhanced CT documents the vascular nature of the lesion (Fig. 8-27A-C). On MRI, the prominent arterial structures may be seen feeding the dilatated vein. There is often associated hydrocephalus. Most vein of Galen malformations are treated by arterial embolization. Untreated cases usually result in death.

SEQUELAE OF IN UTERO INSULTS

In contrast to developmental abnormalities that result from abnormal formation, other congenital abnormalities may arise from destruction of already developed structures. Most commonly, they are related to vascular ischemia and infarction that can be caused by a number of underlying causes. The most commonly encountered lesions are porencephaly, encephalomalacia, and hydranencephaly.

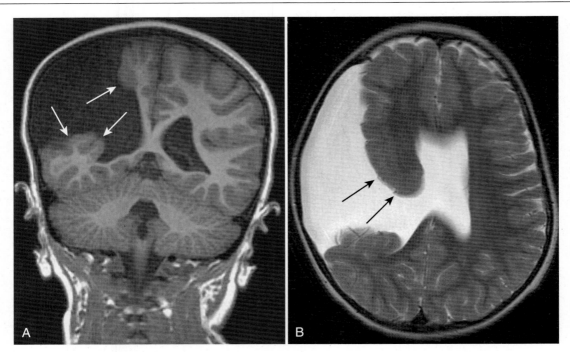

FIGURE 8-24. Schizencephaly. **A,** Coronal T1-weighted image shows large fluid-filled space that is in communication with the right lateral ventricle. The communication is lined by gray matter *(arrows)*, consistent with schizencephaly. **B,** Axial T2-weighted image again shows large fluid-filled space that is in communication with the right lateral ventricle. The communication is lined with gray matter *(arrows)*.

Porencephaly and Encephalomalacia

Prior to the end of the second trimester, parenchymal injury does not result in glial scar formation.

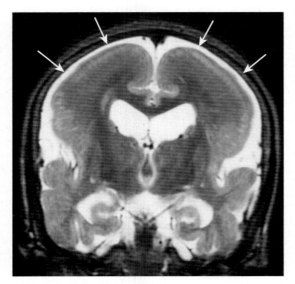

FIGURE 8-25. Agyria (lissencephaly) in a 10-year-old girl with seizures and developmental delay. Coronal T2-weighted image shows the smooth surface of the bilateral frontal lobes *(arrows)*, without formation of sulci and gyri.

During this early time period, focal injury results in the development of a fluid-filled space. When such a cyst communicates with the ventricles, it is called a porencephalic cyst. On imaging, this cyst appears as thin-walled CSF-containing cysts, communicating directly with the ventricles (Fig. 8-28). There are no septations. During the third trimester, parenchymal injury incites glial scar formation. During this period, brain injury results in encephalomalacia. Encephalomalacia appears as areas of high T2-weighted signal with multiple septations in the region of injury.

Hydranencephaly

Hydranencephaly is the destruction of the majority of the cerebral hemispheres secondary to a massive ischemic event thought to be related to bilateral internal carotid artery occlusion. Large thin-walled cystic structures are seen in place of the cerebral parenchyma (Fig. 8-29). The occipital lobes, inferior temporal lobes, thalami, brainstem, and cerebellum are typically intact. These structures remain because they are supplied by the vertebrobasilar arterial system. The presence of the falx cerebri and the separation of the thalami seen in hydranencephaly help to differentiate this

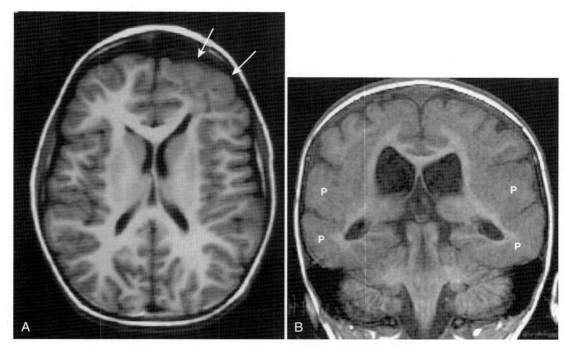

FIGURE 8-26. Pachygyria in two patients. **A,** Axial T1-weighted MRI shows poorly defined, thickened gyri *(arrows)* within the left frontal lobe. **B,** Coronal T1-weighted MRI shows all gyri to be abnormal. The most strikingly thickened, broad gyri are denoted *(P).*

disorder from severe (alobar) holoprosencephaly. It is sometimes impossible to differentiate hydranencephaly from severe hydrocephalus.

NEUROCUTANEOUS SYNDROMES

The neurocutaneous syndromes (phakomatoses) are a group of related diseases that affect tissues of ectodermal origin, primarily the skin and nervous system. Some of the more common phakomatoses that present in childhood include neurofibromatosis, tuberous sclerosis, and Sturge-Weber syndrome.

Neurofibromatosis

Neurofibromatosis is the most common of the phakomatoses and is divided into a number of subcategories, of which neurofibromatosis type 1 (NF-1) and neurofibromatosis type 2 (NF-2) are the most common.

NF-1 is an autosomal dominant disorder. Diagnostic criteria for NF-1 are listed in Table 8-4. The neuroimaging manifestations of NF-1 are multiple. The most common lesions (as many as 95% of patients with NF-1) of the central nervous system (CNS) are the "NF-1 spots" that appear as high T2-weighted lesions in the globus pallidus (Fig. 8-30), cerebellum, brainstem, internal capsule, splenium, and thalami. The lesions typically arise at 3 years of age, increase in number and size until 12 years of age, and then regress. Other lesions of NF-1 include optic tract gliomas (Fig. 8-31), cerebral astrocytomas, hydrocephalus, vascular dysplasia (including aneurysms and moyamoya secondary to stenosis), dural ectasia, and sphenoid wing dysplasia. Patients with NF-1 can develop cranial nerve schwannomas, peripheral neurofibromas, plexiform neurofibromas (Fig. 8-32A, B), and malignant peripheral nerve sheath tumors. Plexiform neurofibromas are locally aggressive masses that are histiologically more disorganized than typical neurofibromas. In the head and neck, they often involve the scalp and orbit. They are often monitored by imaging to evaluate for findings suspicious for malignant degeneration. Spinal manifestations include posterior vertebral scalloping (resulting from dural ectasia or neurofibromas), scoliosis, and lateral meningoceles.

NF-2 is characterized by the presence of bilateral acoustic schwannomas (Fig. 8-33).

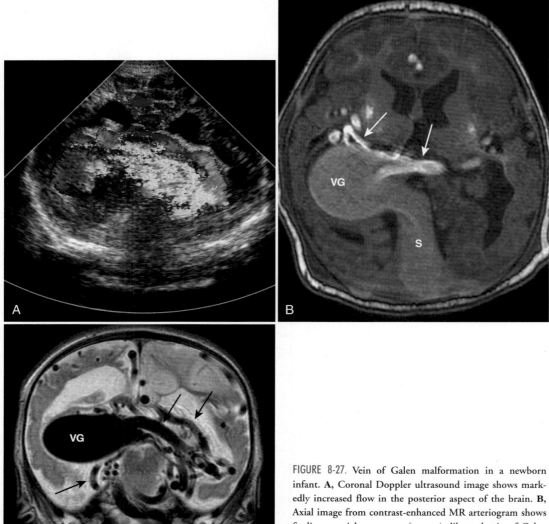

FIGURE 8-27. Vein of Galen malformation in a newborn infant. **A,** Coronal Doppler ultrasound image shows markedly increased flow in the posterior aspect of the brain. **B,** Axial image from contrast-enhanced MR arteriogram shows feeding arterial structures *(arrows)*, dilatated vein of Galen *(VG)*, and dilatated draining straight sinus *(S)*. **C,** Coronal T1-weighted MR image shows multiple arterial feeders *(arrows)*, and dilatated vein of Galen *(VG)*. Note that there is cortical loss, cortical edema, and dilatated ventricles.

Other associated lesions include meningiomas, gliomas and neurofibromas. Patients most commonly present in adulthood.

Tuberous Sclerosis

Tuberous sclerosis is an autosomal dominant syndrome associated with a classic triad of seizures, mental retardation, and adenoma sebaceum (a facial rash that is an angiofibroma of the skin). The disease affects the skin, CNS, skeletal system, and abdominal organs.

The most common neuroimaging finding is the presence of tubers. These are hamartomatous lesions that appear as subependymal masses. They typically occur along the lateral ventricles (Fig. 8-34A-C). The signal characteristics are variable and are related to age. In older patients, tubers are often calcified. In older children, the lesions tend to be isointense to gray matter. Most tubers do not enhance. Interval growth and development of contrast enhancement are findings that are associated with malignant degeneration, a rare occurrence. However, enhancement in itself does not imply malignancy. When a tuber

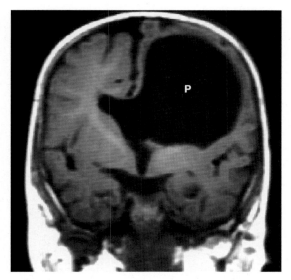

FIGURE 8-28. Porencephalic cyst shown on coronal T1-weighted MRI as a large CSF cyst *(P)* that is contiguous with the left lateral ventricle. The communication is not lined by gray matter.

Table 8-4. Diagnostic Criteria for Neurofibromatosis Type 1

Two or more of the following:
1. Six or more café-au-lait macules
2. Two or more neurofibromas or one plexiform neurofibroma
3. Axillary or inguinal freckles
4. Bilateral optic nerve gliomas
5. Two hamartomas of the iris (Lisch nodules)
6. Parent, sibling, or child with NF-1

within the white matter secondary to areas of abnormal glial cells (see Fig. 8-34).

Visceral manifestations of tuberous sclerosis include renal cysts, renal angiomyolipomas, cardiac rhabdomyomas, and hamartomas of other organs.

Sturge-Weber Syndrome

Sturge-Weber syndrome, or encephalotrigeminal angiomatosis, is characterized by a low-flow vascular malformation in the distribution of the trigeminal nerve, both intracranially

near the foramen of Monroe rapidly enlarges, it is referred to as a giant cell tumor. Such giant cell tumors frequently lead to hydrocephalus. Patients with tuberous sclerosis can also have areas of abnormal high T2-weighted signal

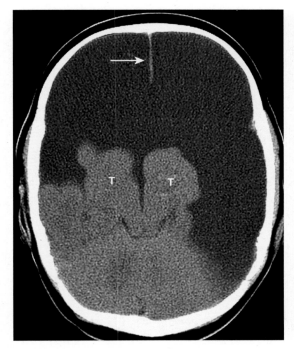

FIGURE 8-29. Hydranencephaly. Axial noncontrast-enhanced CT shows most of cerebrum replaced by CSF space. The thalami *(T)* are present bilaterally and are not fused. A falx cerebri *(arrow)* is present.

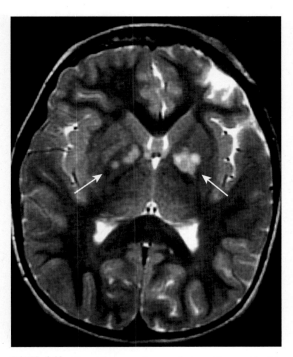

FIGURE 8-30. Neurofibromatosis type 1 in a 3-year-old girl. Axial, T2-weighted MR image shows NF-1 spots as abnormal increased signal within the globus pallidi bilaterally *(arrows)*. There is also cortical dysplasia in the left frontal lobe.

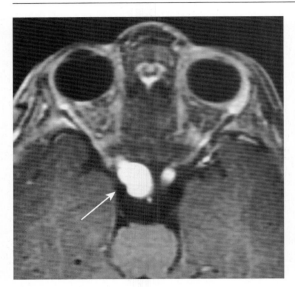

FIGURE 8-31. Optic nerve glioma in a patient with NF-1. Contrast-enhanced, fat-saturated T1-weighted MR image shows enlargement and enhancement of the posterior right optic nerve *(arrow)*.

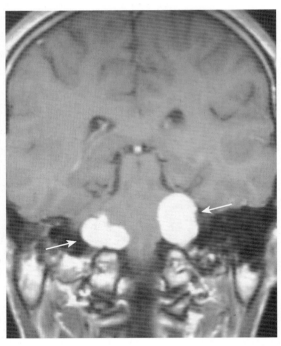

FIGURE 8-33. NF-2 with bilateral acoustic schwannomas. Coronal, postcontrast MR image shows bilateral high signal masses *(arrows)* consistent with bilateral acoustic schwannomas.

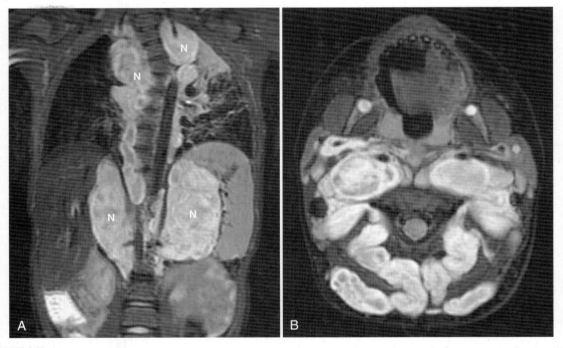

FIGURE 8-32. Plexiform neurofibroma in a child with NF-1. **A,** Coronal T2-weighted image shows multiple retroperitoneal masses *(N)* consistent with plexiform neurofibromas. **B,** Axial T2-weighted image of neck, in same patient, shows multiple high-signal lesions consistent with plexiform neurofibromas. In both A and B, note lower signal, rounded areas within the masses. These are typical for plexiform neurofibromas.

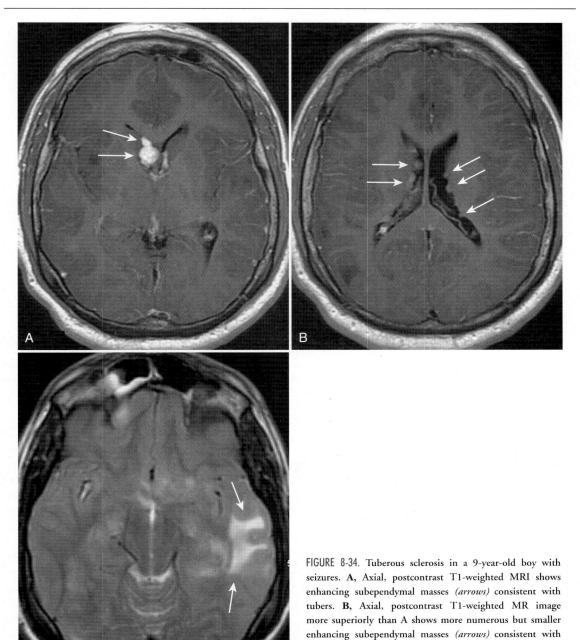

FIGURE 8-34. Tuberous sclerosis in a 9-year-old boy with seizures. **A,** Axial, postcontrast T1-weighted MRI shows enhancing subependymal masses *(arrows)* consistent with tubers. **B,** Axial, postcontrast T1-weighted MR image more superiorly than A shows more numerous but smaller enhancing subependymal masses *(arrows)* consistent with tubers. **C,** Axial T2-weighted MRI shows areas of abnormal high signal *(arrows)* in the white matter, typical of tuberous sclerosis.

and extracranially. The syndrome manifests as abnormalities of the skin (port wine nevus), leptomeninges, and underlying brain. The altered flow results in chronic ischemic injury to the affected underlying brain. On CT imaging, there is serpiginous calcification, abnormal enhancement, and atrophy of the involved gyri (Fig. 8-35A, B). The cranium is commonly thickened adjacent to the brain abnormalities.

Clinical manifestations include seizures, mental retardation, and hemiparesis.

NORMAL MYELINATION

Great changes in the myelination of the brain occur during the first 24 months of life. Prior to myelination, white matter is hydrophilic and, because it

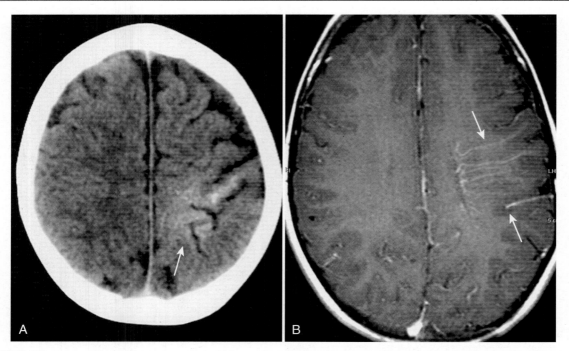

FIGURE 8-35. Sturge-Weber syndrome in a 7-year-old boy with seizures. **A,** Noncontrast-enhanced CT shows abnormal calcifications *(arrow)* within the left parietooccipital region. There is associated atrophy of the left-sided gyri. **B,** Axial, contrast-enhanced T1-weighted MRI shows asymmetric, increased deep medullary veins *(arrows).*

contains water, appears high in signal on T2-weighted images and low in signal on T1-weighted images (Fig. 8-36). With myelination, the white matter becomes hydrophobic and, because it contains less water, appears low in signal on T2-weighted images and high in signal on T1-weighted images (see Fig. 8-36). Myelination progresses from caudal to cranial, paralleling neurologic development. During the first 3 months of life, there is progressive myelination of the spinal cord and brainstem, followed by myelination of the cerebellar white matter. The corpus callosum begins to myelinate in the splenium (posterior part) at 2 to 3 months of age, proceeds anteriorly, and is completely myelinated through the rostrum (anterior part) by 6 to 8 months of age. The adult pattern of myelination is complete by 18 to 24 months of age.

Abnormal myelination is a nonspecific finding and can be secondary to a number of causes, including metabolic disease, infection, trauma, hypoxia-ischemia, and malformative syndromes.

METABOLIC AND DEGENERATIVE DISORDERS

A large number of metabolic, degenerative, and toxic disorders can result in abnormal

myelination patterns. Most of these diseases are rare and untreatable. Categories of disease include lysomal storage disorders, mitochondrial disorders, peroxisomal disorders, and amino acid disorders, among others. On MRI, these disorders typically demonstrate abnormally increased T2-weighted signals involving portions of white matter, gray matter, or a combination of the two. There may be associated atrophy of the involved structures. The distribution of the abnormal signal can be helpful in narrowing the differential diagnosis (Figs. 8-37A-C through 8-39). MR spectroscopy can also provide helpful information. The most specific case is marked increased NAA in Canavan disease. Representative disorders and the associated distribution of abnormalities as demonstrated on MRI are listed in Table 8-5.

INFECTION

Many of the imaging findings in CNS infection (meningitis, cerebritis, empyema, encephalitis, and parenchymal abscess) are similar in children and adults and are not emphasized here. This section focuses on several of the issues unique to children.

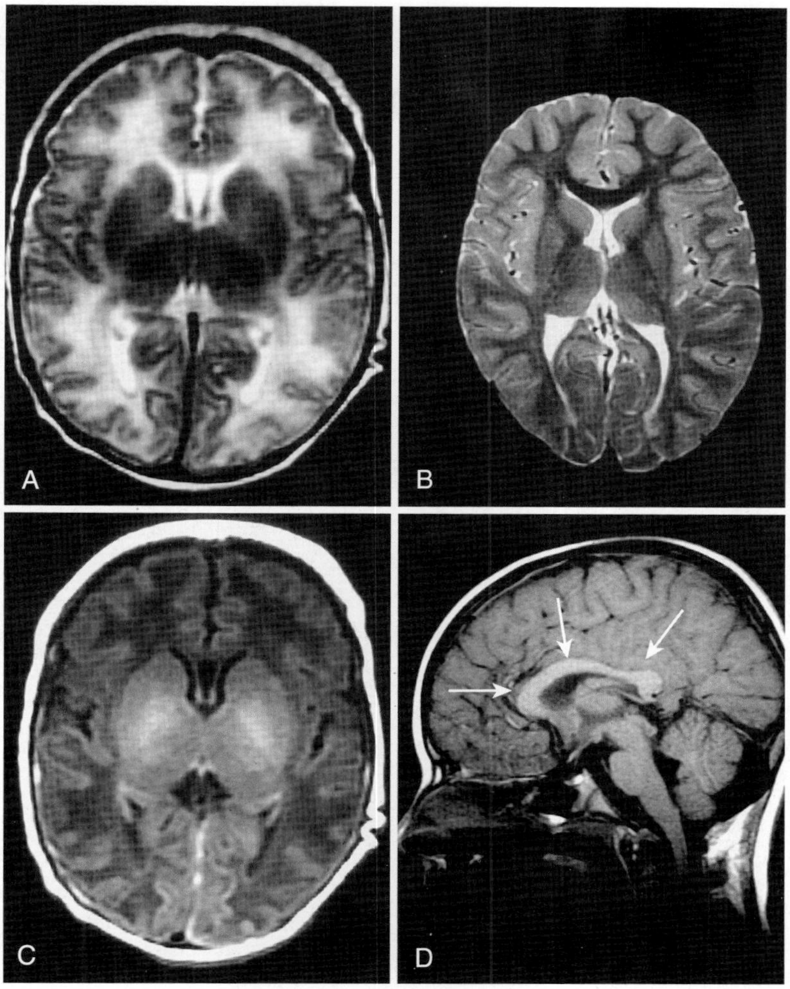

FIGURE 8-36. Normal age-related change in appearance on MRI of white matter related to myelination. **A,** Premyelination T2-weighted appearance in an 8-day-old infant. Axial, T2-weighted MR image shows white matter to be diffusely high in signal. **B,** Postmyelination T2-weighted (adult) appearance in an 8-year-old child. Axial, T2-weighted MR image shows white matter to be diffusely low in signal. **C,** Premyelination T1-weighted appearance in same 8-day-old infant as shown in A. Axial, T1-weighted MR image shows white matter to be diffusely low in signal. **D,** Postmyelination T1-weighted (adult) appearance in same 8-year-old child as shown in B. Sagittal, T1-weighted MR image shows white matter to be higher in signal. Note high signal in corpus callosum *(arrows)*.

Congenital Infections

There are a number of in utero infections (toxoplasmosis, other [syphilis], rubella, cytomegalovirus, herpes; TORCH; see Chapter 7) that can affect the CNS. They demonstrate unique findings as compared to CNS infections that occur later in life because in utero infections can affect brain development. The severity of the abnormality commonly reflects the time period during which the infection occurred.

Infection by cytomegalovirus is the most common TORCH infection to involve the CNS. Imaging findings include periventricular calcifications, migrational abnormalities (cortical dysplasia), cerebellar hypoplasia, and ventricular enlargement (Fig. 8-40). Clinical manifestations include microcephaly, hearing impairment, mental retardation, and developmental delay.

Toxoplasmosis is the second most common TORCH infection to involve the CNS. The parenchymal calcifications seen in toxoplasmosis are more variable in location than those seen with cytomegalovirus. Other manifestations include hydrocephalus and, in severe cases, hydranencephaly.

With congenital infection by the human immunodeficiency virus (HIV), CNS abnormalities can be related to primary HIV involvement and to secondary complications, such as infection and tumor. However, secondary infection and tumor are much less commonly seen in children than in adults. The majority of children with congenital HIV infection have CNS manifestations, typically progressive encephalopathy. Imaging findings include diffuse atrophy, delayed myelination, and calcifications. These calcifications most commonly occur within the basal ganglia and subcortical white matter of the frontal lobes.

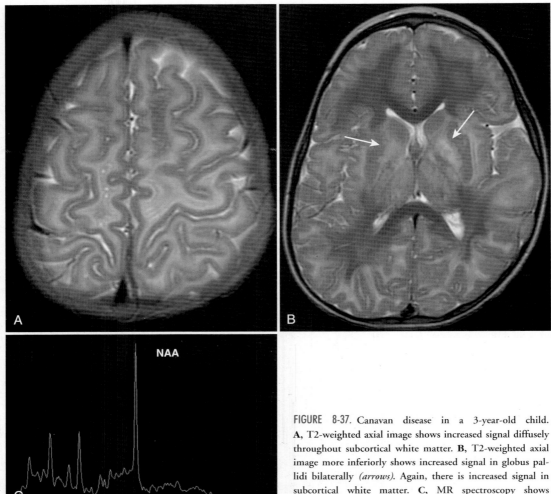

FIGURE 8-37. Canavan disease in a 3-year-old child. **A,** T2-weighted axial image shows increased signal diffusely throughout subcortical white matter. **B,** T2-weighted axial image more inferiorly shows increased signal in globus pallidi bilaterally *(arrows)*. Again, there is increased signal in subcortical white matter. **C,** MR spectroscopy shows increased NAA peak.

Encephalitis

Encephalitis is inflammation of the brain, sometimes seen in conjunction with meningeal inflammation. It can occur secondary to direct viral infection, can be associated with an autoimmune response to a virus or immunization, or can be the extension of a meningeal infection. Children typically present with seizures, lethargy, or focal neurologic deficits. Several types of encephalitis occur predominantly during childhood.

1. **Herpes simplex-1 virus** can lead to necrotizing meningoencephalitis. When it occurs secondary to the reactivation and migration of a previous, latent infection via the branches of the trigeminal nerve, it typically affects one or both temporal lobes (Fig. 8-41A, B). On MRI, high signal is seen within the cortex of one or both temporal lobes. There are often areas of hemorrhage within the affected areas.

In a neonate who acquires a systemic infection during birth, any portion of the brain can be affected.

2. **Subacute sclerosing panencephalitis** is thought to be an encephalitis that occurs secondary to reactivation of latent measles infection. It is a disease of childhood. Imaging demonstrates nonspecific atrophy and increased T2-weighted signal within the cerebral white matter (Fig. 8-42).

3. **Acute disseminated encephalomyelitis (ADEM)** is an immunologic disease that occurs in response to a recent viral infection or immunization. It typically occurs days to weeks after the preceding stimulus. On MRI, areas of increased T2-weighted signal are typically seen in the white matter (Fig. 8-43), the brainstem, and the cerebellum. The treatment is steroids, and some children may completely recover.

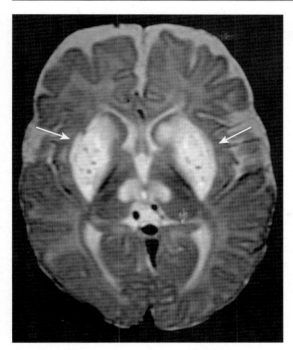

FIGURE 8-38. Leigh disease in a 5-month-old boy. Axial, T2-weighted MR image shows abnormal increased signal within the deep white matter of the basal ganglia (arrows). There is also atrophy within the frontal lobes.

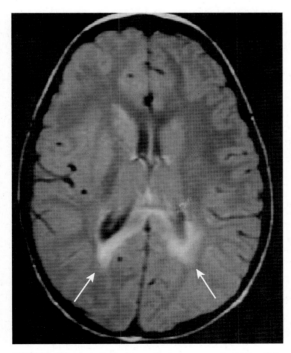

FIGURE 8-39. Adrenoleukodystrophy in a 9-month-old boy failing milestones. Axial, T2-weighted MR image shows abnormal increased signal *(arrows)* in the central white matter posteriorly.

TUMORS

Tumors of the CNS are the most common solid malignancies of childhood. The imaging approach to differential diagnosis is based on the categorization of the tumors according to their anatomic location: posterior fossa, supratentorial (cerebral or region of third ventricle), extraaxial, or head and neck.

Posterior Fossa Tumors

Tumors of the posterior fossa are more common in childhood than in adulthood. The most common posterior fossa tumors in children include cerebellar astrocytoma, medullablastoma, brainstem glioma, and ependymoma (Table 8-6). As previously discussed, other non-neoplastic conditions that are associated with a posterior fossa mass include Dandy-Walker malformation, arachnoid cyst, and mega cisterna magna. Extraaxial tumors such as meningiomas can also occur in the posterior fossa. Posterior fossa tumors often present with obstructive hydrocephalus secondary to compression of the fourth ventricle.

CEREBELLAR ASTROCYTOMA
Cerebellar astrocytoma is the most common type of posterior fossa tumor. It is a low-grade malignancy (pilocytic subtype) and has the best prognosis of any CNS malignancy. Most require only surgical resection. The lesions occur in the vermis or cerebellar hemispheres. There is a wide spectrum of appearances on imaging. Cerebellar astrocytomas can be predominantly cystic or completely solid in appearance (Fig. 8-44A, B). There can be an enhancing mural nodule associated with the cystic lesions (Fig. 8-45). The margins of the lesions are usually well defined. The fourth ventricle is displaced anteriorly, and the margin between the lesion and the fourth ventricle is typically also well defined (see Fig. 8-44). Unlike medulloblastomas and ependymomas, cerebellar astrocytomas usually do not demonstrate areas of calcification or hemorrhage. The solid lesions enhance heterogeneously (see Fig. 8-44).

MEDULLOBLASTOMA
Medulloblastoma is the second most common posterior fossa tumor in children and is the most malignant. It is considered a primitive neuroectodermal tumor (PNET) and typically arises

Table 8-5. **Metabolic and Degenerative Disorders of the Central Nervous System**

Disorder	Category of Disease	Primary Distribution of Abnormality on MRI
Leigh disease	Disorder of mitochondria	Deep gray matter
Kearns-Sayre disease	Disorder of mitochondria	Deep gray (primarily globus pallidus) + white matter
Adrenoleukodystrophy	Peroxisomal disorder	White matter (initially central white matter)
Phenylketonuria	Amino acid disorder	White matter (initially central white matter)
Maple syrup urine disease	Amino acid disorder	Deep gray (primarily globus pallidus) + white matter
Mucolipidosis	Lysosomal storage disorders	Cortical gray matter
Mucopolysaccharidosis	Lysosomal storage disorders	Cortical gray matter + white matter
Metachromatic leukodystrophy	Lysosomal storage disorders	White matter (initially central white matter)
Krabbe disease	Lysosomal storage disorders	White matter (initially central white matter)
Canavan disease	Miscellaneous metabolic disorders	Deep gray (primarily globus pallidus) + white matter (initially peripheral white matter)
Alexander disease	Miscellaneous metabolic disorders	White matter (initially peripheral white matter)

from the granular layer of the inferior medullary velum of the vermis. The neoplasm occupies the fourth ventricle. On imaging, the lesion appears as a poorly defined mass filling the fourth ventricle (Fig. 8-46). Because it arises from the roof of the fourth ventricle, the border between the vermis and lesion as seen on a sagittal MRI is poorly defined (see Fig. 8-46). On CT, the lesion may appear hyperdense and enhance

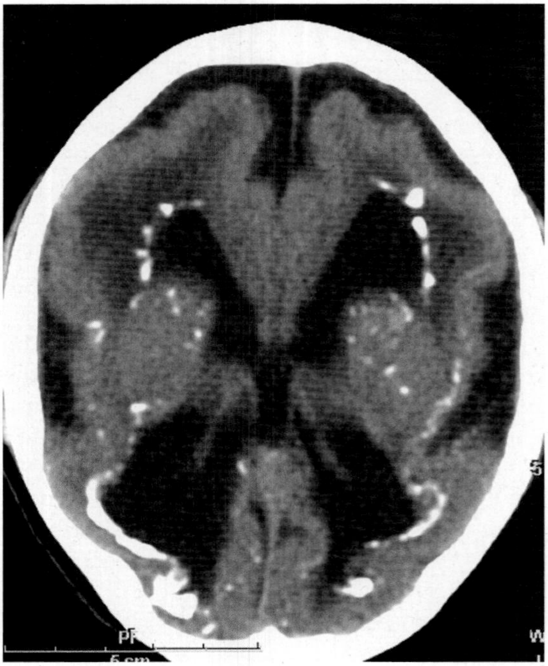

FIGURE 8-40. **Sequelae of cytomegalovirus infection. CT shows marked periventricular calcifications and dilatation of the ventricles. The brain parenchyma has lack of normal gyri formation, resulting in a smooth appearance consistent with lissencephaly.**

diffusely and homogeneously. On MRI, the lesions tend to be more homogeneous in signal than cerebellar astrocytomas or ependymomas. Medulloblastomas tend to be hypointense to mildly hyperintense on T2-weighted images. There is a propensity for seeding within the intracranial and intraspinal CSF spaces. Unlike other posterior fossa tumors, medulloblastomas are hypercellular and as a result show restricted diffusion on DWI sequences.

BRAINSTEM GLIOMA

Brainstem gliomas are most commonly astrocytomas of moderate aggressiveness. They occur most commonly in the pons. Unlike other posterior fossa masses, the lesions tend to present with cranial nerve abnormalities, pyramidal tract signs, or cerebellar dysfunction, rather than with signs of hydrocephalus. The lesions may cause circumferential enlargement of the brainstem (Fig. 8-47A-D) or grow in an exophytic fashion. On MRI, the lesions tend to demonstrate a homogeneous high signal on T2-weighted images (see Fig. 8-47). Prior to treatment, enhancement is rare, with the exception of exophytic lesions. Approximately 10% have a cystic component. If displaced, the fourth ventricle is pushed posteriorly (see Fig. 8-47). In many of these tumors, complete surgical resection is not possible. Radiation therapy remains the primary mode of therapy.

EPENDYMOMA

Ependymomas are relatively slow-growing, typically benign tumors that arise from the ciliated ependymal cells that line the ventricles.

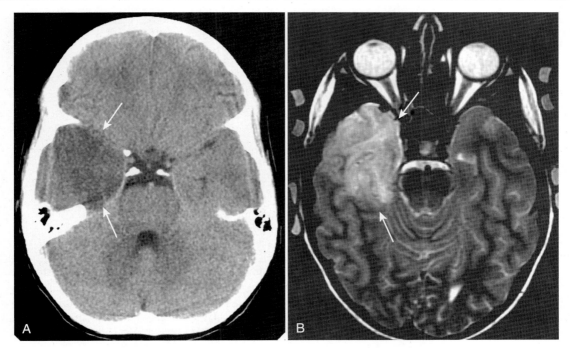

FIGURE 8-41. Herpes encephalitis. **A,** CT shows region of low attenuation in the right temporal lobe *(arrows)*. **B,** Axial T2-weighted MR image shows abnormal increased signal in the right temporal lobe *(arrows)*.

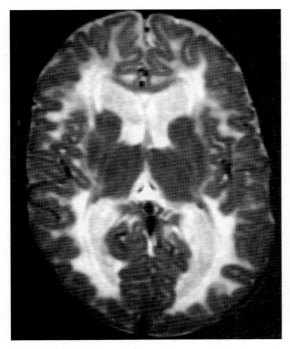

FIGURE 8-42. Subacute sclerosing panencephalitis. Axial, T2-weighted MR image shows abnormal increased signal throughout periventricular white matter. There is associated volume loss and dilatation of the lateral ventricles.

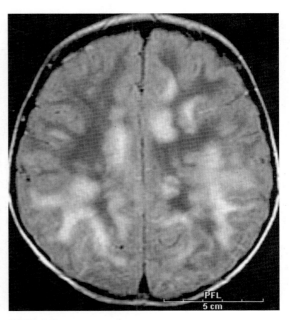

FIGURE 8-43. Acute disseminated encephalomyelitis (ADEM) in a 4-year-old child with seizures and a history of respiratory illness. Axial, FLAIR MR image shows abnormally increased signal in the white matter, more prominent posteriorly. Note that the normal white matter is low in signal.

Table 8-6. Posterior Fossa Tumors

Tumor	Imaging Characteristics
Cerebellar astrocytoma	Cystic or solid Mural nodule common when cystic Solid; heterogeneous signal/density Well defined Fourth ventricle displaced anteriorly, with well-defined interface No calcification or hemorrhage
Medulloblastoma	Arises from roof of fourth ventricle; poorly defined interface Homogeneous signal on MRI Poorly defined CSF metastasis Restricted diffusion on DWI sequences
Brainstem glioma	Circumferential enlargement or exophytic mass of brainstem (most commonly pons) Nonenhancing Fourth ventricle pushed posteriorly Hydrocephalus uncommon
Ependymoma	Arises from floor of fourth ventricle; poorly defined interface Heterogeneous on CT and MRI (hemorrhage, necrosis) Well-defined lobulated margins Calcifications in 70%

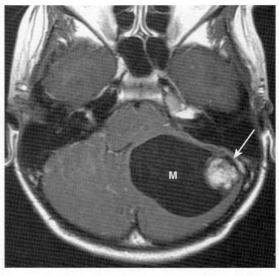

FIGURE 8-45. Cerebellar astrocytoma. Contrast-enhanced T1-weighted MR image shows predominantly cystic mass *(M)* in the left cerebellar hemisphere. There is an enhancing mural nodule *(arrow)*.

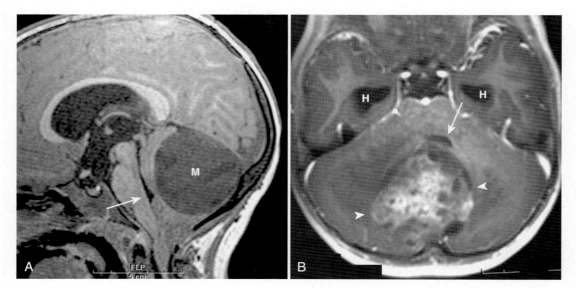

FIGURE 8-44. Cerebellar astrocytoma. **A,** Sagittal, T1-weighted MRI shows large, heterogeneous, relatively low signal mass *(M)* seen within the cerebellar vermis. Note anterior displacement of fourth ventricle *(arrow)*. Note that the third ventricle is dilatated secondary to obstructive hydrocephalus. **B,** Axial, postcontrast T1-weighted MRI shows heterogeneous enhancement of mass *(arrowheads)* and anterior displacement of fourth ventricle *(arrow)*. Note the dilatated temporal horns of lateral ventricles *(H)*, consistent with secondary obstructive hydrocephalus.

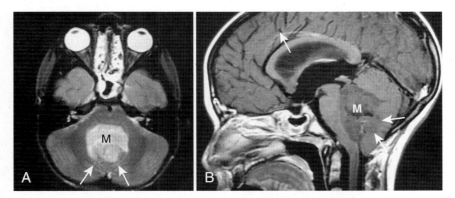

FIGURE 8-46. Medulloblastoma in an 11-year-old boy. **A,** Axial, T2-weighted MR image shows homogeneous high-signal mass filling the fourth ventricle. The border between the mass *(M)* and the vermis is poorly defined *(arrows)*. **B,** Sagittal, T1-weighted MR image shows the mass filling the fourth ventricle. The poorly defined border *(arrows)* between the mass *(M)* and the vermis is more easily appreciated.

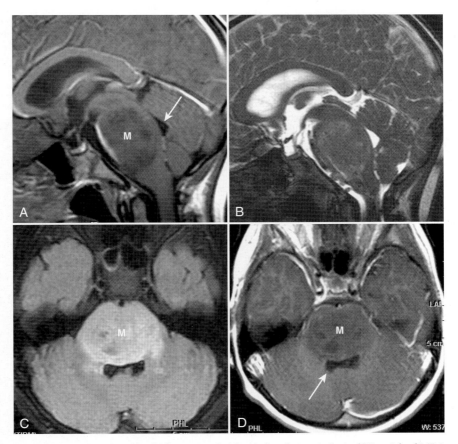

FIGURE 8-47. Brainstem glioma in a 9-year-old girl who presented with gait disturbance. **A,** Sagittal T1-weighted MR image shows mass *(M)* within brainstem. The mass is relatively low in signal. The fourth ventricle *(arrow)* is displaced posteriorly. **B,** Sagittal T2-weighted MR image shows homogeneous high-signal mass in pons. **C,** Axial FLAIR MR image shows lesion *(M)* to occupy the majority of the pons and to be high in signal. **D,** Postcontrast T1-weighted MR image shows minimal enhancement of lesion *(M)*. Note the posteriorly displaced fourth ventricle *(arrow)*.

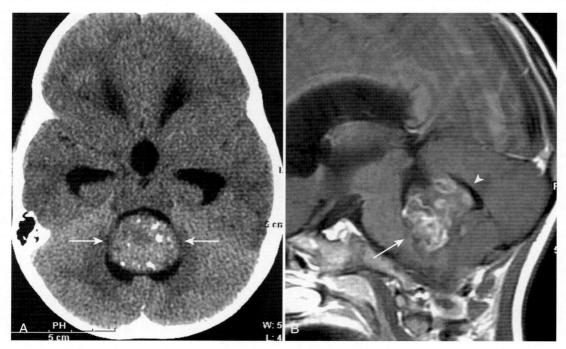

FIGURE 8-48. Ependymoma in a 2-year-old child with headaches. **A,** Axial, noncontrast CT shows heterogeneous but well-defined mass *(arrows)* with calcifications filling the fourth ventricle. **B,** Sagittal contrast-enhanced T1-weighted MR image shows mass with heterogeneous enhancement. The border between the brainstem and the mass *(arrow)* is poorly defined whereas the outline of the roof of the fourth ventricle *(arrowhead)* is well defined.

Two thirds occur in the fourth ventricle. When they occur in the fourth ventricle, ependymomas arise from and have a broad connection with the floor of the fourth ventricle, opposite from the roof involvement seen in medulloblastoma. Therefore, the border between the lesion and the floor of the fourth ventricle is often poorly defined (Fig. 8-48A, B). The lesions may fill and grow out of the fourth ventricle via the foramina into the cisterna magna and spinal canal. The lesions appear very heterogeneous and enhance heterogeneously on CT and MRI. They have well-defined, lobulated margins. Calcifications are seen on CT in 70% of cases (see Fig. 8-48).

Cerebral Tumors

In children, cerebral tumors are much less common than those of the posterior fossa. Most cerebral tumors affecting children are glial in origin (astrocytoma, oliogodendroglioma, glioblastoma). These tumors range in appearance from well circumscribed to infiltrative (Fig. 8-49). Imaging appearance does not always correlate with histologic grade. Less common tumors include embryonal tumors (PNETs), ependymoma, and choroid

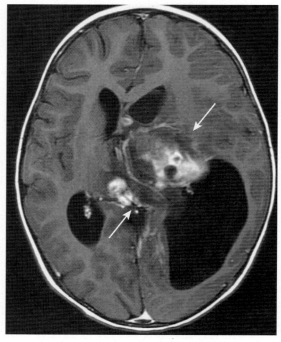

FIGURE 8-49. Supratentorial desmoplastic infantile ganglioglioma in a 3-year-old child. Axial, postcontrast T1-weighted image shows heterogeneously enhancing centrally located mass *(arrows)*. There is marked obstructive hydrocephalus.

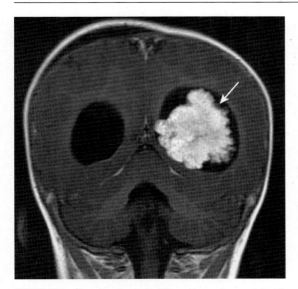

FIGURE 8-50. Choroid plexus papilloma in an 8-year-old girl. Coronal postcontrast T1-weighted image shows homogeneously enhancing mass *(arrow)* distending the left lateral ventricle. There is hydrocephalus.

plexus tumors. Choroid plexus tumors occur most commonly in the lateral ventricles. They are benign and slow growing in most cases. However, there are malignant choroid plexus sarcomas (Fig. 8-50). These lesions are markedly vascular and demonstrate marked enhancement at imaging (see Fig. 8-50).

Suprasellar and Other Tumors Around the Third Ventricle

Tumors that occur in the region of the third ventricle include those that arise in the suprasellar region as well as pineal-region tumors, and intraventricular tumors. Although there is a long list of tumors that can occur in this region, the most common in children include optic glioma, hypothalamic glioma, craniopharyngioma, and germ cell tumor. There are also several pineal tumors that are unique to childhood.

OPTIC GLIOMA

Optic glioma is one of the most common suprasellar tumors in childhood. Optic gliomas are typically astrocytic tumors and can involve any or all portions of the visual pathways: optic nerves, chiasm, and hypothalami. Lesions range from benign hamartomas to aggressive malignancies. There is an increased incidence in patients with NF-1. Optic nerve involvement is demonstrated as bulbous enlargement of the optic nerves on MRI (see Fig. 8-31). It is often difficult to differentiate optic gliomas of the chiasm from hypothalamic gliomas on MRI. Tumors arising in either location commonly extend into the other location. Both hypothalamic and optic nerve gliomas tend to be hyperintense on T2-weighted images and demonstrate diffuse enhancement with gadolinium.

GERM CELL TUMORS

Germ cell tumors of the CNS most commonly occur in the region of the pineal gland, hypothalamus, or third periventricular region. The most common histiologic type is germinoma. Other types include teratoma, embryonal carcinoma, and choriocarcinoma. There may be hemorrhage in the lesions, and the MR signal and CT density are variable. Teratomas may demonstrate fatty tissue or calcifications related to bone or teeth in the tumor.

PINEAL TUMORS

Primary pineal tumors range from benign pineocytomas to pineoblastomas. Pineoblastomas are highly malignant tumors, histologically similar to PNETs. They occur almost exclusively in childhood. On imaging of both pineocytoma and pineoblastoma, an enhancing pineal mass is seen. There is almost always hydrocephalus (Fig. 8-51A, B).

CRANIOPHARYNGIOMA

Craniopharyngiomas arise from the persistence and proliferation of squamous epithelial cells within the tract of an embryologic structure, the craniopharyngeal duct. They account for 7% of all intracranial tumors in children and are benign and slow-growing lesions. Typically, they are intrasellar and suprasellar in location (Fig. 8-52A, B). Calcifications are present in up to 80% of cases. Typically, CT shows a large calcified suprasellar mass with both cystic portions and solid enhancing portions. On MRI the cystic components tend to be high signal on all sequences, because they contain proteinaceous and cholesterol-laden fluid (see Fig. 8-52). The signal characteristics of the solid portions are variable on MRI.

TRAUMA

The evaluation of significant pediatric head trauma should be performed by CT. Skull radiographs obtained to rule out skull fracture are grossly overused and result in increased cost

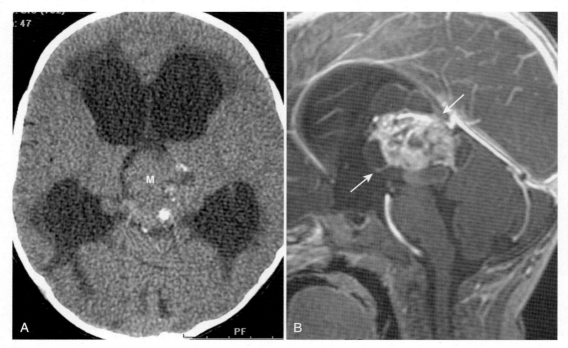

FIGURE 8-51. Pineoblastoma in an 11-year-old boy. **A,** Noncontrast CT shows heterogeneous mass *(M)* with some calcifications in the pineal region and secondary obstructive hydrocephalus. **B,** Sagittal contrast-enhanced T1-weighted MR image shows heterogeneously enhancing mass *(arrows)* with some associated cysts.

and radiation and little useful information. The presence of a skull fracture does not necessarily indicate intracranial injury, and the absence of a skull fracture certainly does not exclude it. Finally, the presence or absence of a skull

fracture usually does not affect the management of a child with head trauma.

Most of the CT findings in intracranial trauma, including subdural hematoma, epidural hematoma, subarachnoid hemorrhage, and

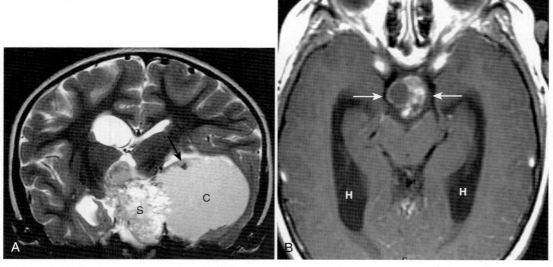

FIGURE 8-52. Craniopharyngioma: imaging findings in two patients. **A,** Coronal T2-weighted image shows heterogeneous signal mass in the suprasellar region. There are cystic *(C)* and solid *(S)* components. There is a low-signal area consistent with calcification *(arrow)*. There is hydrocephalus. **B,** Axial, contrast-enhanced, T1-weighted MR image in a different patient shows heterogeneously enhancing suprasellar mass *(arrows)* and secondary hydrocephalus *(H)*.

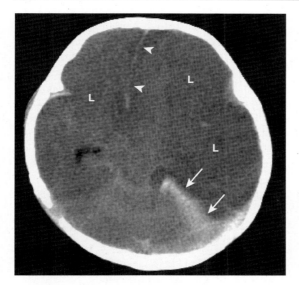

FIGURE 8-53. Fatal child abuse in an infant. Nonenhanced CT shows diffuse low-attenuation *(L)* throughout the majority of the brain, consistent with edema and infarction resulting from strangulation. There is resultant rightward midline shift. Note the rightward displacement of the falx cerebri *(arrowheads)*. There is also high attenuation along the falx *(arrows)*, consistent with subarachnoid hemorrhage.

parenchymal contusion, are similar in appearance in adults and children.

Abuse

For the most part, the imaging appearance of intracranial trauma that occurs secondary to abuse is similar to that seen with accidental trauma. Intracranial injury is the number one cause of death in abused children. Types of injury that should increase the degree of suspicion for abuse include interhemispheric subdural hematoma (caused by shaking) and the combination of a traumatic subdural or subarachnoid hematoma with anoxic-ischemic injury (a result of suffocation or strangulation; Fig. 8-53). Subdural hemorrhages of varying ages as demonstrated by fluid characteristics on CT or MRI are also suggestive (Fig. 8-54A, B).

HYDROCEPHALUS AND VENTRICULOPERITONEAL SHUNTS

Hydrocephalus is a problem commonly encountered in pediatric neuroimaging. It can occur

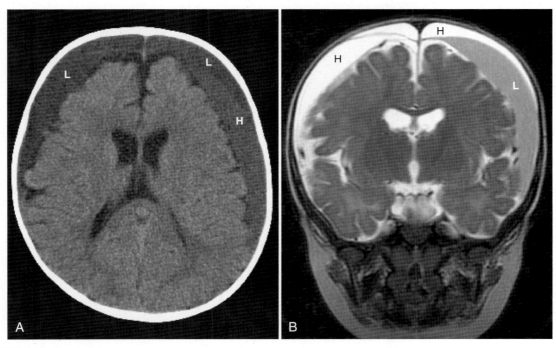

FIGURE 8-54. Child abuse in an infant. **A,** Noncontrast CT shows bilateral subdural hematomas. Note that the subdural hematomas are of varying attenuation, with some areas higher in attenuation *(H)* and some lower in attenuation *(L)*, consistent with subdural hematomas of varying age. **B,** Coronal T2-weighted image shows bilateral subdural hematomas. The subdurals are of varying signal intensities, with some high in signal *(H)* and some low in signal *(L)*, consistent with subdural hematomas of varying age.

secondary to one of the many problems previously listed in this chapter: developmental anomaly, hemorrhage, infection, or tumor. These patients are often treated by the placement of ventricular shunts. The most commonly used shunt is the ventriculoperitoneal shunt (VPS), in which the proximal portion of the shunt is positioned in one of the lateral ventricles, and the distal end is positioned in the peritoneal cavity. When a patient with a VPS presents with headaches, vomiting, or lethargy, increased intracranial pressure resulting from VPS malfunction should be investigated. Imaging includes radiographs of the shunt from cranium to abdomen to ensure that there is no evidence of shunt disconnection or kinking. The most common site for shunt dislocation is at the connection between the shunt tubing and the shunt chamber (Fig. 8-55A-D), which usually overlies the cranium. Familiarity with

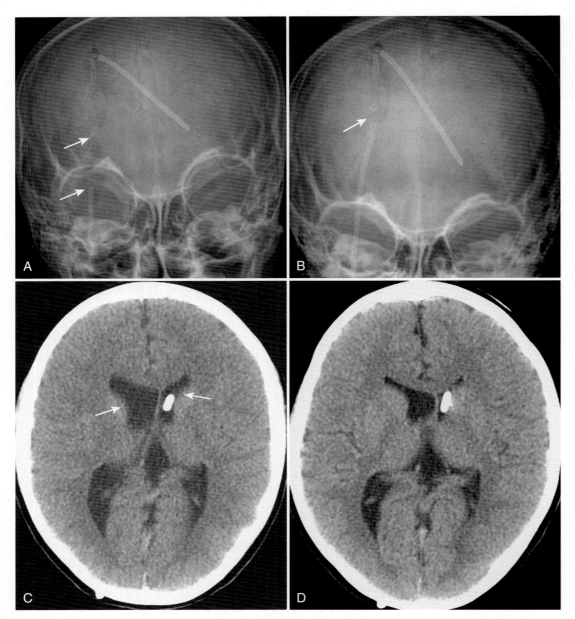

FIGURE 8-55. Ventriculoperitoneal shunt malfunction in a vomiting child. A, Frontal view of skull from shunt series shows a gap *(arrows)* between the shunt reservoir and the more distal tubing. B, Previous comparison radiograph shows reservoir and tubing to have been contiguous previously *(arrow)*. C, CT at time of presentation shows interval increase in size of lateral ventricles, particularly in frontal horns *(arrows)*, consistent with increased hydrocephalus. Note the VPS tip in the left frontal horn. D, Previous baseline CT shows the smaller size of the ventricles.

the various types of commercially available shunts is important because some types have radiolucent portions that could be mistaken for areas of disconnection.

A head CT is also obtained to evaluate for any interval change in the size of the cerebral ventricles (see Fig. 8-55). Symptoms are most often related to insufficient shunting and interval increase in ventricular size but can occasionally be secondary to overshunting, which produces slitlike ventricles. It is always important to evaluate the scout image from the CT for evidence of shunt dislocation or kinking. An abdominal pseudocyst surrounding and obstructing the intraabdominal tip of the VPS is also a possibility. This may be suspected when interval radiographs demonstrate a static position of the distal shunt tubing. Further investigation for VPS pseudocyst is usually performed using ultrasound.

CRANIOSYNOSTOSIS

Craniosynostosis is premature closure of the sutures of the skull. It can occur as an idiopathic, primary condition or it can be secondary to a number of genetic or metabolic disorders. Primary craniosynostosis is typically present at birth and occurs more commonly in boys than in girls. The sagittal suture is most commonly involved. Because the skull stops growing in the direction of the closed suture and continues to grow in the directions of the open sutures, craniosynostosis of a particular suture leads to a predictable head shape on physical exam and radiography. With sagittal suture synostosis, the head becomes long and narrow (dolichocephaly; Fig. 8-56). With coronal suture synostosis, the head becomes short from anterior to posterior and is wide from left to right (brachycephaly). The orbits assume an oval, oblique lateral margin that is referred to as a harlequin-eye appearance. With metopic suture craniosynostosis, the forehead assumes a pointed or triangular appearance (trigonocephaly; Fig. 8-57). Synostosis of all of the sutures results in cloverleaf skull (Kleeblattschädel). There is severe deformity of the skull, with bulging in the squamosal areas and in the bregma. It is associated with thanatophoric dwarfism.

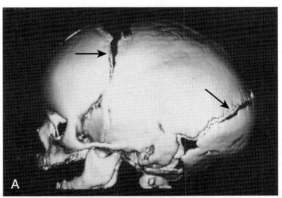

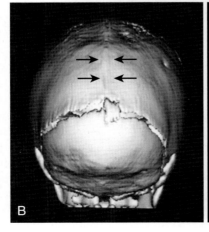

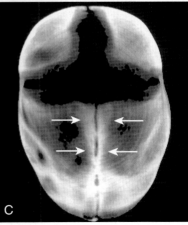

FIGURE 8-56. Sagittal suture synostosis in a 6-week-old boy with dolichocephaly. **A,** Lateral-surface-rendered three-dimensional CT shows a long, narrow skull (dolichocephaly). The coronal and lambdoid sutures *(arrows)* are patent. **B,** Posterior-surface-rendered three-dimensional CT shows fusion of the sagittal suture *(arrows).* **C,** Maximum-intensity-rendered image, as shown from above, demonstrates narrowing of the posterior portion of the sagittal suture with perisutural sclerosis *(arrows).*

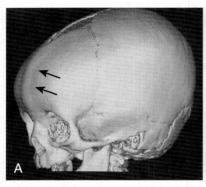 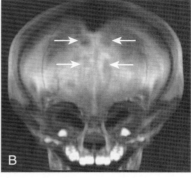

FIGURE 8-57. Metopic suture synostosis in an 8-week-old boy with trigonocephaly. **A,** Lateral surface rendered three-dimensional CT shows a pointed appearance *(arrows)* of the forehead (trigonocephaly). The metopic suture is not visualized as a patent space. **B,** Maximum-intensity-rendered image, as shown from the front, demonstrates narrowing of the metopic suture with perisutural sclerosis *(arrows).*

The screening examination for craniosynostosis remains radiography. In addition to the characteristic skull shapes, radiographs may demonstrate bony bridging, perisutural sclerosis, or narrowing of the involved suture. Many institutions perform three-dimensional helical CT of the head (see Figs. 8-56, 8-57) using surface-rendered or maximum-intensity-projection three-dimensional images.

LACUNAR SKULL

Lacunar skull, also known as Lückenschädel, is a defect in the mesenchymal formation of the skull that is associated with myelomeningocele. The radiographic findings include multiple oval lucencies that occur secondary to the thinning of the inner table of the skull (Fig. 8-58) and are more prominent in the occipital and parietal regions. It is present in all patients with myelomeningocele under 3 months of age; the imaging findings typically resolve by 6 months of age. It is always associated with myelomeningocele. It is said that lacunar skull should not be confused with the skull changes related to increased intracranial pressure (Fig. 8-59). With increased intracranial pressure, there is marked accentuation of the normal convolutional markings. The appearance has been likened to hammer-beaten silver. Personally, I think that they appear rather similar, with lacunar skull appearing more severe. Other radiographic findings of increased intracranial pressure include sutural diastasis, sellar enlargement, and demineralization.

ORBITAL CELLULITIS

Orbital cellulitis is the most common abnormality of the pediatric orbit. It is most commonly a bacterial infection and arises from extension of a sinus infection. The more common infectious agents include staphylococcus, streptococcus, and pneumococcus organisms. Orbital cellulitis is categorized anatomically as being preseptal or postseptal on the basis of the relationship between the inflamed tissue and the orbital septum. When inflammation extends posterior to the septum, it is considered to be postseptal and is typically extraconal and subperiosteal in location (Fig. 8-60). Almost all cases of postseptal cellulitis are associated with ethmoid sinus disease. The inflammatory process should be categorized as cellulitis or abscess. The presence of a drainable abscess is suggested on CT when rim enhancement is present surrounding an area of fluid attenuation or gas. Drainable abscesses are typically treated surgically. Cellulitis is treated with antibiotics alone.

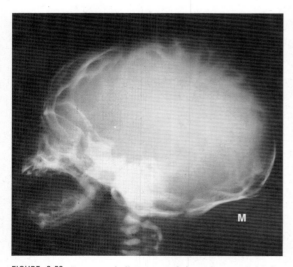

FIGURE 8-58. Lacunar skull in an infant with encephalocele. Radiograph shows multiple oval lucencies. The encephalocele can be seen as a subtle posterior soft tissue mass *(M).*

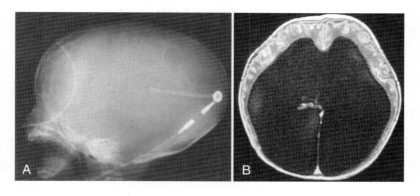

FIGURE 8-59. Skull changes in increased intracranial pressure. **A,** Radiograph shows accentuation of convolutional markings. Note the ventriculoperitoneal shunt. **B,** Axial, T1-weighted MRI shows massive dilatation of the lateral ventricles.

RETINOBLASTOMA

Retinoblastoma is a tumor that arises in the retina. It typically presents in children younger than 5 years of age. It is bilateral in as many as 25% of cases and can also rarely involve the pineal region (triretinoblastoma). In bilateral cases, there is often a genetic predisposition. Patients with retinoblastoma are also predisposed to secondary osteosarcoma after radiation therapy. On CT, retinoblastoma typically appears as a calcified intraocular mass (Fig. 8-61A, B). MRI demonstrates a heterogeneous intraocular mass of variable enhancement. There are a variety of other causes of intraorbital

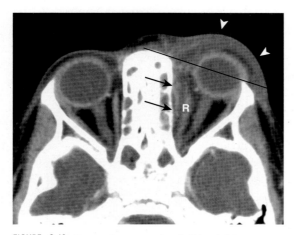

FIGURE 8-60. Pre- and postseptal cellulitis. Axial, contrast-enhanced CT shows marked asymmetric thickening of the left preseptal soft tissues *(arrowheads).* A line drawn through the anterior bony confines of the orbit defines tissue as pre- and postseptal. There is abnormal extraconal soft tissue *(arrows)* between the medial rectus muscle *(R)* and the bony wall of the orbit, displacing the medial rectus muscle. There is no evidence of drainable abscess. There is ethmoid sinus opacification bilaterally.

masses, the most common of which are listed in Table 8-7. The differential diagnosis can be limited on the basis of the location of the mass: global, intraconal, or extraconal.

NECK MASSES

There are a large number of causes of pediatric neck masses (Table 8-8). The most common cause is suppurative lymphadenitis (Fig. 8-62). This can occur secondary to systemic viral infection or focal bacterial infection. Lymph nodes larger than 1 to 1.5 cm in the neck are considered abnormal. Sometimes a purulent lymph node develops into a drainable abscess.

Of pediatric malignancies, 5% occur in the head and neck. Most malignant lesions present as painless masses. The head and neck area is one of the most common sites, along with the genitourinary tract, for rhabdomyosarcoma to occur. Rhabdomyosarcoma typically presents in the preschool age child. In older children, lymphoma is the most common cause of malignant lymphadenopathy (Fig. 8-63).

A number of congenital lesions can present with palpable neck masses, including branchial cleft cyst (Fig. 8-64); thyroglosssal duct cyst (Fig. 8-65); lingual thyroid; laryngocele; and dermoid/epidermoid. Branchial cleft cysts can persist from any of the developmental branchial arches, but those arising from the second branchial cleft are the most common. Typically, second branchial cleft cysts occur at the angle of the mandible (see Fig. 8-64). Midline neck masses are most likely to be dermoid/epidermoid, thyroglossal duct cysts (see Fig. 8-65), mucous retention cysts, or lymph nodes. Off-midline masses are more likely to be branchial cleft cysts.

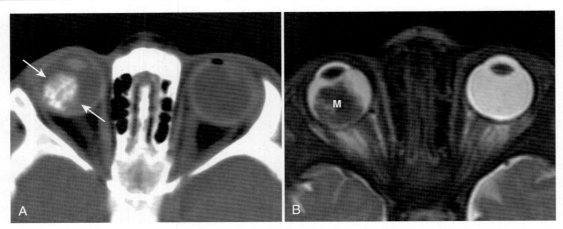

FIGURE 8-61. Retinoblastoma. **A,** CT shows calcified mass *(arrows)* within the posterior aspect of the right globe. **B,** Axial, T2-weighted MRI shows low-signal right intraocular mass *(M)*.

CONGENITAL VERTEBRAL ANOMALIES

A number of fairly common anomalies of the vertebral bodies occur as the result of abnormal development (see Fig. 7-59). There may be lack of fusion of the two cartilaginous centers of the vertebral bodies that results in a cleft in the sagittal plane. This is referred to as a butterfly vertebra. When one of the lateral cartilaginous centers fails to form, a hemivertebra results. It may be associated with scoliosis, rib anomalies, and other vertebral anomalies. Anterior and posterior hemivertebrae are also possible. If there is failure of separation of two or more adjacent vertebral bodies, a block vertebra is formed. The fusion of multiple cervical vertebral bodies can be seen in Kippel-Feil syndrome. A number of other associated anomalies may be seen in Klippel-Feil syndrome: a low posterior hairline, a short webbed neck, genitourinary anomalies, and congenital heart disease.

A Sprengel deformity (high-riding scapula) in association with a bridging omovertebral bone is present in 25% of patients with Klippel-Feil syndrome.

SPINAL DYSRAPHISM

Spinal dysraphism is a group of disorders of the spine in which the posterior bony and neuronal tissues fail to fuse (Table 8-9). The abnormalities are categorized as open (neural tissue exposed through bone and skin defect; spina bifida aperta) or closed (abnormality covered by skin; spina bifida occulta). Spinal dysraphism is the most common congenital abnormality of the CNS.

The most common of the open dysraphisms are meningoceles and myelomeningoceles. The lesions are defined by the contents of the herniated sac. Meningoceles contain meninges but not neural tissue (Figs. 8-66, 8-67).

Table 8-7. Common Causes of Pediatric Orbital Masses (Extra-ocular)

Orbital cellulitis/abscess
Orbital pseudotumor
Hemangioma
Lymphatic/venous malformation
Optic nerve glioma
Rhabdomyosarcoma
Lymphoma/leukemia
Retinoblastoma
Langerhans cell histiocytosis
Metastatic neuroblastoma
Hematoma

Table 8-8. Common Causes of Pediatric Neck Masses

Congenital	Thyroglossal duct cyst
	Branchial cleft cyst
	Lingual thyroid
	Dermoid/epidermoid
Inflammatory	Suppurative lymphadenitis
	Abscess
	Inflamed salivary gland
	Ranula
Neoplastic	Rhabdomyosarcoma
	Lymphoma
	Metastatic disease
Vascular	Venous malformation
	Lymphatic malformation

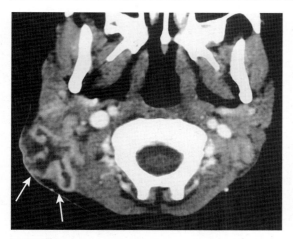

FIGURE 8-62. Suppurative lymphadenitis with abscess formation. Contrast-enhanced CT shows matted lymph nodes with area of fluid attenuation and rim enhancement *(arrows).*

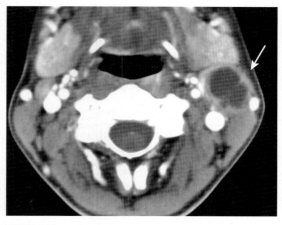

FIGURE 8-64. A second branchial cleft cyst in an 18-year-old girl with a tender mass. CT shows a low-attenuation cystic lesion *(arrow)* just inferior to the left angle of the mandible. The lesion has an enhancing rim.

Myelomeningoceles contain portions of the spinal cord or nerve roots. Although the lesions are most common in the lower lumbar spine, they can occur at any level. Encephaloceles occur through defects in the cranium (Fig. 8-68). Myelomeningoceles are associated with multiple other congenital anomalies. As previously discussed, essentially all patients with myelomeningoceles (but not meningoceles) have associated Chiari II malformations and 90% have hydrocephalus. Hydrosyringomyelia or dilatation of the central canal of the spinal cord is also often present. On radiography, the posterior elements of the spine are absent, and there is widening of the spinal canal and interpediculate distances (Fig. 8-69). There may be associated congenital

vertebral anomalies. Typically, multiple contiguous vertebral levels are involved. MRI is often used to look for delayed complications such as syrinx, dermoid, or postoperative tethering.

With closed dysraphisms, children may be asymptomatic or may present with subcutaneous masses or dermal tracts, bladder dysfunctions, lower-extremity neurologic abnormalities, or orthopedic deformities of the feet or legs. The closed dysraphisms may be associated with tethered cord, congenital dermal sinus, and lipomyelomeningocele.

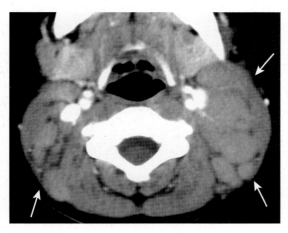

FIGURE 8-63. Lymphoma in a 5-year-old boy. Contrast-enhanced CT shows bulky lymphadenopathy *(arrows)* bilaterally, greater on the left than on the right.

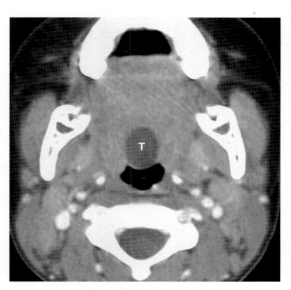

FIGURE 8-65. Thyroglossal duct cyst in a 2-year-old boy. Contrast-enhanced CT shows well-defined, nonenhancing mass *(T)* in the midline, just inferior to the base of the tongue.

Table 8-9. Common Types of Spinal Dysraphism

Open spinal dysraphism	Myelomeningocele Myelocele
Closed (occult) spinal dysraphism	Lipomyelomeningocele Dermal sinus tract Tethered cord syndrome

In infants who demonstrate a sacral dimple, patch of hair, or other findings suspicious for an occult dysraphism, the initial screening examination is often ultrasound. In a normal infant, the conus medullaris is located superior to or at the level of L2-L3 (Fig. 8-70). The cord and nerve roots are seen to be freely moving during real-time ultrasound evaluation. In tethered cord syndrome, the tip of the spinal cord is low-lying, below the level of L2-L3 (Fig. 8-71A, B). Tethered cord may occur as a primary problem or in association with other components of spinal dysraphism, such as lipomyelomeningocele, hemangioma, or a dermoid tract. With a tethered cord, the filum terminale may be short and abnormally thick (>2 mm). On real-time ultrasound examination, the cord and nerve roots do not float freely in the CSF space and may be positioned posteriorly.

When ultrasound evaluation of the spine is performed, posterior developmental masses should also be excluded. These include

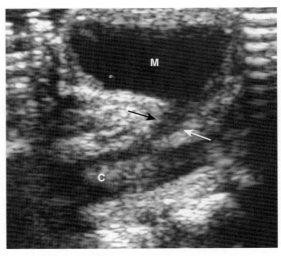

FIGURE 8-67. Meningocele in a newborn. Midline sagittal ultrasound shows a meningocele as a cystic structure *(M)*. There is a hypoechoic tract *(arrows)* connecting the cyst to the spinal canal *(C)*.

lipomyelomeningocele, a contiguous dermal sinus tract, or others, such as lipoma or dermoid. Lipomyelomeningocele is the most common of the occult myelodysplasias. When present, a lipomatous mass extends inferiorly and posteriorly from the incompletely fused spinal cord through a defect in the dura and bone and is contiguous with the subcutaneous fat. A palpable mass may be present but the overlying skin is intact. A dermal sinus is an epithelium-lined tract that extends from the skin to the deep soft tissues. It may connect to the spinal canal or end in a dermoid, epidermoid, or lipoma.

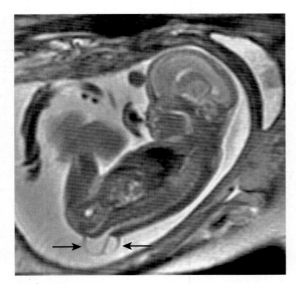

FIGURE 8-66. Meningocele demonstrated on fetal MRI. Image with fetus in sagittal view shows cystic area *(arrows)* posterior to the lumbar spine and contiguous with the spinal canal, consistent with a meningocele.

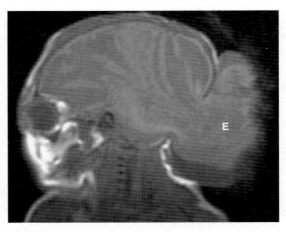

FIGURE 8-68. Encephalocele. Off-midline, sagittal T1-weighted image shows a large area of brain *(E)* protruding outside of the cranium through a defect in the skull. Note that white matter tracts extend intracranially to extracranially.

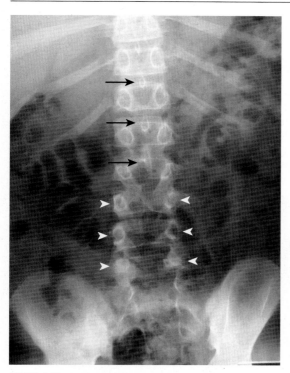

FIGURE 8-69. Dysraphic changes within the lumbar and sacral spine. Radiograph shows absence of the posterior elements and widening of the interpeduncular distance *(arrowheads)*. The posterior elements superior to the level of the dysraphism appear normal *(arrows)*.

The tracts are usually identifiable on ultrasound and appear as low-signal-intensity tracts on T1-weighted MR images. When findings of occult dysraphism are found on ultrasound or are highly suspected clinically, definitive evaluation is performed using MRI.

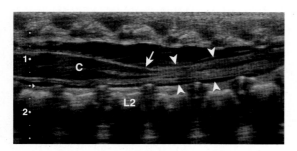

FIGURE 8-70. Normal infant spinal ultrasound. Midline sagittal image shows tip of conus medullaris *(arrow)* to be located at the level of *L2*, which is normal position. The cord *(C)* is shown as a hypoechoic structure, and the surrounding nerve roots *(arrowheads)* are more echogenic. Note that the cord and nerve roots lay anteriorly, with gravity. On real-time ultrasound in a normal patient, the cord and nerve roots float freely in the CSF and show motion.

SPINAL TRAUMA

Injury to the spine is much less common in infants and young children than it is in adults. Most injuries that occur in older children and teenagers have the same appearances and locations as those seen in adults and are not discussed here. In infants and young children, the majority of cervical spine injuries involve the superior cervical spine, as opposed to the lower cervical spine injuries seen in adults. This is thought to be related to the relatively large head size of young children and the immaturity of the spinal column. As with all cervical spine trauma, one must be diligent concerning the technical factors and the interpretation of radiographs.

Fractures of the upper cervical spine in infants and young children often involve the atlas and axis. With flexion injuries, there can be a fracture through the base of the dens (at the synchondrosis between the dens and body of C2; Fig. 8-72). With this injury, there is typically anterior displacement of C1 in association with soft tissue swelling. Extension injuries in this region may result in fractures of the posterior arch of C1 or of the dens or in a "hangman fracture" (a fracture through the posterior arch of C2; Fig. 8-73). Atlantooccipital dislocations can also occur (Fig. 8-74). The atlantooccipital dislocation is a severe injury that commonly results in death. On radiographs, the distance between the occiput and C1 is increased and there is marked soft tissue swelling. Atlantoaxial instability can also occur and is discussed subsequently.

Lap belt injuries occur in children who are restrained by lap belts but not by shoulder belts. Anterior compression fractures of the lumbar vertebral bodies may occur in association with disruption of the posterior processes (Chance fractures; Fig. 8-75A, B). These fractures are not commonly associated with neurologic injury but are frequently associated with intraabdominal injuries, particularly bowel injuries.

NORMAL VARIANTS AND CONGENITAL ANOMALIES OF THE CERVICAL SPINE

Another difficulty in the interpretation of pediatric cervical spine radiographs in cases of trauma is recognizing normal variants and differentiating them from trauma. One of the more common

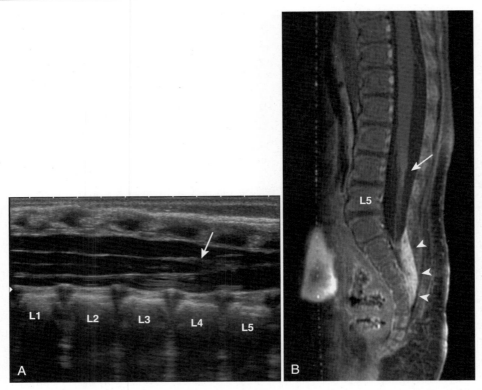

FIGURE 8-71. Tethered cord with associated hemangioma. **A,** Sagittal ultrasound shows the tip of the conus medullaris *(arrow)* to lie abnormally low, at the level of L4. The cord and nerve roots appear to be taut (posteriorly tethered) and in a straight line and do not fall anteriorly with gravity. No motion was seen in real time. **B,** Sagittal postcontrast T1-weighted MR image shows the abnormally low level of the conus medullaris *(arrow)* at L4. There is also an enhancing mass *(arrowheads)* posterior to the sacrum, adjacent to the filum terminalis, consistent with an associated hemangioma.

normal variants that may lead to confusion is cervical pseudosubluxation. In normal children, there may be a slightly anterior position of C2 in relation to C3 (Fig. 8-76). However, in contrast to ligamentous injury, with pseudosubluxation the posterior cervical line (a line drawn along the anterior aspect of the posterior processes) remains straight. Pseudosubluxation may also be seen at the C3 to C4 level.

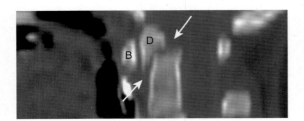

FIGURE 8-72. Fracture through base of dens. Sagittal reconstructed CT shows fracture line *(arrow)* through base of dens with anterior displacement of dens *(D)* and anterior button of C1 *(B)* in relationship to the base of C2.

There are a number of age-related variations in C1 and C2. The three ossification centers that make up the atlas fuse posteriorly by 1 year of age and laterally by 3 years of age. Prior to fusion, a lucent synchondrosis is seen radiographically. In addition, there may be a congenital defect in the posterior portion of C1 that should not be confused with a fracture (Fig. 8-77). C2 also has multiple ossification centers. These nonossified synchondroses should not be mistaken for fractures. The synchondrosis between the dens and body of C2 typically fuses between 3 and 6 years of age. Prior to fusion, the lucent synchondrosis is seen through the base of the dens. The ossiculum terminale (tip of the dens) fuses to the body of the dens by 12 years of age. The dens may also be normally tilted slightly posteriorly in young children.

ATLANTOAXIAL INSTABILITY

The atlantoaxial joint, or the articulation between the C1 and C2 vertebral bodies, is a

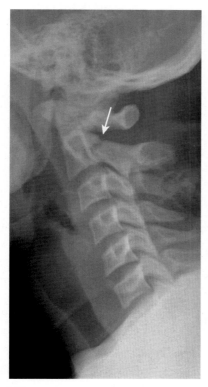

FIGURE 8-73. Hangman fracture. Radiograph shows linear fracture *(arrow)* through the posterior elements of C2.

unique joint that allows for lateral rotation of the cervical spine. The joint is stabilized by a number of ligaments. The transverse ligament is responsible for stabilizing the relationship between the dens of C2 and the anterior arch of C1. In children, the space between the dens and the anterior arch of C1 should not exceed 5 mm. Atlantoaxial subluxation leads to an abnormal increase in this distance (Fig. 8-78). Unfortunately, it also leads to a decrease in the diameter of the spinal canal and can cause cord compression (see Fig. 8-78). Causes of atlanto-axial instability include trauma, inflammation (juvenile rheumatoid arthritis, retropharyngeal abscess), and congenital predisposition (Down syndrome, hypoplasia of the dens, absence of the anterior arch of C1). Patients with Down syndrome are typically screened for atlantoaxial instability prior to participation in physical activities.

SPONDYLOLYSIS AND SPONDYLOLISTHESIS

The most common abnormality identified on radiography in children who present with lower back pain is spondylolysis. Spondylolysis refers to a defect in the pars interarticularis of the posterior vertebral arch. It usually occurs bilaterally and at a single level. The overwhelming majority of cases (93%) occur at the L5-S1 level; the second most common location is L4-L5. It is a common lesion, affecting approximately 7.1% of adolescents. Symptoms usually present in late childhood, although many of these children are asymptomatic. There is debate concerning whether the cause is traumatic, congenital, or some combination of the two.

Spondylolisthesis refers to anterior displacement of the more superior vertebral body onto the inferior vertebral body (Fig. 8-79). Spondylolisthesis is graded from 1 through 5 on

FIGURE 8-74. Craniocervical dislocation in a 5-year-old boy after a high-speed collision. **A,** Radiograph shows increased distance between the skull base and C1 vertebral body. **B,** Sagittal T2-weighted MR image shows high signal within the cord *(C)*, representing a cord contusion. There is high-signal edema within the posterior soft tissues *(arrows)* secondary to ligamentous injury.

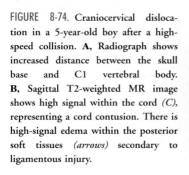

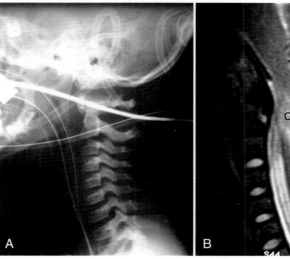

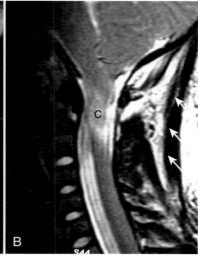

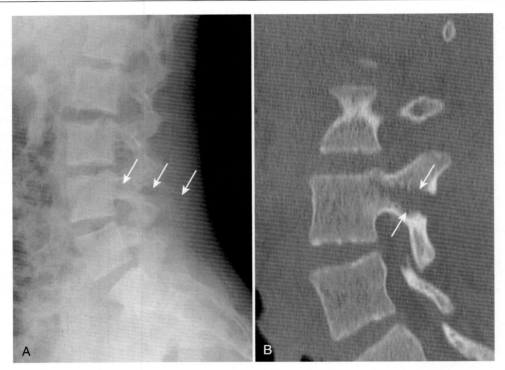

FIGURE 8-75. Chance fracture. **A,** Radiograph shows fracture *(arrows)* through posterior elements of the spine. **B,** CT better shows the fracture through the posterior elements *(arrows)*.

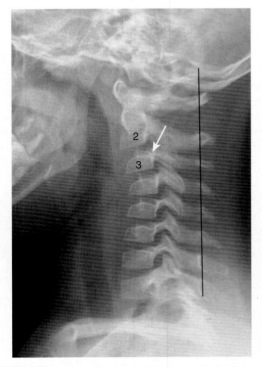

FIGURE 8-76. Pseudosubluxation of C2 onto C3. Radiograph shows that the posterior aspect of C2 vertebral body is slightly more anteriorly positioned than is that of C3 *(arrow)*. However, the posterior cervical line shows that the posterior elements of C2 are not more anterior than the posterior elements of C3, consistent with pseudosubluxation rather than true injury.

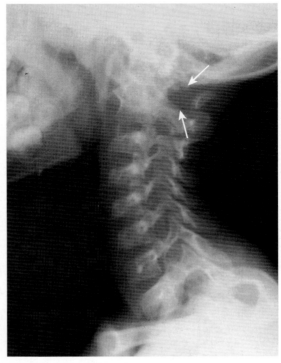

FIGURE 8-77. Congenital absence of the posterior portion of C1 is shown in the lucent area *(arrows)* on radiography.

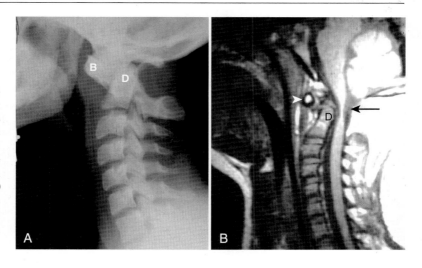

FIGURE 8-78. Atlantoaxial instability in a 20-year-old patient with Down syndrome. **A,** Radiograph shows increased distance between the anterior button of C1 *(B)* and the dens of C2 *(D).* **B,** Sagittal T1-weighted MR image again shows increased distance between the anterior button of C1 *(arrowhead)* and the dens of C2 *(D).* There is also marked narrowing of the spinal canal and severe spinal cord compression *(arrow).*

the basis of increments of one quarter of the vertebral body. Grade 1 refers to anterior displacement of up to one quarter of the superior vertebral body beyond the anterior border of the inferior vertebral body. In grade 2, the displacement is up to one half; in grade 4, it is the entire vertebral body. Grade 5 is complete anterior displacement and inferior migration such that the superior vertebral body is anterior to the inferior vertebral body.

On lateral radiographs, spondylolysis appears as a lucent defect through the region of the pars, with or without associated anterior slippage. Oblique views demonstrate the lucency through the pars. The pars defect has been likened to a lucent, broken neck of what appears to look like a Scottish terrier on the oblique views (see Fig. 8-79). Personally, I think the defect is often easier to see on the straight lateral films. In cases where confirmation is necessary, CT can be used.

Suggested Readings

Ball WS Jr: *Pediatric neuroradiology,* Philadelphia, Lippincott-Raven, 1997.

Barkovich A:. *Diagnostic imaging: pediatric neuroradiology,* Salt Lake City. UT, Amirsys, 2007.

Cecil KM, Jones BV: Magnetic resonance spectroscopy of the pediatric brain, *Top Magn Reson Imaging* 12: 435-452, 2001.

Roberts TPL, Simon-Schwarts E: Principles and implementation of diffusion-weighted and diffusion tensor imaging, *Pediatr Radiol* 37:739-748, 2007.

Robertson RL, Glaisier CM: Diffusion-weighted imaging of the brain in infants and children, *Pediatr Radiol* 37: 749-768, 2007.

Rollins NK: Clinical applications of diffusion tensor imaging and tractography in children, *Pediatr Radiol* 37: 769-780, 2007.

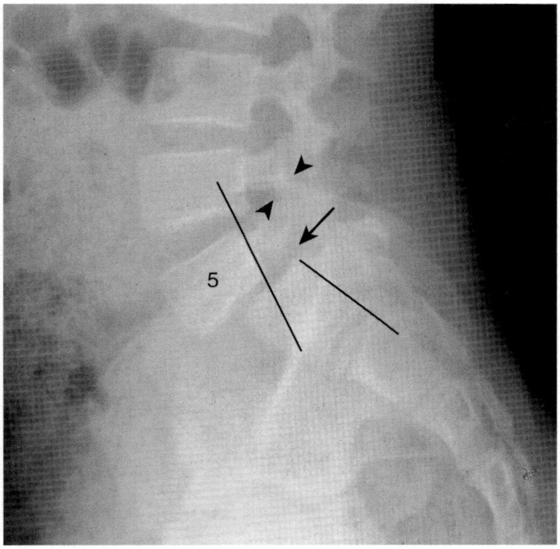

FIGURE 8-79. L5-S1 spondylolysis with grade 2 spondylolisthesis. Lateral radiograph shows anterior displacement of L4 vertebral body in relationship to the S1 vertebral segment. Lines are drawn parallel to the posterior aspect of L5 and S1, demonstrating the anterior displacement of L5. The normal, intact pars is seen at L4 *(arrowheads)* and resembles a "dog collar on a Scotty dog." There is lucency through the pars *(arrow)* at the L5 level, consistent with the spondylolysis.

Index

Note: Page numbers followed by f indicate figures; those followed by t indicate tables.